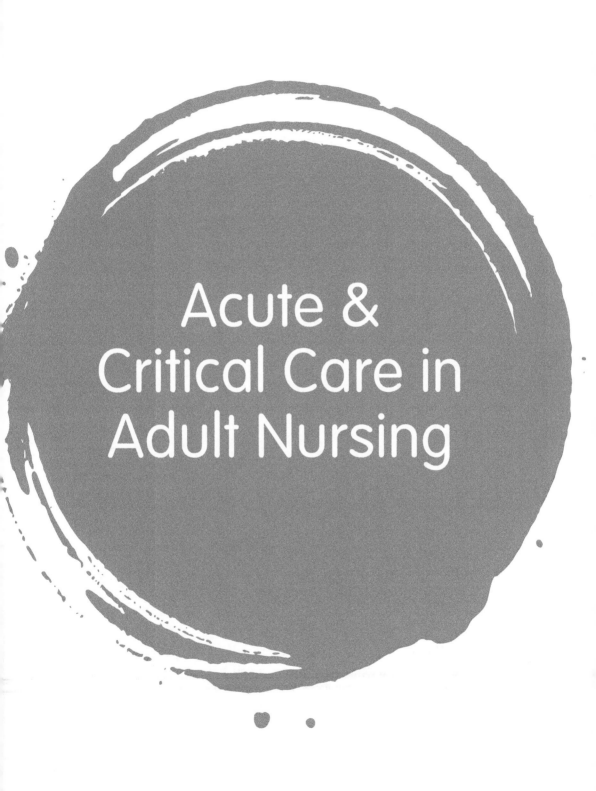

Acute &
Critical Care in
Adult Nursing

Sara Miller McCune founded SAGE Publishing in 1965 to support the dissemination of usable knowledge and educate a global community. SAGE publishes more than 1000 journals and over 800 new books each year, spanning a wide range of subject areas. Our growing selection of library products includes archives, data, case studies and video. SAGE remains majority owned by our founder and after her lifetime will become owned by a charitable trust that secures the company's continued independence.

Los Angeles | London | New Delhi | Singapore | Washington DC | Melbourne

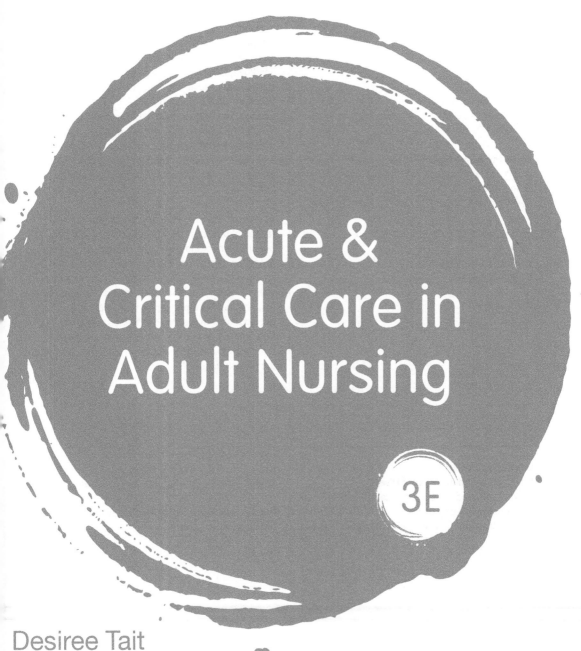

Acute & Critical Care in Adult Nursing

3E

Desiree Tait
Catherine Williams
David Barton
Jane James

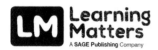
A SAGE Publishing Company

Learning Matters
A SAGE Publishing Company
1 Oliver's Yard
55 City Road
London EC1Y 1SP

SAGE Publications Inc.
2455 Teller Road
Thousand Oaks, California 91320

SAGE Publications India Pvt Ltd
B 1/I 1 Mohan Cooperative Industrial Area
Mathura Road
New Delhi 110 044

SAGE Publications Asia-Pacific Pte Ltd
3 Church Street
#10-04 Samsung Hub
Singapore 049483

Editor: Laura Walmsley
Development Editor: Eleanor Rivers
Senior project editor: Chris Marke
Cover design: Wendy Scott
Typeset by: C&M Digitals (P) Ltd, Chennai, India

Library of Congress Control Number: 2021947643

British Library Cataloguing in Publication Data

A catalogue record for this book is available from the British Library

ISBN 978-1-5264-4467-7
ISBN 978-1-5264-4468-4 (pbk)

Contents

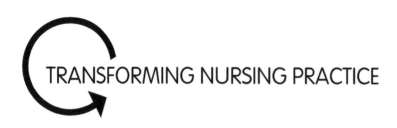

TRANSFORMING NURSING PRACTICE

Transforming Nursing Practice is a series tailor made for pre-registration student nurses.
Each book addresses a core topic and is:

 Clearly written and
easy to read

 Full of case studies
and activities

 Mapped to the NMC Standards of
proficiency for registered nurses

 Focused on applying theory to
everyday nursing practice

Each book addresses a core topic and has been carefully developed
to be simple to use, quick to read and written in clear language.

An invaluable series of books that explicitly relates to the NMC standards. Each book covers a different topic that students need to explore in order to develop into a qualified nurse... I would recommend this series to all Pre-Registered nursing students whatever their field or year of study.

LINDA ROBSON,
Senior Lecturer at Edge Hill University

Many titles in the series are on our recommended reading list and for good reason - the content is up to date and easy to read. These are the books that actually get used beyond training and into your nursing career.

EMMA LYDON,
Adult Student Nursing

ABOUT THE SERIES EDITORS

DR MOOI STANDING is an Independent Academic Nursing Consultant (UK and international) responsible for the core knowledge, personal and professional learning skills titles. She has invaluable experience as an NMC Quality Assurance Reviewer of educational programmes, and as a Professional Regulator Panellist on the NMC Practice Committee. Mooi is also a Board member of Special Olympics Malaysia.

DR SANDRA WALKER is a mental healthcare innovator and clinical academic, responsible for the mental health nursing titles in the series. A practising mental health nurse for over 30 years, Sandy also lecturers at Portsmouth University, is Director of SanityCo and Co-Founder/Director of the Good Mental Health Cooperative.

BESTSELLING TEXTBOOKS

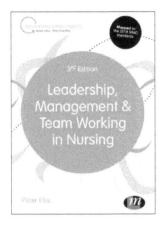

3rd Edition

Leadership, Management & Team Working in Nursing

Peter Ellis

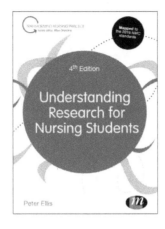

4th Edition

Understanding Research for Nursing Students

Peter Ellis

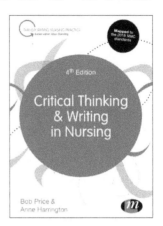

4th Edition

Critical Thinking & Writing in Nursing

Bob Price & Anne Harrington

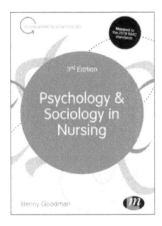

3rd Edition

Psychology & Sociology in Nursing

Benny Goodman

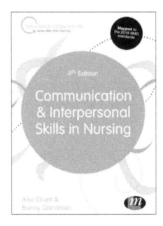

4th Edition

Communication & Interpersonal Skills in Nursing

Alec Grant & Benny Goodman

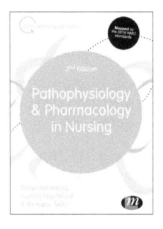

2nd Edition

Pathophysiology & Pharmacology in Nursing

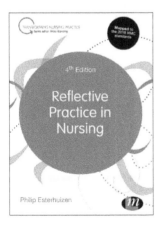

4th Edition

Reflective Practice in Nursing

Philip Esterhuizen

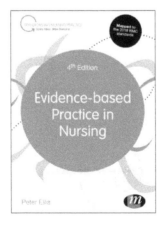

4th Edition

Evidence-based Practice in Nursing

Peter Ellis

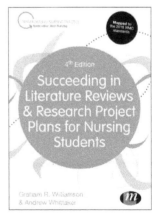

4th Edition

Succeeding in Literature Reviews & Research Project Plans for Nursing Students

Graham R. Williamson & Andrew Whittaker

You can find a full list of textbooks in the *Transforming Nursing Practice* series at
uk.sagepub.com/TNP-series

About the authors

Desiree Tait PhD, DNSc, MSc Nursing, DNE, DN, RGN is Principal Academic in Adult Nursing at the Faculty of Health and Social Sciences, Bournemouth University.

David Barton PhD, MPhil, BEd, RNT, DipN, RGN was Academic Lead in the Department of Nursing, College of Human and Health Sciences in Swansea University until his retirement.

Thomas C. Barton MSc Advanced Clinical Practice in Healthcare, DipN, RGN is an Advanced Nurse Practitioner working for Abertawe Bro Morgannwg University Health Board in Neath Port Talbot Hospital as part of the Advanced Practice Team clinically staffing the inpatient wards.

David Blesovsky MN, RGN, PGCE(A), DPSN was a Senior Lecturer in Adult Nursing and Admission Tutor in the College of Human and Health Sciences in Swansea University.

Jane James MSc Nursing, PGCE, RNT, RGN was a Senior Lecturer in Adult Nursing and Admissions Tutor in the College of Human and Health Sciences in Swansea University.

Catherine Williams MSc Nursing, BSc (Hons) Nursing, PGCE, RNT, RN is the Undergraduate Programme Director BSc Nursing at the College of Human and Health Sciences.

Acknowledgements

The authors and publishers wish to thank Alison Buckley and Denise Brooks for their invaluable feedback on draft chapters of this new edition. Their thoughtful engagement with the material and generosity in sharing their expertise are greatly appreciated.

Introduction

About this book

The student and newly qualified nurse and/or nursing associate continue to be able to demonstrate their development towards professional accountability through clinical decision making, collaborative working, and clinical leadership or integrated care (NMC, 2018a, b). A person can become critically ill in any clinical or home setting and prompt assessment and management of their condition can reduce the risk of further deterioration and death. The purpose of this book continues to be to provide you with the knowledge and professional guidance you will need to assist you in developing the clinical decision-making skills and self-confidence required to care for patients who are unstable, deteriorating or critically ill, regardless of their location.

Each chapter focuses on the development of key clinical assessment and decision-making skills that will support your learning in the second and/or third year of pre-registration study in nursing and following qualification. The core element of each chapter continues to be to assist you in the development of skills in rapid assessment and response to clinical deterioration. Its coverage of the provision and monitoring of care makes the book a helpful read for trainee nursing associates too.

Requirements for the NMC Standards of Proficiency for Registered Nurses

The book is structured so that it will help you to understand and meet the proficiencies required for entry to the NMC register; each chapter begins by linking the aim and objectives to the NMC (2018a) Standards of Proficiency for Registered Nurses. In this third edition of the book, we have revisited the existing chapters and updated them according to the latest evidence. It is important to recognise, however, that evidence-based practice is, by its very nature, subject to review and change, and we urge you to ensure that you focus on the most recent evidence to support your decision making.

Learning features

All chapters have been updated and continue to be focused on the reader putting themselves in the role of the decision maker as each person's clinical story unfolds. Each chapter is person-centred and includes the integration of applied pathophysiology to assessment, risk assessment, and management of care. Quick reference guides are used throughout to assist you with the clinical decision-making activities found in the chapters and, where appropriate, you will be asked to reflect on your experiences in practice. Feedback on the activities can be found at the end of each chapter.

Book structure

In Chapter 1 you are given an overview of why patients deteriorate, together with the knowledge and skills required to assess, recognise, and respond to acute and critical illness. The chapter introduces you to the levels of dependency for acute and critically ill patients as well as providing quick guides for rapid assessment and response to changes in the patient's condition. The quick reference guides can be applied to all subsequent chapters, giving you opportunities to rehearse the process, apply and refine your skills.

In Chapter 2 you are introduced to the breathless patient and are guided through how to undertake a respiratory assessment and the care of patients with type I and type II respiratory failure. The chapter includes an introduction to acid-base balance and the interpretation of arterial blood gases. Patient conditions such as heart failure, pneumonia, and chronic obstructive pulmonary disease are discussed and applied to patient stories.

Chapter 3 builds on the content presented in Chapter 2 and explores the assessment and management of patients who need advanced respiratory support and the assessment and monitoring of people who require non-invasive and invasive respiratory support. In this chapter you are introduced to Jenny Matthews, who is experiencing an acute asthma attack.

In Chapter 4 you are introduced to assessing and prioritising care for people with chest pain, and you will be guided through the process of chest pain assessment and management according to national guidelines. A range of causes of chest pain are introduced, including respiratory and musculoskeletal, gastrointestinal, and cardiac, with a focus on the need for a rapid and full assessment prior to determining the focus of collaborative care.

Chapter 5 focuses on the patient in pain and explores the significance of pain in relation to the patient experience and the impact of pain on the development of critical illness. Pain assessment and management is considered in the context of holistic and collaborative care.

In Chapter 6 you will be guided through the process of assessing, recording, and responding to patients in shock. There is also an opportunity for you to practise risk assessment and early recognition of patients in shock and to take steps to prevent the progression of shock.

Chapter 7 focuses on the risk assessment and management of patients at risk of developing sepsis and the management of patients with sepsis and septic shock. You will be guided through how to use sepsis screening and care bundles in the context of patient scenarios.

In Chapter 8 you are introduced to patients with delirium. The chapter focuses on the risk assessment of patients who have the potential to develop delirium and how to plan ways in which to prevent and/or manage patients in a state of delirium. You have an opportunity to reflect on patients you have nursed and how you may influence practice development in the care of patients with delirium.

Chapter 9 focuses on the risk assessment for, and prevention of, acute kidney injury in individuals in a variety of critical care settings. You will have an opportunity to recognise the difference between acute kidney injury and chronic kidney disease as well as the relationship between them in the context of caring for people with multiple co-morbidities.

In Chapter 10 you are introduced to the assessment and management of patients who have experienced physiological trauma. The chapter links well with Chapter 6 and includes the care of patients with soft tissue injuries, including burns as well as patients with traumatic fractures.

Chapter 11 focuses on explaining the causes and management of the unconscious patient. The focus is on prioritising care and reducing the risks of side effects associated with loss of consciousness. Neurological assessment is discussed, together with an evidence base for practice. Opportunities to practise neurological assessment and recognition of clinical deterioration in levels of consciousness are included.

In Chapter 12 you are introduced to people living with endocrine disorders. The dominant feature of this chapter concerns the risk assessment and management of patients experiencing hypoglycaemic episodes, diabetic ketoacidosis, and hyperosmolar hyperglycaemic state. The scenarios included give you an opportunity to focus on the clinical decision-making skills required to maintain patient safety and reduce the risk of morbidity and mortality for people living with both type 1 and type 2 diabetes, and other acute endocrine disorders.

The book concludes by offering a summary of lessons learned and an action plan for practice. You will be able to consider how you can develop either a career in acute and critical care and/or continue to utilise the lessons learned in both hospital and community-based care. We hope you find the chapters a useful contribution to your own clinical and professional development.

Chapter 1

Assessing, recognising, and responding to acute and critical illness

Desiree Tait

NMC Future Nurse: Standards of Proficiency for Registered Nurses

This chapter will address the following platforms and proficiencies:

Platform 3: Assessing needs and planning care

Registered nurses prioritise the needs of people when assessing and reviewing their mental, physical, cognitive, behavioural, social and spiritual needs. They use information obtained during assessments to identify the priorities and requirements for person-centred and evidence-based nursing interventions and support. They work in partnership with people to develop person-centred care plans that take into account their circumstances, characteristics and preferences.

At the point of registration, the registered nurse will be able to:

3.2   demonstrate and apply knowledge of body systems and homeostasis, human anatomy and physiology, biology, genomics, pharmacology and social and behavioural sciences when undertaking full and accurate person-centred nursing assessments and developing appropriate care plans.

3.9   recognise and assess people at risk of harm and the situations that may put them at risk, ensuring prompt action is taken to safeguard those who are vulnerable.

Platform 6: Improving safety and quality of care

Registered nurses make a key contribution to the continuous monitoring and quality improvement of care and treatment in order to enhance health outcomes and people's experience of nursing and related care. They assess risks to safety or experience and take appropriate action to manage those, putting the best interests, needs and preferences of people first.

(Continued)

(Continued)

At the point of registration, the registered nurse will be able to:

6.2   understand the relationship between safe staffing levels, appropriate skills mix, safety and quality of care, recognising risks to public protection and quality of care, escalating concerns appropriately.

6.5   demonstrate the ability to accurately undertake risk assessments in a range of care settings, using a range of contemporary assessment and improvement tools.

Chapter aims

By the end of this chapter, you should be able to:

*   identify the terms used to define patient acuity and levels of acute and critical care;
*   describe how to undertake a rapid assessment and risk assessment of a changing clinical situation;
*   describe how to collate accurate data from a variety of sources and analyse the results;
*   demonstrate how to communicate the findings to staff at the appropriate level.

Introduction

Within this chapter you will be introduced to Sally Smith. We will explore her clinical assessment and highlight the core skills required for recognising and interpreting, communicating, and acting on an episode of clinical deterioration. As a student you can observe, learn, and practise clinical decision-making skills under supervision before you embrace them as a registered and accountable practitioner. While this book cannot equip you with all these skills, it does highlight core skills and landmarks to guide you towards competent practice. This chapter gives you an overview of how to recognise deterioration, assess and prioritise care, and communicate your concerns. We will begin by thinking about why a person might deteriorate and how this links to the chapters included in this book.

Why do patients deteriorate?

A person is at risk of clinical deterioration in any situation where damage to the body's cells, organs, and systems is left unchecked. Causes of cellular injury can be varied but generally relate to damage to cells, tissues, and organs as a result of deficiency, such as reduced oxygen and/or nutrients; damage through intoxication such as infection or poisoning; or trauma. Cell injury occurs when the cell is no longer able to maintain homeostasis and normal function. If the cause of the injury is identified in a timely manner the cell(s) may recover and the injury can be reversed. However, if the injury is sustained for a prolonged period cell death will occur, leading to permanent damage to tissues and organs (McCance and Huether, 2019). Timing is of the essence, and you will be reminded of this in numerous chapters! The list below links the causes of cell injury to chapters included in this book:

- damage as a result of a deficiency in oxygen and/or nutrients as illustrated in patients with hypoxia (Chapters 2, 3, 4, 9, and 11);
- patients in shock, leading to reduced cellular perfusion of oxygen and nutrients (Chapters 5, 6, 7, 9, and 11);
- patients with ketoacidosis, hyperglycaemia, hypoglycaemia, and/or an electrolyte imbalance (Chapters 8 and 12);
- damage through intoxication including drugs, alcohol, and infection (Chapters 7 and 9);
- damage through trauma or injury (Chapters 9, 10, and 11).

In the scenario below, Sally Smith is introduced through the eyes of a student nurse. Sally's story will continue to be analysed in the context of this chapter and, where appropriate, linked to other chapters in the book.

Scenario: Sally Smith

I am a second-year student and this is my first day on the acute medical admissions unit. Up until now my only experience has been working in a nursing home and on a surgical day unit. I arrived just as a new patient was being admitted; her name was Sally Smith, and she was 67 years old. She was being admitted with a six-day history of malaise, vomiting, falls, and confusion. Her husband was with her and he seemed very anxious. He suggested we call his wife Sally because she seemed to respond better to that name. We transferred Sally onto the bed, and I was asked to make sure she kept her oxygen mask on while she was assessed. We uploaded her vital signs onto the computer database and her NEWS2 (National Early Warning Score 2) was recorded as seven. This was the first time that I had looked after someone with a score higher than three and I began to feel very anxious about the situation. What does seven mean, what was going to happen, what was I going to do? I looked at the patient as if for the first time. The medical team had been informed that the patient was now in the ward and a nurse from the critical care outreach team had arrived to assess her. The outreach nurse began asking Sally's husband questions about the last week and was able to obtain detailed information about the progression of Sally's illness and how she had come to be admitted. At the same time, an airway, breathing, circulation,

(Continued)

(Continued)

disability, and exposure (ABCDE) assessment and interventions were being completed and fluid balance monitored. All the time, the outreach nurse remained calm and continued to observe Sally very closely, while quietly reminding me to help Sally to keep the oxygen mask on. I felt completely out of my depth but was reassured by the calm efficiency of my mentor and the outreach nurse. I had a lot to learn!

Within five minutes we had obtained the following data:

Situation: Sally Smith, age 67 years, is presenting with hypoxia and confusion; she has two Red Flags for sepsis together with a recent history of a urinary tract infection.

Background: Sally has been ill for six days, provisionally with a three-day history of decreasing appetite and vomiting, diagnosed by her GP as viral gastritis. By day five the patient was still unable to tolerate food but was able to take sips of water. She was also complaining of loin pain when trying to pass urine. According to her husband, Sally had fallen twice when attempting to get to the bathroom and had periods when 'she didn't seem to make sense'. As a consequence, on day five Sally received a home visit from her GP, who diagnosed a urinary tract infection. He asked Sally's husband to send a urine sample from his wife to the pathology department in the local hospital and prescribed a broad spectrum antibiotic. Twenty-four hours later the patient was not improving, and she was admitted as an emergency at the GP's request. She has a past medical history of hypertension diagnosed 10 years ago and controlled by lisinopril 20 mg.

Next of kin: Husband, no children. Sally is for active resuscitation.

Assessment

Airway: Patent; patient confused; GCS 14/15; no evidence of nausea.

Breathing: R 22/minute; oxygen saturation (SpO_2): 92% (receiving oxygen 40% prescribed in the emergency unit to maintain SpO_2 at >94%).

Circulation: P 94/minute; sinus rhythm; BP 120/75 mmHg; T: 37.4 °C; cool hands and feet; has not passed urine for approximately six hours, urethral catheter inserted, 70 ml drained and a sample was sent for culture and sensitivity. Infusion of 0.9% saline commenced in the emergency department at 125 ml/hr.

Biochemistry:

- Arterial blood gases:
  - pH: 7.32 (acidosis)
  - PaO_2: 8.5 kPa; (low oxygen)
  - $PaCO_2$: 5.8 kPa; (elevated carbon dioxide)
  - HCO_3: 26 mmol/L
  - High risk of respiratory failure
- Lactate: 1.9 mmol/L
- WBC: 18.2×10^9/L

- Hb: 106 g/L
- CRP: 20 mg/dL
- Na: 132 mmol/L
- K: 5.0 mmol/L
- Urea: 12.5 mmol/L
- Creatinine: 160 micromol/L

Disability: Confused; GCS: 14/15, glucose: 6.5 mmol/L.

Exposure: Skin appears dry to touch; weight 73 kg (11 st 7 lb) prior to her illness; height 1.6 m (5 ft 4 in); she has a red area over her right hip.

NEWS2 = 10

Recommendation from the outreach nurse:

- Initiate the Sepsis Six protocol (Chapter 7).
- Continuous oxygen therapy to maintain SpO_2 at >94%.
- Blood cultures taken together with a second arterial blood for analysis, and venous blood for full biochemical analysis.
- Administer IV antibiotics according to Trust Protocol.
- Administer a fluid challenge of 500 ml.
- Continuous assessment and monitoring of the patient's vital signs, fluid, and electrolyte balance.
- Review the effect of administering the Sepsis Six protocol at the end of the first hour.

What Sally's story illustrates is that assessing, risk assessing, and managing care can require complex skills and a multidisciplinary approach that combines knowledge and experience of the following:

- the patient as a person;
- biopsychosocial systems;
- clinical assessment and interpersonal skills;
- relevant clinical experience;
- the ability to interpret complex patterns of illness and behaviour;
- the ability to interpret and manage care in rapidly changing situations.

Why is the nursing assessment and monitoring of care important?

Assessing and monitoring of the patient's condition has been a central role of the nurse for 150 years, and nurses are in the privileged position of providing 24-hour care to people in a variety of clinical and community-based settings. With the correct skill mix of registered nurses to patients, nurses can improve the quality of care and reduce patient morbidity and mortality (Aiken et al., 2017; Griffiths et al., 2018). In Aiken et al.'s (2017) study, they were also able to demonstrate that a reduction in nursing skill mix can have the opposite effect, leading to an increase in patient morbidity and mortality. Registered nurses are key to providing safe and effective care, and yet in the last 25 years there has been a growing body of evidence that nurses and other health-care practitioners have been unable to provide safe and consistent standards of care for acutely ill adults. This has resulted in evidence of unnecessary distress and patient deaths on an international scale. A review of these findings is included in the research summary below.

Research summary: suboptimal care recognition and action

Empirical evidence of suboptimal care can be traced back to the 1990s. In the USA, Franklin and Matthew (1994) undertook a retrospective study of patient signs and symptoms before cardiac arrest and demonstrated that in 25% of the 150 cases studied there was evidence that the nurse had documented deterioration but failed to inform the medical team. They also found significant failings in the medical management of the patients. In the UK, case studies of patients admitted to intensive care from the ward by McQuillan et al. (1998) and McGloin et al. (1999) found evidence of suboptimal care in 50% and 30%, respectively, of the cases studied. Both studies identified that nursing and medical staff had failed to recognise and/or report the urgency of the situation, and that there was evidence of lack of continuity of care, poor supervision of junior staff, and other organisational failings. The National Patient Safety Agency (NPSA) Report (2007b) further reinforced the concerns by publishing that out of 425 reported deaths in acute care, 64 (15%) were related to patient deterioration not being recognised or acted upon. All these research findings are based on retrospective analysis of case studies and cannot be considered to be gold standard evidence, but the nature and implications of the findings have triggered a national and international campaign to improve the recognition of and response to clinical deterioration (Institute for Healthcare Improvement (IHI), 2011; NICE CG50, 2020; RCP, 2012). Proposed solutions included: measuring levels of patient acuity and aligning this to the skill mix required (Mark and Harless, 2011); physiological track and trigger tools and weighted response systems (RCP, 2017, 2012); communication tools such as 'SBAR' (Merten et al., 2017); and the development of critical care outreach or medical emergency teams (Tirkkonen et al., 2017). Studies of the sensitivity and clinical effectiveness of these various tools and frameworks have been difficult to evaluate due to several factors. These include: lack of standardisation of the tools used in research studies making comparison and meta-analysis of the findings difficult to achieve (Downey et al., 2017); difficulties associated with measuring the impact of a defined variable on patient outcome when there are extraneous variables influencing patient outcome (Churpek et al., 2017;

Downey et al., 2017; Smith et al., 2013); and recognising that the roles and responsibilities of healthcare practitioners are managed in complex organisational systems which impact on patient outcome. Such system factors include the presence of person-centred care, the presence of continuity of care, the knowledge and experience of the workers, skill mix, education, communication processes, organisational culture, and availability of resources (White and Tait, 2019; Dalton et al., 2018; McGaughey et al., 2017; Massey et al., 2016).

The assessment, recognition, communication, and management of patients with clinical deterioration is a vital part of the nurse's role and supports collaborative practice. According to Coulter Smith et al. (2014), recognising and responding to clinical deterioration requires not only physiological measurement but the combination of rapid, detailed assessment and skilled clinical judgement concerning the history and context of the person's illness. By highlighting the key factors that influence the quality of care provided when patients deteriorate cited by Dalton (2018); Massey et al. (2016); McGaughey et al. (2017), and White and Tait (2019), we can begin to unpick the optimum skills, organisational culture, and resources required to manage the care of deteriorating patients safely and effectively, as well as anticipating and preventing those conditions that lead to deterioration. These key factors are:

- person-centred care and continuity of care;
- knowledge and experience of the nurse and other healthcare workers in the team;
- nursing skill mix;
- communication;
- clinical and self leadership;
- team working and mutual reciprocity;
- organisational culture and management strategies;
- strategic planning and availability of resources.

In the remainder of the chapter, we will begin to explore these factors by focusing on how you can provide a safe but rapid assessment and response to patients with acute and critical illness by using physiological measurement, clinical judgement, and effective communication in a variety of organisational settings.

Knowing and understanding the acutely ill patient

The World Health Organization's (WHO) global goal for humanising healthcare focuses on the person and their family as being central to the process of care,

> *The overall vision for people-centred healthcare is one in which individuals, families and communities are served by and are able to participate in trusted health systems that respond to their needs in humane and holistic ways.*

(WHO, 2007, p7)

This goal does not change just because a person's condition changes, and should be recognised as the minimum standard required for all aspects of healthcare. Person-centred care puts the patient at the centre of care and prioritises the human connection between the patient and the carer (Sharp et al., 2015). There is a growing body of evidence that person-centred care enhances the quality of patient care and has the potential to improve patient outcomes through improvements in a person's self-efficacy, better communication and psychological support for recovery, and an improved ability to meet the patient's needs (Edvardsson et al., 2017; Etkind et al., 2015; Pirhonen et al., 2017; Sharp et al., 2015). The better you know a person, the more able you are to see subtle changes in their behaviour and form an overview of the clinical picture. In this way you can work to prevent further deterioration rather than wait for it to occur (White and Tait, 2019). In the absence of person-centred practice, dehumanisation of care and objectification of the person occurs, leading to suboptimal care and patient harm, as evidenced in the Report on Mid Staffordshire Healthcare Foundation Trust (Francis, 2013).

In 2000, the Department of Health set out guidance for managing patient dependency in relation to skill mix and location. These guidelines have subsequently been updated by the Intensive Care Society (ICS, 2021) and describe ward-level patients up to those requiring advanced level 3 critical care, listed in Table 1.1. These levels of care have been used to assist in the risk assessment of patients as well as in the identification and justification of decisions made about the skill mix requirements for individual wards and units (NICE, 2007; Smith, 2009).

When we return to Sally's story, we can see that she meets the criteria for level 1, with the potential to require level 2 patient care, for the following reasons.

- Sally's NEWS2 score = 10.
- Sally meets two Red Flags for sepsis (see Chapter 7).
- She is receiving continuous oxygen therapy for impaired respiratory function.
- She requires fluid resuscitation.
- She is at risk of acute kidney injury.
- Initially, she required the support of the outreach nurse.

We shall return to Sally's story later in the chapter.

Level of critical care criteria	Patient/clinical examples
Ward care Requires hospitalisation: needs can be met through normal ward care. • Patients recently discharged from higher levels of care. • Person who can be managed clinically on a ward but remains at risk of clinical deterioration.	• Jennifer Harris is admitted for routine surgery. Her planned length of stay is two days, and she will need post-operative monitoring and intravenous therapy for 24 hours during her stay. • Fred Johnson has been discharged to your care from the high dependency unit, where he received respiratory support and interventions for acute respiratory failure.
Level 1 Enhanced care • Patients in need of more detailed observations and interventions. • Those stepping down from higher levels of care. • Patients requiring ongoing critical care outreach service support. • Patients requiring enhanced pre-operative care to optimise their post-operative recovery.	• A patient requiring close physiological monitoring after major surgery – may have additional monitoring devices in situ, e.g. arterial line. • A patient requiring vasopressor support (peripheral or central) but otherwise stable who requires monitoring of BP. • A patient requiring non-invasive ventilation/continuous positive airways pressure (NIV/CPAP) for single organ failure. For example, acute heart failure with pulmonary oedema, acute respiratory failure. • Patients requiring ongoing interventions from critical care outreach teams in their active management.
Level 2 Critical care • Patients needing extended post-operative care. • Patients stepping down from level 3 to level 2 care. • Patients needing monitoring and support of two or more organ systems. • Patients requiring enhanced nursing assessment and interventions that cannot be met elsewhere. • Patients receiving advanced cardiovascular/renal/neurological/dermatological support.	• Mr Brown needs stabilisation and invasive monitoring of his cardiac and haemodynamic function prior to receiving a general anaesthetic for planned surgery. He has an arterial and central venous line. • Mary Simpson was admitted to critical care for 24 hours following a surgical carotid endarterectomy to remove plaque from the carotid artery. She required a prolonged period in recovery following post-operative haemodynamic instability. The surgery carries a risk of stroke and haemorrhage, and Mary required hourly invasive haemodynamic monitoring and cardiovascular support together with neurological assessment and monitoring.

(Continued)

Table 1.1   (Continued)

Level of critical care criteria	Patient/clinical examples
	• Harry Green has a history of mental health disease and COPD. Following an acute exacerbation of his COPD he required 14 days of invasive ventilation in intensive care. He is now being weaned from full respiratory support to spontaneous breathing with the help of non-invasive ventilation. He is confused at times and tires quickly.
	• Jane Morris has been admitted with sepsis and requires invasive haemodynamic support, fluid resuscitation and oxygen therapy as part of her ongoing care.
	• Paul Stone was admitted following a road traffic incident. He had sustained bruises to his sternum and left lower ribs, bilateral fractured shafts of femur, and a fractured pelvis. He requires oxygen therapy, advanced cardiovascular support, and pain relief following emergency surgery to stabilise the fractures with internal fixation.
Level 3 Critical care • Patients receiving advanced respiratory support alone or support for a minimum of two organs. • Patients with chronic impairment of one or more organ systems sufficient to restrict daily activities (co-morbidity) and who require support for an acute reversible failure of another organ system. • Patients who experience delirium in addition to requiring level 2 care. • Complex patients requiring support for multiple organ failures.	• Ben Williams was transferred from an acute medical ward after showing signs of clinical deterioration. He is diagnosed with pneumonia, acute respiratory distress syndrome, septic shock, and acute kidney injury. He requires invasive ventilation, invasive haemodynamic support, and renal replacement therapy.

Table 1.1   Defining levels of critical care informed by the Intensive Care Society Consensus Statement on Levels of Adult Critical Care

Source: ICS, 2021.

During handover

Knowing and understanding your patient can begin before you meet them and, in some cases, begins with the patient's handover, followed by meeting and assessing the patient and ensuring continuity of patient-centred care. The levels of patient dependency also allow you to risk assess from a distance and monitor the potential for patient deterioration. If the patient's dependency level is noted during handover, then you have already started to prioritise your patient's needs. Other related factors, identified during handover and/or during the patient assessment, may influence the potential for the patient to deteriorate (Elliot et al., 2014). These include the following:

- *Age*: increasing age in the older adult is associated with increased vulnerability to co-morbidities, infection, and the need for multiple medications.
- *Hydration*: over- or under-hydration can increase the risk of clinical deterioration.
- *Nutrition*: malnutrition can prolong recovery, wound healing, and increase the risk of infection.
- *Pain*: a patient in pain is likely to have impaired mobility and increased risk of venous thrombosis, chest infection, and a longer length of stay in hospital.
- *Mobility*: reduced mobility increases the risk of pressure ulcers, venous thrombosis, sepsis, and lethargy.
- *Mood/psychological*: anxiety, fear, and low mood can negatively impact on the speed and progress of a patient's recovery.
- *Mental health*: knowledge and understanding of patients' mental health problems can enhance your understanding of their ability to cope with other health problems.
- *Learning difficulties*: knowledge of underlying physiological disorders related to their learning difficulties can be crucial and vital for risk assessment of these patients.
- *Co-morbidities and medication*: the presence of combined biopsychosocial problems such as diabetes, heart disease, and the patient's requirement for a hip replacement will increase the risks associated with surgery. Drugs such as prednisolone are steroids that, when prescribed, can lead to a suppressed immune response, hypertension, and raised blood glucose. There is also an increased risk of acute kidney injury and/or chronic kidney disease (see Chapter 9 for further details).
- *Previous admission to ITU*: The patient that has been previously admitted to intensive care during this hospital stay will have increased vulnerability to infection, haemodynamic instability, weakness, and lethargy.

Recognising the significance of these factors in patients will alert you to the potential for deterioration.

Meeting and assessing the patient

This should always begin with a rapid assessment of your patient's safety (illustrated in Table 1.2). If you are concerned, complete the rapid assessment, and report your concerns without delay (NICE, 2007 [reviewed without change in 2016]; NPSA, 2007a; RCP, 2017). The difference between a routine assessment and a rapid assessment of a patient's condition is the ability to anticipate, recognise, and respond in a timely manner to any aspect of concern you have for the patient's condition. As a student or junior nurse, the use of clinical guidelines will provide a safe starting point for you to recognise and manage concern and, as you develop your level of expertise and experience, you will begin to develop the core skills required for the nurses' professional gaze. The professional gaze (Tait, 2009, cited by White and Tait, 2019) can be described as including a continuous process of scanning: Having sideways vision while at the same time concentrating on the particulars of practice … the visual thing (Tait, 2009, p235).

The professional gaze also includes using the senses of sight, hearing, smell, and touch to perceive and selectively attend to changes in the patient's condition, described by Resuscitation Council UK (2015) as look, listen, and feel. The knowledge and skills that a nurse utilises to perform the professional scan include the following:

- clinical, historical, and experiential knowledge of the person, his/her condition, and the clinical situation;
- the ability to balance the subjective, contextual, and objective data collected in order to collate and understand the data;
- the use of previously learned clinical cues and pattern recognition that act as shortcuts to a provisional diagnosis;
- focused observation when data are interpreted in the context of all available clinical information and results of investigations leading to a diagnosis;
- communication with the patient, family, and clinical colleagues;
- initiating clinical actions required to manage the patient's situation in collaboration with others;
- continued scanning and monitoring of the patient's condition for signs of change.

Regardless of your level of skill, the National Institute for Health and Care Excellence (NICE, 2007) recommends that if you are concerned about a patient, you should initiate and perform the admissions, recognition, and response bundles and monitor the patient's condition as illustrated in Table 1.2.

Central to the use of these bundles is the integration of the physiological track and trigger score, and the use of emergency outreach teams for the provision of patient and staff support. The National Early Warning Score (NEWS) was developed to standardise risk assessment across the UK (RCP, 2012). The Royal College of Physicians (RCP) proposes that standardising the numerical score and tracking the changes in the patient's condition provides objective evidence of deterioration, justifies calling the rapid response team for support, and optimises standards for education and training of all healthcare staff. However, a systematic review of the effectiveness of

Bundle of care	Bundle purpose	Interventions
Admission bundle: multidisciplinary	To achieve a baseline of patient data within two hours of admission, collected and communicated to the medical team.	1. Minimum data to collect on admission to your practice area: T, P, R, BP, level of consciousness, oxygen saturation (SpO_2). 2. Document a clear monitoring plan including the type and frequency of observations to be undertaken. 3. Ensure that all members of the multidisciplinary team know and agree the monitoring plan.
Recognition bundle	Early identification and risk assessment of the deteriorating patient.	1. Monitor physiological signs at least 12 hourly for all patients. 2. Record track and trigger score. 3. Perform risk assessment according to the assessment and trigger score. 4. Consider the possibility of sepsis. 5. Communicate the information to the medical team.
Response bundle	Optimal and timely treatment of the at-risk patient.	1. If there is clinical concern. The RCP (2017) recommend: 2. If the trigger score is low (1–4), ask a registered nurse to assess the patient and make a clinical decision to either increase the frequency of the observations and/or escalate care requirements. 3. If the trigger score is YELLOW (a score of 3 in a single parameter) increase observations to hourly and a registered nurse should contact the patient's medical team for review. 4. If the trigger score is AMBER (a total of 5 or more) increase observations to hourly/continuous and the registered nurse will immediately inform the medical team and contact the critical care outreach team urgently. 5. If the trigger score is RED (a total of 7 or more) commence continuous monitoring, and the registered nurse will contact the medical team, critical care outreach team, and consider transfer to HDU/ICU. 6. In all cases communicate and document communication using the SBAR (situation, background, assessment, recommendation) tool.

Table 1.2 Rapid response to acute illness: admission, recognition, and response bundles

Source: NICE, 2007.

physiological track and trigger tools by Gao et al. (2007) concluded that the validity, reliability, and sensitivity of the tools in use were poor when used as a single indicator for evidence of deterioration. However, Smith et al. (2013) found that NEWS has a greater ability to discriminate patients at risk of deterioration than 33 other early warning scoring systems. Further evaluation of NEWS has highlighted its value in several settings including pre-hospital care and emergency departments (Bilben et al., 2016; Keep et al., 2016; Silcock et al., 2015). However, concerns have been raised about the potential overuse of oxygen for patients with hypercapnic respiratory failure increasing the risk of further deterioration for this patient group (Kane et al., 2012). A study by Ludikhuize et al. (2012) highlights another area of concern that relates to evidence of incomplete documentation. They found that in a retrospective study of 204 patients in an acute hospital the collection of vital signs and track and trigger scores was incomplete in most cases they reviewed. This suggests that future studies need to focus on measuring the effectiveness of NEWS implementation and the use of clinical judgement in recognising and responding to clinical deterioration. These findings prompted some amendments to NEWS when it was evaluated in 2015 by the NEWS Review Group. These evidence-based changes were published in December 2017 and launched in 2018 by the RCP and have been incorporated in this textbook in relevant chapters (RCP, 2017).

Clinically effective detection and management of clinical deterioration therefore begins with nurses being alerted to or recognising signs of clinical deterioration and using a systematic, comprehensive, and holistic approach to managing care.

When meeting and assessing the patient, it is important not to make assumptions about your patient's biopsychosocial and spiritual needs until you have verified this with the patient and the healthcare team. Has your patient made a choice about resuscitation? Does your patient have an advance directive? According to joint guidance from the British Medical Association (BMA), Resuscitation Council (UK), and the Royal College of Nursing (RCN) (2016), the provision of patient-centred care should consider patients' individual needs and wishes where possible. You should be encouraging patients to make informed decisions about their care, and this includes advanced care planning for decisions about cardiopulmonary resuscitation when it is appropriate to do so, as illustrated, for example, in the following patient case study.

Case study: Tom Romano

Tom is 74 years old and has a 20-year history of chronic respiratory disease. For the last ten years he has been admitted to level 2 and/or 3 care for management of acute exacerbations of his chronic respiratory problem during the winter months. Last year he was in hospital for a period of 12 weeks, four weeks of which were in intensive care. Tom has made it clear to his family and the nursing team that he does not want to go through 'that torture' again. He has expressly wished that he does not want to be '**intubated** and put on a **ventilator**'. A collaborative team meeting with Tom and his family resulted in clear documented guidelines for active treatment of his chest infection with a ceiling of treatment noted: 'He will receive active and full support for his condition including non-invasive respiratory support but excluding **invasive respiratory support of any kind and cardiopulmonary resuscitation**.' The documentation was agreed and signed, with review dates and criteria agreed with the patient and family.

Knowledge of your patient will enable you to make informed decisions about your patient's progress. Where possible, plan for continuity of care using a collaborative team approach to organising person-centred care with clear lines of responsibility.

Evidence-based rapid assessment and interpretation of the patient's condition

The purpose of undertaking a rapid assessment and interpretation of a patient's condition is to:

- anticipate potential risks;
- prevent deterioration;
- ensure timely interventions to provide optimal outcome.

The Airway – Breathing – Circulation – Disability – Exposure 'ABCDE' approach to assessment advocated by the Resuscitation Council (UK) (2015) provides a simple but systematic and priority-driven approach that focuses initially on assessing patient safety and then provides a focus for more in-depth assessment once the patient's safety has been established. When the ABCDE approach is combined with clinical assessment processes – including look, listen, feel, measure, monitor, collate evidence, and finally respond – you will have the basis of preliminary but detailed assessment data that can be used to communicate and collaborate with the medical team to achieve an effective response (Zinchenko, 2018).

This chapter and subsequent chapters introduce you to the ABCDE algorithm and encourage you to apply this in the context of patient assessment, clinical interpretation, and management of care. In the remainder of this chapter, you will be taken through the rapid assessment process by using the core skills: look, listen, feel, measure, monitor and collate evidence, and respond.

Each element of the process is summarised in table format and provides a working guide that you can apply to scenarios in this book and in clinical practice. In the following tables each assessment activity is prioritised and listed using A-B-C-D-E; there are columns that illustrate normal and abnormal signs, and tips for drawing conclusions and acting.

It is important to note that while, for the purpose of this book, these core skills have been listed in separate tables, in practice you will be using these skills concurrently and consistently to manage patient care.

Assessing your patient: Look/Listen/Feel

When assessing a person, it is often the first look or sound that alerts you to their condition and helps you to start focusing on your priorities. This is often before a formal assessment has been made.

Look: As you approach the patient, your initial observation of them begins and your priority is to look and assess for any evidence of patient distress. Nurses often say that 'they only have to look at a patient to know there is something wrong': what they are doing is using their skills of visual perception, combined with knowledge and clinical experience, to interpret a picture of the patient before them (Tait, 2009; Thompson and Dowding, 2002).

Listen: Once you have approached the patient, the second sense to use is listening. This includes listening for signs of a patient's physiological distress such as noisy and laboured breathing and/or signs of psychological distress such as crying. Assessment skills related to listening include the active process of gathering verbal data from the patient and/or relatives, receiving handover from clinical staff, and the process of linking relevant data to form clinical judgements.

Feel: The use of touch in professional caring can be involved with functional nursing activities related to physical aspects of care, as well as therapeutic nursing activities related to communication and psychological care. When undertaking a rapid assessment of a patient, your priority is to focus on factors affecting circulation. This includes assessing for evidence of cardiac activity and changes to the patient's circulation that affect the colour and warmth of the skin.

Airway

Assessment data	Normal signs	Abnormal signs	Drawing conclusions/taking action
Are they breathing?	Quiet regular respiratory pattern: 10–20/min.	Absent breathing; no rise and fall of the chest or abdomen. No response to verbal stimulation.	Absent breathing (apnoea). If the patient does not respond and is not breathing normally after you have opened the airway and checked for airway obstruction then follow the guidelines for basic life support (Resuscitation Council (UK), 2015).
Is there an airway obstruction?	Regular rise and fall of the chest.	Laboured breathing. Choking behaviour. Irregular pattern of breathing with paradoxical chest movements (see-saw respirations). Unequal chest expansion (may be a sign of a pneumothorax or haemothorax).	Untreated airway obstruction leads to a lowered level of oxygen in the arterial circulation (hypoxia) and increases the risk of hypoxic damage to the brain, kidneys, and heart. This situation can lead to cardiac arrest and death. Open the patient's airway, suction, and consider the use of an oropharyngeal airway. Anticipate the need for tracheal intubation in a medical emergency. Commence high-flow oxygen using a mask with an oxygen reservoir. Aim for oxygen saturations of 94–98% if the patient does not have pre-existing COPD and 88–92% if the patient is at risk of hypercapnic respiratory failure (RCP, 2017).
Is there potential for airway obstruction?	Alert Glasgow coma score (GCS) = 15	Evidence of a deteriorating level of consciousness. Reduced level of consciousness and vomiting. Evidence of blood loss that may obstruct the airway. GCS of 8 or less.	Open the patient's airway, suction, and consider the use of an oropharyngeal airway. Anticipate the need for tracheal intubation in a medical emergency. If GCS is 8 or less the airway is compromised: intubate. Commence high-flow oxygen using a mask with an oxygen reservoir. Aim for oxygen saturations of 94–98% if the patient does not have pre-existing COPD and 88–92% if the patient is at risk of hypercapnic respiratory failure (RCP, 2017).

Table 1.3 Quick guide to rapid assessment and response to clinical deterioration: Look/Listen/Feel: Airway

Breathing			
Assessment data	**Normal signs**	**Abnormal signs**	**Drawing conclusions/taking action**
Is the breathing noisy?	Quiet relaxed respirations.	Respiratory stridor indicates narrowing or partial obstruction to the upper airways. Respiratory wheeze is consistent with narrowing of the bronchi due to bronchospasm. Rattle indicates sputum or liquid in the apices of the lung.	For airway obstruction see Table 1.3. Assess the patient history for a diagnosis of asthma or chronic obstructive pulmonary disease (COPD). Aim for oxygen saturations of 94–98% if the patient does not have pre-existing COPD and 88–92% if the patient is at risk of hypercapnic respiratory failure (RCP, 2017).
Does the patient have a cough?	No cough.	Cough present. Dry cough. Chesty cough. Productive cough with sputum.	If the cough is dry and wheezy this may indicate an acute asthma attack. If the patient is producing yellow/green sputum this may indicate an infection. Obtain a sputum sample for microbial culture.
		Sputum green/yellow/black/pink/thick, tenacious, copious amounts (fills a tissue in one cough). Rapid shallow breathing	If the sputum is black and there is a recent history of exposure to fire this may indicate inhalation of smoke/inhalation burns. Frothy pink sputum may indicate pulmonary oedema. Rapid shallow breathing may be related to diabetic ketoacidosis, sepsis, and/or exhaustion.
Is there evidence of abdominal breathing or use of accessory muscles to breathe?	Quiet relaxed respirations.	Use of accessory muscles indicates there is increased work of breathing. The use of abdominal breathing without chest expansion may indicate an injury to the cervical spine.	Does the patient have a history of chronic respiratory disease? Have you checked for signs of airway obstruction? Does the patient have a pneumothorax or fluid obstructing the lung space in the thorax? Risk assess for and assume spinal injury in the presence of abdominal breathing until this cause has been ruled out or confirmed. Aim for oxygen saturations of 94–98% if the patient does not have pre-existing COPD and 88–92% if the patient is at risk of hypercapnic respiratory failure (RCP, 2017).

Table 1.4 Quick guide to rapid assessment and response to clinical deterioration: Look/Listen/Feel: Breathing

Circulation

Assessment data	Normal signs	Abnormal signs	Drawing conclusions/taking action
What can you interpret from looking at and feeling the skin?	Skin is pink or brown with pink mucosa. Skin is warm to touch and well perfused. Capillary refill time (CRT) of 2 seconds.	Skin is pale. Lips and mucosa pale blue or purple. Skin shows signs of central cyanosis. Cold hands and feet with a blue tinge to the skin on fingers and toes. Skin shows signs of peripheral cyanosis. Skin is warm, flushed, and red. One or more limbs pale and cold with absent pulses. Prolonged capillary refill.	Pale skin may indicate early signs of shock. Central cyanosis is an indication of severe hypoxia. Peripheral cyanosis may indicate poor peripheral perfusion/peripheral shutdown and, in the presence of other clinical factors such as a fall in BP, may indicate shock (Chapter 6). A flushed skin indicates peripheral vasodilation, present in anaphylaxis. A patient with sepsis may present with warm flushed skin because of distributive shock (Chapter 7). Localised peripheral changes may indicate localised trauma and loss of circulation, such as in compartment syndrome (Chapter 10). Prolonged peripheral capillary refill time (CRT) of more than 2 seconds is suggestive of peripheral vasoconstriction in the presence of other indicators for shock (Chapter 6) and/or hypothermia. CRT of less than 1 second is indicative of a hyperdynamic state such as systemic inflammation, sepsis, distributive shock and/or hyperthermia.
Pulse?	Pulse is present and regular. Pulses present in the peripheral pulse points.	Carotid pulse is absent. Pulse is weak and thready. Pulse is full and bounding. Pulse is irregular. Pulse is absent or altered in one or more of the following: pedal, radial, and femoral.	If the patient has no carotid pulse and cardiac output is absent follow the Resuscitation Council (UK) (2015) algorithm on basic life support or in-hospital life support. A weak thready pulse indicates reduced cardiac output. A full and bounding pulse may indicate sepsis. A rapid irregular pulse indicates an increased risk of embolus development and/or a failing cardiac output. Localised peripheral changes may indicate localised trauma and loss of circulation.

Table 1.5 Quick guide to rapid assessment and response to clinical deterioration: Look/Listen/Feel: Circulation

Disability			
Assessment data	**Normal signs**	**Abnormal signs**	**Drawing conclusions/taking action**
Is the patient alert and responding?	The patient is alert and responding to questions in a logical manner when assessed using the ACVPU algorithm (Alert/ new Confusion/ responds to Voice/responds to Pain/ Unresponsive) (RCP, 2017).	The patient responds to voice, pain or is unconscious. Evidence of new confusion. Evidence of: • response to voice • response to pain. Unresponsive GCS <15.	Consider possible causes including: • hypoxia • ketoacidosis (smell the breath for the presence of ketones – pear drops) • head injury • drugs • stroke. Place patient in the recovery position unless a spinal injury is suspected. If you suspect the person may have a cervical spine injury, open the airway using a jaw thrust rather than a head tilt (Resuscitation Council (UK), 2015). Open the patient's airway, suction, and consider the use of an oropharyngeal airway. Anticipate the need for tracheal intubation in a medical emergency. If GCS is 8 or less: intubate. Commence high-flow oxygen using a mask with an oxygen reservoir. Aim for oxygen saturations of 94–98% if the patient does not have pre-existing COPD and 88–92% if the patient is at risk of hypercapnic respiratory failure (RCP, 2017).

Table 1.6 Quick guide to rapid assessment and response to clinical deterioration: Look/Listen/Feel: Disability

Exposure/examination			
Assessment data	**Normal signs**	**Abnormal signs**	**Drawing conclusions/ taking action**
Is there evidence of trauma/injury?	No signs of physical damage to the person, comfortable in any position. Calm facial expression.	Unresponsive patient with facial grimacing, frowning. Signs of bruising, physical trauma, foreign object in the person, abnormal movement of the chest, immobility.	Attempt to open the airway where safe and possible for the patient. If you suspect the person may have a cervical spine injury, open the airway using a jaw thrust rather than a head tilt (Resuscitation Council (UK), 2015).

		Exposure/examination	
Assessment data	Normal signs	Abnormal signs	Drawing conclusions/ taking action
			Protect the patient's airway to maintain ventilation.
Is there evidence of factors that may be related to the patient's condition?	A safe environment.	Causes of injury or trauma include: empty medication packets, empty bottle of alcohol, sharp objects, etc.	Look for causes of injury or trauma. Ensure patient and personal safety.
Is there evidence of fluid loss, blood loss?	No signs of loss of body fluids.	Evidence of vomiting and/or diarrhoea. Blood loss. Loss of fluid through burns.	Risk assess for hypovolaemic shock (see Chapters 6 and 10).

Table 1.7 Quick guide to rapid assessment and response to clinical deterioration: Look/Listen/Feel: Exposure

The process of collating additional information begins with your rapid assessment of the patient and becomes a vital part of the data-collection process that informs your decision making and that of the healthcare team. This includes collating a record of the patient's recent history, past medical and social history as well as spiritual needs and agreed existing treatment plans. Table 1.8 gives you some pointers for what you should be asking and analysing.

Assessment data	Normal signs	Abnormal signs	Drawing conclusions/ taking action
Have you listened to the patient's or relative's story of events?	Patient is able to give you a clear account of their problem and history.	Patient is unable to respond, unconscious, confused, and unable to give appropriate answers. A relative or others are able to give an account of the events.	Always listen and be alert to information regardless of the source: it may be important!
Do you know the patient?	The patient has a named nurse.	Patient has been admitted in the last 24 hours and has no prescribed limiting directives.	If the patient is not for resuscitation this does not mean that active treatment has been withheld.
	The patient is registered 'do not resuscitate'	Patient is not known by the staff.	Therefore, always check to obtain a collaborative agreement of the patient's care plan.

(Continued)

Table 1.8 (Continued)

Assessment data	Normal signs	Abnormal signs	Drawing conclusions/ taking action
	and this has been dated and signed with an agreed time frame.		If the patient is a recent admission and no information is available, then assume that all active treatment continues.
			If the patient does not have a recent history of continuous care by the nursing staff then ensure that a baseline of assessment details is recorded for comparison.

Table 1.8 Quick guide to additional information gathering when undertaking a rapid assessment and response to clinical deterioration

The use of 'Look: Listen: Feel' is often the initial assessment that focuses on safety and preservation of life and this process runs concurrently with 'measure, monitor, and collate evidence'. Table 1.9 identifies objective measures that can be interpreted in the context of data already collected to create a more detailed and comprehensive presentation of the patient's condition.

Measure and collate evidence of clinical change

The core assessment skills of 'Look: Listen: Feel' can be completed within a few minutes of meeting the patient. The process of measuring and collating evidence for clinical change involves bringing together the objective data that can be collected on a patient through the assessment of vital signs, blood glucose, fluid and electrolyte balance, and other relevant investigations. This process also begins when you meet the patient and runs concurrently with the 'Look: Listen: Feel' assessment. According to Adam et al. (2010), there is strong evidence to suggest that changes in respiratory rate are associated with clinical deterioration, along with a decline in patient oxygen saturation levels, changes in pulse and blood pressure, and level of consciousness. It is at this stage that evidence of your concerns becomes apparent and, if necessary, triggers the next step. See Table 1.10.

Assessment data	Normal signs	Abnormal signs	Drawing conclusions/taking action
Airway	Patient alert. GCS >8.	New confusion. Responding to: • voice • pain. Unconscious. GCS <8.	If the person is confused this may be associated with reduced oxygen levels (dysoxia) and increases the risk to the patient's airway. Assess in conjunction with the 'Look: Listen: Feel' assessment. If GCS is 8 or less the person is unconscious and their airway is at risk: a skilled practitioner should intubate. Commence high-flow oxygen using a mask with an oxygen reservoir. Aim for oxygen saturations of 94–98% if the patient does not have pre-existing COPD and 88–92% if the patient is at risk of hypercapnic respiratory failure (RCP, 2017). Link assessment to risk of head injury (Chapter 11), endocrine causes of altered consciousness (Chapter 12), respiratory disease (Chapters 2 and 3), shock (Chapters 6 and 7).
Respiration (R)	R: 12–20/min	R: <12, >20	Assess the patient in context: are you concerned about your patient? Is there evidence to support this from your 'Look: Listen: Feel' assessment? If so, what information is there, and can you see a pattern or trend in deterioration? Has the NEWS2 score changed? Is there evidence of respiratory failure? (see Chapters 2 and 3) Is there evidence of sepsis? (see Chapter 7) Is there a recent history of head trauma? (Chapter 11) Is there evidence of a cardiac problem? (Chapter 4)

(Continued)

Table 1.9 (Continued)

Assessment data	Normal signs	Abnormal signs	Drawing conclusions/taking action
Oxygen saturation (SpO$_2$)	SpO$_2$: 94–100% in a person **without** hypercapnoea and/or COPD. SpO$_2$: 88–92% in a person **with** hypercapnoea and/or COPD. Does not need supplemental oxygen to maintain SpO$_2$ within the normal range.	SpO$_2$: <94% SpO$_2$: <88% Requires supplemental oxygen therapy to support SpO$_2$.	

Arterial blood gas analysis (ABG)	ABG:
	• pH: 7.35–7.45;
	• PaO$_2$: 11.5–13.5 kPa;
	• PaCO$_2$: 4.5–6.0 kPa;
	• HCO$_3$: 24–27 mmol/L.
		ABG
		• Respiratory acidosis:
		  o pH: <7.35;
		  o PaCO$_2$: >6.0 kPa.
		• Respiratory alkalosis:
		  o pH: >7.45;
		  o PaCO$_2$: <4.5 kPa.
		• Metabolic acidosis:
		  o pH: <7.35;
		  o HCO$_3$: <22 mmol/L.
		• Metabolic alkalosis:
		• pH: >7.45;
		• HCO$_3$: >26 mmol/L.	

Pulse (P) rate	P: 51–90/min	P: <50, >90/min	
Blood pressure (BP)	BP: 110/70–140/90 mmHg	BP: <110/70 mmHg, >140/90 mmHg	

Assessment data	Normal signs	Abnormal signs	Drawing conclusions/taking action
Electrocardiogram (ECG)	Sinus rhythm.	Evidence of any abnormal-looking complexes and irregularities in rate. For example: ectopic beats, atrial fibrillation, and elevation of the ST segment in some ECG leads.	
Urine output	>0.5 ml/kg body weight/hr >1000 ml/24hrs.	Urine output: • oliguria (acute kidney injury): <0.5 ml/kg body weight/hr; • polyuria (diabetes, diabetes insipidus). Negative urine balance despite rigorous fluid replacement.	If the person has oliguria, investigate serum creatinine levels – does the patient have acute kidney injury? If polyuria, assess blood glucose levels for signs of diabetes (Chapter 12). Has there been a recent head injury that may have damaged the hypothalamus? (Chapter 11).
Fluid balance	Fluid balance should be equal (=) based on a minimum input of 2 L/24hrs.	Fluid balance < or > = based on a minimum input of 2 L/24hrs.	Is there evidence of shock? Is there evidence of fluid overload, oedema?
Central venous pressure (CVP)	Mid-axilla: 2–6 mmHg (5–10 cm water).	Mid-axilla: • hypovolaemia. CVP: <2–6 mmHg; • hypervolaemia/cardiac failure. CVP: >2–6 mmHg.	CVP is an indicator of circulating volume and right sided cardiac function. Consider shock if low or, if high, consider fluid overload or heart failure.
Capillary refill time (CRT)	<2 seconds	>2 seconds	Is the person dehydrated? Are they hypovolaemic with evidence of peripheral shutdown?
Level of consciousness (LOC)	ACPVU score: A Alert/new Confusion/responds to Voice/responds to Pain/Unresponsive) (RCP, 2017). GCS score: 15	ACPVU score indicating CPVU. GCS: <15	If confusion is apparent, consider respiratory failure, head injury. Other causes of altered consciousness (Chapters 2, 11). GCS of <8 means that the airway is compromised.

(Continued)

Table 1.9 (Continued)

Assessment data	Normal signs	Abnormal signs	Drawing conclusions/taking action
Pain assessment	Pain managed effectively.	Elevated pain score.	Utilise a comprehensive pain assessment tool, PQRST (Chapter 5).
Blood results			Any changes in serum results should be assessed in context of the person's other clinical signs and communicated to the medical team.
Glucose	Glucose: 4–8 mmol/L	Glucose: <4 or >7.7 mmol/L	
Urea and creatinine	Urea: 3.5–6.5 mmol/L	Urea: <or >3.5–6.5 mmol/L	
Electrolytes	Creatinine: 60–120 micromol/L	Creatinine: >60–20 micromol/L	
Haematology	Na: 135–145 mmol/L	Na: < or >135–145 mmol/L	
Microbiology	K: 3.5–4.5 mmol/L	K: < or >3.5–4.5 mmol/L	
C-reactive protein (CRP) (inflammatory marker)	Mg: 1.25–2.5 mmol/L	Mg: < or >1.25–2.5 mmol/L	
Erythrocyte sedimentation rate (ESR)	Cl: 95–108 mmol/L	Cl: < or >95–108 mmol/L	
	Haemoglobin:	Haemoglobin:	
	Male: 130–170 g/L	Male: < or >130–170 g/L	
	Female 110–150 g/L	Female: < or >110–150 g/L	
	WCC: 4–12 109/L	WCC: <4 or >12 109/L	
	CRP: <3 mg/L	CRP: >3 mg/L	
	Erythrocyte sedimentation rate (ESR): 15-30 mm/hr	ESR > 30 mm/hr	

Table 1.9 Quick guide to rapid assessment and response to clinical deterioration using objective clinical measurement

Date and time of initial call:	Patient's name: *Sally Smith aged 67 years*	
05/11/18 at 18.00 hrs Date and time of response: *05/11/18 at 18.05 hrs*	Nurse's name: *Susan Brown* Name of person called: *Specialist registrar (Brian James)*	
Situation: reason for the call	*I am concerned about Sally Smith; she was admitted today at 16.00 hrs after being diagnosed with dehydration, possible urinary tract infection and sepsis. Her condition has deteriorated after initiation of the Sepsis Six criteria 1 hour ago.*	
Background	*Past medical history: hypertension controlled by lisinopril 20 mg but she has been unable to take her medication for six days.*	
Assessment	*Previous assessment data: 17.00 hrs* **Airway:** *patent* **Breathing:** *R: 22/min;* *SpO_2: 92% on 40% O_2* **Circulation:** *P: 94/min;* *sinus rhythm;* *BP 120/70 mmHg;* *T: 37.4 °C; cool hands and feet.* *Has not passed urine for approximately six hours.* *Urinary catheter passed 70 ml* *Infusion of 0.9% saline commenced in the emergency unit running at 125 ml/hour and a fluid challenge of 500 ml infused.* *CRP: 20 mg/L* *White cell count 18.2 10^9/L* **Disability:** *Confusion* *Glucose: 6.5 mmol/l* *NEWS = 10*	*New assessment data: 18.00 hrs* **Airway:** *patent* **Breathing:** *R 26/min;* *SpO_2: 89% on 40% O_2* **Circulation:** *P: 100/min;* *sinus tachycardia* *BP 90/50 mmHg;* *T: 37.7 °C; cool hands and feet.* *Urine output 50 ml* *(Urine positive to blood and protein).* *CRP: 30 mg/L* *White cell count 19.2 10^9/L* **Disability:** *responding to Voice.* *Glucose: 7.9 mmol/l* *NEWS = 14*
Recommendations and response	What are you requesting? *Sally Smith requires an urgent review of her sepsis management.* *I have contacted the outreach nurse who reviewed her 1 hour ago and he will meet you on the ward. I am preparing her for possible transfer to ICU.* *Sally's husband is aware of the change in her condition and is with her.* *Is there anything else you would like me to get ready for you?* Action taken and registrar's response: *Thank you. Can you increase the oxygen therapy immediately according to the sepsis guidelines* (see Chapter 7) *and I will come and reassess the patient? Please ensure a second set of blood cultures are taken and initiate a second fluid challenge according to the protocol. I will be on the ward in 2–3 minutes.* Signatures: Signed by both the staff nurse and the registrar following Sally's assessment and management.	

Table 1.10   Communicating concern using the SBAR approach

The outreach nurse in Sally's story was able to demonstrate expertise and clinical reasoning in the context of the clinical situation. This resulted in him being able to quickly obtain a clinical grasp of the situation, and to anticipate and prevent potential problems. This is what Benner et al. (2011, p2) describe as *habits of thought and action* (problem identification, clinical problem solving, anticipating, and preventing potential problems) that rely on a dynamic process of knowledge acquisition, experience, pattern recognition, and critical reflection. The development of these skills occurs over time and is always dependent on the history, knowledge, and experience of the nurse (White and Tait, 2019). In Activity 1.1 you have a chance to practise rapid assessment and management of a patient.

Activity 1.1   Risk assessment and decision making

Isabel Campbell is 85 years old and lives a full and active life. She lives alone but has two adult children living nearby. Isabel routinely takes an **angiotensin converting enzyme** (ACE) inhibitor to control hypertension, and aspirin as a preventer for stroke and heart disease. This evening Isabel has been experiencing some abdominal discomfort and nausea, but she put it down to eating rich food and went to bed. Two hours later she awoke and vomited a large amount of brown liquid over the bed. She felt faint, dizzy, and frightened, so phoned her daughter Holly for help. Holly was too far away to get to her mother quickly and phoned the out of hours service for advice. After some deliberation, a paramedic was dispatched and, following assessment, Isabel was admitted to the local medical assessment unit at 01.00 hours.

1.   What knowledge and skills identified in this chapter would you use to assess Isabel on admission and who would you seek guidance from?

On assessment the following data were collected regarding her condition.

- R 28/min.
- SpO_2 94%.
- Skin pale and cool.
- P 98/min.
- BP 105/93 mmHg.
- Has not passed urine since teatime at home.
- Alert.
- T 37.3 °C.

2.   What concerns would you have and what would you do about your concerns?

There are sample answers to this question at the end of the chapter.

Communicating and collaborating with patients, relatives, and staff to achieve appropriate and timely interventions

Risk assessment is a continuous process. If, however, you are concerned about your patient and you wish to seek advice or help, the next stage of the process is to communicate your concerns to the relevant person or team using the recognition and response bundles (NICE, 2007) referred to in Table 1.2 and supported by the guidance in NEWS2 (RCP, 2017):

- If you have a clinical concern about the patient and the data indicate the patient to be at low risk, then increase the frequency of the observations (minimum 4–6 hourly) and monitor the patient.
- If you have a clinical concern about the patient and the data indicate the patient to be at medium risk, then contact the patient's medical team urgently and monitor the patient at least hourly or more frequently. If necessary, contact the critical care outreach team to get an urgent assessment by a clinician with core competencies to assess the acutely ill patient.
- If you have a clinical concern about the patient and the data indicate the patient to be at high risk, then contact the critical care outreach team urgently and consider transfer to critical care. Provide continuous assessment and monitoring and do not leave the patient unattended.

When communicating with the medical team or critical care outreach team it is vital that the date, time, and nature of your concern are identified and documented. It is this process of documentation that provides a timeline and audit trail for the review of practice.

SBAR is an abbreviation for 'Situation: Background: Assessment: Recommendation' and is a structured communication tool that has been recommended by the Institute for Healthcare Improvement (IHI, 2011) and NICE (2007) for use to improve inter-professional communication and patient safety. A systematic review of the effect of SBAR on patient safety by Müller et al. (2018) highlighted that there was a lack of high-quality research to support its use but did find there was moderate evidence to support its use as a tool to communicate information over the phone. One of the challenges the reviewers met was that the SBAR tool has been modified or adapted to include other elements (for example, ISBAR – where I is identification of the patient and communicator). SBAR has also been adopted as a tool for verbal and written handovers in a variety of clinical settings. According to Dayton and Henriksen (2007), SBAR works because it provides a shared and logical structure for communicating core details of a patient's situation, either verbally or through written communication. This argument is supported by Field et al. (2011), who were able to demonstrate a statistically significant improvement in the management of people requiring regular coagulation monitoring in care homes by using SBAR reporting.

The explanation below focuses on the core elements of SBAR, but the author recognises that adaptations to the tool may be used in practice.

- Situation: identify yourself, your location, and the patient. Describe the problem, your concern, and your reason for calling.
- Background: provide the patient's reason for admission, diagnosis, and relevant medical history and medications.
- Assessment: provide both your subjective concerns and objective data. Offer a provisional diagnosis of the problem or clarify your concern.
- Recommendations: explain what you need, when, and where. Clearly identify your priorities for the patient's care.

In the example in Table 1.10, we have returned to our student nurse Susan and her patient Sally, whom we met at the beginning of the chapter. There has been a change in Sally's condition and, using the SBAR approach, we will recap and see what has changed.

In Sally's case there were several reasons why her condition may have deteriorated. These include:

- dehydration and the resultant hypovolaemia (see Chapter 6);
- her progression to respiratory failure, septic shock, and a high risk of AKI (see Chapters 7 and 9);
- a risk of acute heart failure (Chapter 4).

At this stage of her care the priorities include supporting Sally physiologically and psychologically by:

- supporting her airway, breathing, and circulation in order to reduce the risk of further deterioration;
- continuous monitoring of her condition;
- providing information and reassurance to her and her husband;
- arranging her transfer to ICU.

Providing standardised and optimal care during all stages of the patient's journey

A registered nurse has a professional responsibility to ensure safe and clinically effective care to support an agreed patient outcome and to accurately document any changes in the patient's condition or variance from the care pathway. The adoption of a care pathway and a care bundle approach by NICE (2011) has given all healthcare providers an opportunity to standardise practice while continuing to provide patient-focused care. The emphasis is now on you as a nurse to recognise and adopt the most clinically appropriate pathway of care, but at the same time to recognise, record, and respond to any variances in the care package. In this context, those variances must be justified and evidence-based. The seven points below are a useful guide to what should be provided to ensure the quality of nursing documentation (Jeffries et al., 2010).

Good nursing documentation:

- is patient-centred and includes extracts from the patient's description of their illness experience;
- reflects the objective clinical judgement of the nurse so that every statement has an objective descriptor, for example:
  - o incorrect – subjective comment: the patient seemed a bit tipsy;
  - o correct – objective comment: the patient was walking with an unsteady gait, his speech was slurred and his breath smelled of alcohol;
- contains the actual work of nurses including biopsychosocial interventions;
- is presented in a logical sequence;
- is written as events occur so that it remains up to date;
- records all variances in care, in a clear and concise way without repetition;
- fulfils legal and professional requirements according to *The Code* (NMC, 2018c).

In a busy and acute clinical setting, nurses and healthcare professionals can be easily distracted. However, the safety of patients should be paramount, and the prevention of patient deterioration is a multidisciplinary goal that can only be achieved through assessment, communication, and collaboration between the patient and all professional groups.

Managing and organising care using the appropriate skill mix

The ability to know and understand your patients is dependent on you and your team having a balanced skill mix, evidence of continuity of care, effective communication channels, and effective teamwork so that you can assess and respond to the patient's immediate needs in an emergency (Duffield et al., 2010; Scott, 2003). In relation to skill mix, clinical care is provided in increasingly complex systems and the roles and responsibilities of registered practitioners and unregistered carers such as healthcare assistants (HCA) have become blurred. HCAs are now involved in the assessment, data collection, and monitoring of patients as well as the providers of direct patient care (NPSA, 2007a). This trend is set to continue as HCAs take on more of the caring roles once managed by nurses and has occurred in part because of nursing shortages (RCN, 2017; WHO, 2016). According to Quirke et al. (2011) and James et al. (2010), while HCAs play a significant role in the recognition and monitoring of acutely ill patients, they lack the ability to interpret and manage an effective response to patient deterioration, often relying on the registered nurse or doctor to intervene. Correspondingly, student nurses and registered nurses rely heavily on the contributions made by HCAs, and it is the nurse's responsibility to work collaboratively with and to accept responsibility for the contribution that HCAs make (NMC, 2018c). Furthermore, staffing levels often vary because of staff sickness, unexpected patient turnover, and the use of bank or agency nurses.

According to Aiken et al. (2017), the importance of working collaboratively and balancing skill mix has been identified as being a significant factor in reducing patient morbidity and mortality following admission to hospital. In a study of nursing skill mix in 243 acute hospitals across Europe, Aiken et al. (2017) reported that each 10% reduction in the percentage of professional nurses among the caring personnel was associated with an 11% increase in the odds of patient mortality. Correspondingly, a 10% increase in the percentage of professional nurses was associated with a relative reduction in patient mortality. Skill mix and availability of resources are key to the provision of safe and effective nursing care, and when the levels of registered nurses fall there is a corresponding increase in omissions in fundamental aspects of care, as highlighted by Griffiths et al. (2018).

Within this climate of change in models of healthcare provision, there is evidence to support the use of a collaborative team approach to both health and social care (Zwarenstein et al., 2009). A team may consist of all the providers of care for a group of patients, including nurses, healthcare assistants, medical staff, and other health and social care professionals. Nonetheless, the focus should remain on patient-centred care where continuity of care is provided by the team, with each team member ensuring effective communication. Task-based team nursing, where management of care is based on a series of tasks rather than focusing on patient need, should be avoided as this has been found to reduce the quality of care (Fairbrother et al., 2010).

Activity 1.2   Reflection

Think back to your experiences in the clinical setting.

- Can you identify a situation where you have been unable to understand how the nurse was able to know or anticipate clinical changes in a deteriorating patient?
- If you can, write down the story and look back on the incident after reading this chapter.
- Using the chapter as a guide, try to write down an action plan of how you might manage a similar situation in the future.

Hint: These reflective questions will help you to practise the skills of rapid assessment and management of a patient.

As this answer is based on your own reflection, there is no outline answer at the end of the chapter.

Chapter summary

Within this chapter we have introduced you to the skills and processes involved in the rapid assessment of, and response to, deteriorating patients. The core skills focus on risk assessment, recognition and prevention of deterioration, and timely intervention of care. The tables included have been designed to provide you with an aide-mémoire that you can apply to the patient examples in the remainder of the book. Key to the process of providing safe and effective care is person-centred care, communication, and collaboration.

Activities: brief outline answers

Activity 1.1: Risk assessment and decision making (pages 32)

1. The knowledge and skills you would use relate to clinical assessment and, in particular, rapid assessment skills. These include using 'ABCDE' as a guide: look at the patient; listen to the patient, family, handover from other staff, listen for physiological signs of distress; feel the patient's skin and note any abnormal signs; measure the patient's physiological signs. Interpret the clinical signs and assess the findings against the normal range. You would need the help of a registered nurse and the medical team to assist with interpretation, particularly if you have had no experience of this type of patient. Always recognise your limitations and communicate your concerns.
2. Increased respiratory rate with a lower than normal SpO$_2$ suggests early signs of respiratory failure and requires immediate action: call for help from a senior member of staff and administer oxygen guided by the local protocol (Chapter 2). Isabel also has signs of haemodynamic insufficiency indicated by rapid respirations, rapid pulse, and low BP. She is considered to be at high risk of deterioration and requires at least hourly observations of vital signs and fluid resuscitation (NEWS2 = 6). She is also at risk of further fluid loss and requires urgent management of a possible peptic ulcer (see Chapter 6).

Further reading

RCN (Royal College of Nursing) (2004) *Nursing Assessment of Older People: RCN Tool Kit.* London: RCN.

This resource provides general guidance and tools for assessing older people and offers useful background detail on collaborative assessment processes. Accessed at: **www.rcn.org.uk/ professional-development/publications/pub-002310**

Rushforth, H (2009) *Assessment Made Incredibly Easy.* London: Wolters Kluwer/Lippincott Williams and Wilkins.

This book provides information on detailed systematic assessment of all clinical situations and is a useful revision guide to assessment skills.

Useful websites

www.rcn.org.uk/employment-and-pay/integrated-care-in-england

This Resuscitation Council website gives access to the many innovations and developments in the integration of care in the UK.

www.resus.org.uk/dnacpr/

This resource provides information and guidance by the Resuscitation Council on ethical decisions related to cardiopulmonary resuscitation.

www.resus.org.uk/resuscitation-guidelines/abcde-approach/

This resource provides a summary by the Resuscitation Council of the ABCDE assessment using a multidisciplinary approach.

www.rcplondon.ac.uk/projects/outputs/national-early-warning-score-news-2

This website provides the resources used to support NEWS2.

Chapter 2 The breathless patient

Desiree Tait and Jane James

NMC Future Nurse: Standards of Proficiency for Registered Nurses

This chapter will address the following platforms and proficiencies:

Platform 3: Assessing needs and planning care

Registered nurses prioritise the needs of people when assessing and reviewing their mental, physical, cognitive, behavioural, social and spiritual needs. They use information obtained during assessments to identify the priorities and requirements for person-centred and evidence-based nursing interventions and support. They work in partnership with people to develop person-centred care plans that take into account their circumstances, characteristics and preferences.

At the point of registration, the registered nurse will be able to:

3.2   demonstrate and apply knowledge of body systems and homeostasis, human anatomy and physiology, biology, genomics, pharmacology and social and behavioural sciences when undertaking full and accurate person-centred nursing assessments and developing appropriate care plans.

3.3   demonstrate and apply knowledge of all commonly encountered mental, physical, behavioural and cognitive health conditions, medication usage and treatments when undertaking full and accurate assessments of nursing care needs and when developing, prioritising and reviewing person-centred care plans.

3.5   demonstrate the ability to accurately process all information gathered during the assessment process to identify needs for individualised nursing care and develop person-centred evidence-based plans for nursing interventions with agreed goals.

Annexe B: Nursing procedures

8.   Use evidence-based, best practice approaches for meeting needs for respiratory care and support, accurately assessing the person's capacity for independence and self-care and initiating appropriate interventions.

(Continued)

(Continued)

8.1 observe and assess the need for intervention and respond to restlessness, agitation, and breathlessness using appropriate interventions.

Chapter aims

By the end of this chapter, you should be able to:

- identify causes of breathlessness;
- describe the clinical features of breathlessness in relation to cardiac failure, type I and II respiratory failures, pneumonia, chronic obstructive pulmonary disease (COPD), and asthma, and the clinical implications for the patient;
- demonstrate awareness of how to undertake respiratory assessment using look, listen, feel, and measure, together with ABCDE;
- diagnose and differentiate between possible causes of patient deterioration and identify appropriate interventions;
- reflect on clinical examples illustrated in the chapter and relate to your own clinical practice.

Introduction

Breathlessness or **dyspnoea** relates to a feeling of difficulty in breathing; an uncomfortable need to breathe (Innes and Tiernan, 2018, p77), and is a sensation experienced by people in many circumstances during health and illness. In health, during exercise for example, it is normal to feel breathless as the body works to increase the amount of oxygen required to meet demand. During ill health, feelings of breathlessness can be associated with several causes. This chapter gives an overview of some of the possible causes of breathlessness that are included in Table 2.1 and examines in detail the care of people experiencing breathlessness related to:

- cardiac failure;
- pneumonia;
- COPD;
- asthma.

Underlying physiology, social psychology, and ethical implications in the management of individuals diagnosed with these conditions will be discussed in the context of risk assessment and collaborative management and care.

Cardiac	Lung	Neuromuscular	Other
• Heart failure • Angina pectoris • Myocardial infarction • Abnormal heart rhythms such as atrial tachycardia • Cardiac tamponade (blood or fluid in between the pericardium and myocardium, squashing the heart and reducing cardiac output)	• Lung infections such as pneumonia • Pneumothorax (air trapped between the parietal and visceral pleura, reducing lung expansion) • Pulmonary embolism (blockage of an artery in the lungs) • Pleural effusion (fluid trapped between the parietal and visceral pleura) • Chronic obstructive pulmonary disease (COPD) • Asthma • Emphysema (damaged alveoli that have weakened and ruptured producing large inefficient air spaces) • Carcinoma of the lung tissue or bronchus • Fibrotic lung disease (stiff lungs)	• Pain such as rib fractures • Myasthenia gravis (chronic autoimmune neuromuscular disease) • Muscular dystrophy (group of diseases that cause progressive muscle weakness) • Kyphoscoliosis (abnormal curvature of the spine)	• Exercise • Anaemia leading to reduction in haemoglobin and oxygen-carrying capacity • Systemic infection • Distended abdomen that presses on the diaphragm • Allergy/anaphylaxis due to inflammation and swelling of the airways • Metabolic causes such as acidosis associated with sepsis • Stress, anxiety, fear • Brain injury that affects the respiratory centre

Table 2.1   Some conditions that cause breathlessness

The chapter begins with the case study of a patient with cardiac failure, followed by an explanation of breathlessness. This leads to an overview of the knowledge and skills required to recognise, assess, prioritise, and manage care for patients with breathlessness. You will see how the degree of breathlessness represents the severity of the circumstances and thus dictates the level and speed of response required. This chapter focuses on the importance of a detailed respiratory assessment, including arterial blood gas analysis, and supportive nursing interventions, while Chapter 3 focuses on patients who need advanced respiratory support.

Case study: Breathlessness associated with cardiac failure

Susan (a second-year student nurse) had been allocated a small caseload of patients to visit while on her community placement under the supervision of her practice assessor. One of her patients was 76-year-old Charlie Morris, who had been having a chronic leg wound

(Continued)

(Continued)

redressed twice weekly. When Susan arrived at his house on her second visit, she found Mr Morris sitting in a chair dressed in his pyjamas. He said he was having trouble getting going and was very tired because he had not slept very well. His wife added that he had woken several times during the night short of breath, had sat on the edge of the bed and asked her to open the window. He seemed better once morning came, and he was sat in the chair. Mr Morris said that this happened to him sometimes, but not usually this badly. He normally rested and felt better after a while.

When Susan went to look at Mr Morris's wound, she found the leg of his pyjamas was very tight. In helping her to access his wound, he struggled to remove his pyjamas, becoming more breathless and needing time afterwards to get his breath back. Susan also found the wound bandage was constricting Mr Morris's leg, which appeared swollen; his toes were cold and pale. She wondered if she had applied the bandage too tightly on her previous visit and contacted her practice assessor, Bridget, to ask for advice.

Bridget called by and assessed Mr Morris. First, she checked his respirations, pulse, and blood pressure, then asked questions about his regular medication and his fluid intake and output. She felt both Mr Morris' ankles and listened carefully to what Mrs Morris told her. Susan was confused by the fact that Bridget did not seem concerned about Mr Morris's leg wound, but instead requested the GP to visit, saying that she thought he might have an exacerbation of his heart failure.

Susan's experience highlights the fact that patients with chronic conditions often have more than one problem (multiple co-morbidities). Susan thought that she was visiting Mr Morris for a straightforward dressing change, and she had not read the nursing notes before assessing him. If she had, Susan would have known that Mr Morris has chronic heart failure and had been taking ACE inhibitors, beta blockers, and diuretic therapy for several years to manage his symptoms. The fact that Mr Morris was feeling tired and lethargic was not simply due to a poor night's sleep. The reason why his sleep was disturbed was significant in that he was waking up from sleep feeling breathless, and this happened several times. It was also worth noting that his breathlessness worsened on physical exertion and speaking. Breathlessness provoked by lying down at night (orthopnoea) is a feature of heart failure and patients are recommended to sleep in a semi-recumbent position. Paroxysmal nocturnal dyspnoea is described as waking suddenly and gasping for air. On assessment, a person will describe feeling breathless, have a cough, may be expectorating frothy sputum, be pale, sweaty and tachycardic (Mills et al., 2018).

When Bridget heard Mrs Morris's story and saw that Mr Morris was still breathless at rest and had swollen legs, she recognised some important indicators and knew from her experience that it could be a worsening of Mr Morris's heart failure. The presence of breathlessness at rest and bilateral lower leg **oedema**, together with a history of heart failure, is indicative of an acute exacerbation of cardiac failure (Mills et al., 2018) that requires urgent assessment and management from the medical team.

Susan visited Mr Morris to do a dressing but found that he was tired and breathless. His main problem was not his wound but related to his heart. What can we learn from this? The important messages in Susan's story are these:

- Take every opportunity in all clinical settings to assess your patients holistically and systematically (see Chapter 1); assimilate your findings and keep an open mind.
- Listen carefully to your patient's complaints or concerns about things such as breathlessness that affect their daily activities, as these are often significant.
- If you are concerned about your patient, seek advice and support according to the local risk assessment protocol (see Chapter 1).
- The basis of the problem may not necessarily be what you think, and breathlessness, alone or combined with other symptoms, needs further exploration.

Breathing and homeostasis

Breathing is vital for life and is part of the mechanism depended upon to supply oxygen to the tissues. All cells in the human body require a continuous supply of oxygen otherwise they die. As oxygen is used, carbon dioxide is produced as a waste product. While it is important for the body to take in oxygen, it is also important to remove the carbon dioxide at the same rate that oxygen is supplied. Essentially, this is respiration, and it contributes to maintaining homeostasis – a state of balance and stability within the cells to keep them working. Homeostasis was first described by Cannon in 1929 as the maintenance of nearly constant conditions in the internal environment (cited by Hall, 2016, p4). All cells, tissues, and organs in the body work together to maintain constant conditions and contribute to homeostasis. In health and disease, the body will continue to promote homeostasis, including the respiratory system.

Respiration itself comprises four processes: pulmonary ventilation, external respiration, transport of gases, and internal respiration. All these processes are reliant on homeostatic mechanisms to function effectively and interdependently, thus a change in respiratory rate is potentially the first sign of clinical deterioration and a forecaster of events such as cardiac arrest (Cretikos et al., 2008). Table 2.2 describes the processes of respiration and the homeostatic mechanisms that they are dependent on, how they can be assessed, and some clinical examples of where the process has become impaired.

If the cells receive insufficient oxygen due to poor respiration and/or perfusion, they become hypoxic. This state is known as tissue hypoxia. In the presence of reduced oxygen, cells produce energy primarily through the process of glycolysis (anaerobic metabolism) instead of through aerobic metabolism. Aerobic metabolism takes place in mitochondria (the energy packs) of cells and requires the presence of oxygen. The process of glycolysis is less efficient than aerobic metabolism in the mitochondria. It requires glucose and produces a lower percentage of energy in the form of adenosine

The process of respiration	Dependent upon	Assessed and measured by	Clinical examples

• **Pulmonary ventilation:** the movement of air in and out of the lungs.	• Patent airways free from obstruction or narrowing.
	
	• Respiratory centres in the medulla oblongata and pons varolii of the brain stem influence rate, depth, and pattern of respiration.
	
	• Chemo-sensitive areas in the medulla react to changes in carbon dioxide and oxygen levels in the arterial blood identified by chemoreceptors in the aortic and carotid bodies via the vagus and glossopharyngeal nerves (see Figure 6.1).
	
	• Nerves: phrenic and intercostal send the message to breathe to the respiratory muscles.
	
	• Muscles: diaphragm and intercostal perform the work of breathing and when required the work of breathing can be supported by accessory muscles.
	
	• Pressure changes within thoracic cavity. When no air is flowing in or out of the alveoli the air pressure is zero centimetres of water. Inspiration is triggered by contraction of the intercostal muscles and diaphragm thus creating a void (a negative pressure) in the alveoli drawing in air. Expiration occurs following relaxation of the muscles.
	
	• Elasticity (compliance) of the lungs is the extent to which the lungs can stretch to receive air under pressure. The greater the compliance, the greater the stretchability.
	
	• Lung capacity describes the maximum volume of air possible during inspiration and includes the tidal volume (volume in one normal breath) and the inspiratory reserve volume inspired over and above tidal volume. This can be influenced by lung compliance and the structure (shape) of the thoracic cage.
		Airway:
		
		• **Look and feel** for swelling or oedema of the upper airways. Other causes of obstruction to the airway (fluid, foreign body). Abnormal chest movements.
		
		• **Listen** for wheeze, stridor (caused by narrowing), gasping, snoring (unable to maintain own airway, or gurgling).
		
		Breathing (respiratory observations):
		
		• **Look and feel** for signs of respiratory distress (fighting for breath with increased work of breathing and accessory muscle use), lip pursing and/or nasal flaring. Look for evidence of peripheral and central cyanosis, chest X-ray.
		
		• On auscultation **listen** for wheeze (asthma and/or COPD), crackles (pneumonia and heart failure), reduced air entry (pneumothorax or pleural effusion).
		
		• Can the patient speak in complete sentences?
		
		• Measure (Tables 1.3 to 1.8):
		
		  o respiratory rate, rhythm, depth of respiration if spirometry equipment is available
		
		  o oxygen saturations
		
		  o arterial blood gases.
			• Phil was trapped in a fire and inhaled hot smoke, causing pharyngeal oedema and noisy breathing (stridor).
			
			• Diane suffered a head injury which led to cerebral oedema which pressed down on her brain stem, causing an irregular and erratic respiratory pattern. This is called coning.
			
			• Jean has **Guillain Barré syndrome** affecting the nerves supplying her intercostal muscles and reducing the size of her breaths (tidal volume) and causing associated hypoxaemia.
			
			• John has fibrosed lungs due to chronic disease, causing his lungs to be stiff and unable to stretch.
			
			• Peter sustained broken ribs when a tree fell on him, causing pneumothorax and precluding him from taking deep breaths (lung expansion) on the affected side.

The process of respiration	Dependent upon	Assessed and measured by	Clinical examples

External respiration: the exchange of oxygen and carbon dioxide between the alveoli in the lungs and the pulmonary capillaries.	• Tidal volume is greater than the physiological dead space. The physiological dead space is the part of the airways where no gaseous exchange takes place (normally 150 ml of the tidal volume).
	
	• Fresh supply of oxygen to ventilate the alveoli.
	
	• Gas partial pressure changes during inspiration and expiration at normal atmospheric pressure (oxygen and carbon dioxide).
	
	• Presence of blood supply and haemoglobin to transport oxygen (pulmonary capillaries).
	
	• Proximity of pulmonary blood flow to alveoli.
	
	• Diffusion of oxygen into the pulmonary capillaries and carbon dioxide out.
		Breathing (respiratory observations):
		
		• **Look and feel** for signs of respiratory distress (fighting for breath with increased work of breathing and accessory muscle use), lip pursing, and/or nasal flaring, shallow breathing.
		
		• On auscultation **listen** for wheeze (asthma and/or COPD), crackles (pneumonia and heart failure), reduced air entry (pneumothorax or pleural effusion).
		
		• Measure (Tables 1.3 to 1.8):
		  ○ respiratory rate, depth of respiration if spirometry equipment is available
		  ○ oxygen saturations
		  ○ arterial and capillary blood gases.
			• Mary took an overdose of her sleeping tablets, which cause respiratory depression with an excessive dose, and has very shallow breaths.
			
			• Chris was climbing Mount Everest and developed pulmonary oedema due to lower air pressure at altitude.
			
			• Brian has COPD with emphysema and atelectasis.
			
			• Ross was recovering from hip surgery when he suffered a pulmonary embolism, reducing blood supply to the capillary bed surrounding the alveoli.
			
			• Siobhan has pneumonia and secretions have consolidated the bases of both lungs, thus reducing the number of alveoli available for gaseous exchange (increased physiological dead space).

(Continued)

Table 2.2 (Continued)

The process of respiration	Dependent upon	Assessed and measured by	Clinical examples
Transport of gases: the carriage of oxygen from the lungs to the tissues, and carbon dioxide from the tissues to the lungs in the blood.	• Systemic circulation of blood and cardiac output. • Patency of arteries and veins. • Uninterrupted blood flow.	• Oxygen saturations. • Haemoglobin. • Full blood count and clotting factors. • Arterial or capillary blood gas analysis (ABG or CBG).	• Charlie has heart failure and reduced cardiac output (reduced capacity to deliver oxygen to the tissues and remove carbon dioxide). • Trudy is anaemic after months of heavy periods. She has reduced haemoglobin and is breathless on exertion, and her SpO_2 is normal. • Margaret had a thrombosis that lodged in her popliteal artery, causing her foot to become cold, pale, and ischaemic.
Internal respiration: the delivery of oxygen to the body cells and the collection of carbon dioxide from the cells.	• Gas pressure changes. • Blood supply to cells. • Correct environment within the cell, including temperature and pH level.	• Lactate levels. • ABGs – level of metabolic acidosis. • Temperature.	• Bob's gas fire was faulty, and he suffered carbon monoxide (CO) poisoning. This occurs when haemoglobin molecules take up CO instead of oxygen, thus causing tissue hypoxia and the production of carboxyhaemoglobin. • Andy fell into the river, lost consciousness, and suffered hypothermia. This slowed his metabolic rate down and reduced the demand for oxygen, and Andy made a full recovery.

Table 2.2 Processes of respiration, homeostatic mechanisms, and respiratory assessment informed by Hall (2016) and Zinchenko (2018).

triphosphate (ATP). A by-product of glycolysis is lactic acid, which can temporarily increase the acidity of cells and lead to an alteration in circulatory pH. When oxygen is re-established in the circulation the lactic acid quickly converts to chemicals that aid aerobic metabolism (Tait and White, 2019; Hall, 2016).

If the carbon dioxide is not removed efficiently through respiration and perfusion, it builds up in the blood (CO_2 retention) creating hypercarbia. This has the effect of creating a respiratory acidosis (Hall, 2016). Acidity and alkalinity, body temperature, and fluid levels are also involved in homeostasis, and respiration plays an important part in controlling and responding to changes in these factors to achieve the narrow range of normality required (Hall, 2016). Adaptations in response from various other body systems also play a part. These include metabolic processes and the circulatory, neuromuscular, and renal systems.

When different factors of homeostasis are disturbed, the body tries to adjust to put things back to normal (compensation). It does this initially by altering the rate and pattern of breathing. So, anyone who is breathless (dyspnoeic) is in the process of trying to normalise their body's internal environment by drawing on compensatory or corrective mechanisms. The degree of breathlessness often indicates the severity of imbalance within their cells and could be caused by problems with any one of the four processes involved in respiration, as shown in the clinical examples in Table 2.2. Clinical measures that support assessment of respiratory processes and homeostatic balance include assessing oxygen levels in the blood (SpO_2) and the interpretation of arterial blood gases when there is evidence of clinical deterioration. We will begin by exploring the significance of arterial blood gas analysis. Later in the chapter we will continue to explore the clinical significance of oxygen when we analyse Siobhan's story.

Why are arterial blood gas results significant for people experiencing clinical deterioration?

The group of clinical measurements described as arterial blood gases (ABGs) refer to a collection of arterial blood results that allow for the interpretation and assessment of two related physiological functions. These are:

- The exchange of gases in the lungs. This is measured by PaO_2 and $PaCO_2$ and indicates the ability of a person's lungs to simultaneously add oxygen (O_2) and remove carbon dioxide (CO_2) from the pulmonary circulation by the process of diffusion.
- The maintenance of homeostasis in relation to the pH of the blood to between 7.35 and 7.45 (acid-base balance).

Both functions are interrelated and changes in the balance of one will impact on the balance of the other. The sampling and interpretation of ABGs are used for people who demonstrate evidence of either or both of the following:

- People living with COPD who are experiencing an acute exacerbation of their condition.
- Any person who is experiencing an acute deterioration in their respiratory and/or circulatory system.

In Chapter 1 we discussed the reasons why people's conditions deteriorate and identified that for the body's cells, tissues, and organs to function effectively there needs to be a continuous supply of oxygen and nutrients and simultaneous removal of the by-products of metabolism. In the body, acids (substances that release hydrogen ions (H^+) in solution) are constantly being produced as by-products of normal cell metabolism. According to McCance and Huether (2019), the acid produced from cell metabolism must be either neutralised or excreted from the body, to maintain homeostasis and a pH of 7.35–7.45. In conjunction with the body's buffer systems, the lungs eliminate carbonic acid as the respiratory gas carbon dioxide (CO_2), and the kidneys eliminate metabolic acids. Carbon dioxide is a volatile gas that is produced as a by-product of oxidative cell metabolism (activity produced with the aid of oxygen). Therefore, when the body's demand for and use of oxygen increases, the amount of CO_2 also increases. Carbon dioxide, in the presence of water (H_2O) and carbonic anhydrase, becomes carbonic acid (H_2CO_3). This process can also be reversed and, in the presence of the enzyme carbonic anhydrase, H_2CO_3 is then converted back to CO_2 and H_2O, and eliminated as part of the process of expiration.

Meanwhile the by-products of cell metabolism such as: sulphuric acid, phosphoric, keto acids, and lactic acid are eliminated via the renal system. The kidney is also responsible for regulating the concentration of bicarbonate ions in the circulation (HCO_3^-). Bicarbonate ions play a significant role in acid-base balance and in the carbonic acid-bicarbonate buffer system. According to McCance and Huether (2019), the relationship between carbonic acid and bicarbonate is a very important factor in how the body regulates the pH (the calculated acidity of the blood) in the circulation, as well as other buffer systems such as occur in the kidney and renal excretion of hydrogen ions. To maintain a pH of 7.4 (normal blood pH) the ratio between carbonic acid and bicarbonate should stay at one part carbonic acid to 20 parts bicarbonate ($1\ H_2CO_3$: $20\ HCO_3^- + H^+$). This means that if the amount of bicarbonate (HCO_3^-) in the blood falls so must the amount of carbonic acid (H_2CO_3) to maintain a ratio of 1 : 20. The body achieves this by increasing the rate and depth of respiration so that more CO_2 is eliminated through respiration and the ratio is maintained. This is called respiratory compensation and can be seen in patients who are producing an excess of metabolic acids, such as lactic acid in situations where there is a reduction in tissue perfusion (Chapters 6 and 7) and ketone acid in diabetic ketoacidosis (Chapters 8 and 12).

As we have seen, the body has several ways of maintaining the acid-base balance in health and these are generally known as buffer systems. Buffer systems are control mechanisms that can either increase or decrease the number of hydrogen ions in a solution in response to changes in acid-base balance (Patton et al., 2016). It is important to note that buffer systems do not prevent an increase or decrease in blood acidity, but they do help to restore the balance once a change in acidity has occurred and thus minimise any fluctuations in pH. Buffer systems function in both intracellular and extracellular fluid compartments and function at different rates although they are the first line of action in responding to changes in acid-base balance (McCance and Huether, 2019) (see Table 2.3). The most important buffer systems are the bicarbonate and carbonic acid buffer system and haemoglobin acting as a protein buffer system. In the circulation it is the bicarbonate buffer system which converts a strong acid that releases large numbers of H^+, to a weak acid that releases much fewer H^+. For example, hydrochloric acid (HCl: strong acid) can be substituted by carbonic acid (H_2CO_3: weak acid), thus reducing the overall H^+:

$$HCl + NaHCO_3 \leftrightharpoons H_2CO_3 + NaCl$$

(sodium bicarbonate)   (sodium chloride)

This equation is reversible and is accelerated by the presence of the enzyme carbonic anhydrase. The carbonic acid produced dissociates into H^+ and HCO_3^- (bicarbonate ions). The H^+ combines with haemoglobin and the bicarbonate diffuses into the plasma, where it continues to participate in buffering acids. Another type of buffering system is referred to as the cellular ion exchange mechanism. For example, during a period of pH imbalance potassium ions will either move in or out of the intracellular space in exchange for hydrogen ions, thus acting as a buffer. This process, however, does increase the risk of cellular potassium imbalance in the form of hyper or hypokalaemia and an increased risk of serious cardiac arrhythmias.

Buffers are the body's first line of action to restore normal pH	The lungs are the body's second line of action to restore normal pH	Ionic shift is the body's third line of action to restore normal pH	The kidneys are the body's fourth line of action to restore normal pH
Action instantaneous within seconds.	Action within seconds to minutes.	Action is measured in hours (2–4 hours).	Action is measured in hours and days.
They remove or release H+ to correct acid-base balance.	They eliminate or retain CO_2 to maintain the ratio of carbonic acid to bicarbonate at 1 : 20.	The exchange of intracellular potassium for hydrogen ions and vice versa.	They have a number of functions: • retention of carbonate ions to provide bicarbonate • elimination of H+ in urine.

Table 2.3 How the body acts to restore alterations in acid-base balance

Left in the circulation, an imbalance in acids or bases would destroy cells and organs, so it is imperative the body has ways to maintain a pH balance at a value of between 7.35 and 7.45 to maintain normal cell function (Hall, 2016). Should the pH value fall above or below this range, the impact on the body can be critical and in extreme cases leads to death.

What should we be measuring?

The results obtained from analysis of arterial blood provides information about several factors involved in the process of acid-base balance as well as information about the amount of oxygen available to the cells. Blood gases alone do not give us a complete picture of how the body is balancing acid-base homeostasis and therefore the results should be analysed in the context of the wider physiological picture obtained from the following:

- pH value of arterial blood;
- the amount of O_2 in arterial blood (expressed as the partial pressure of oxygen or PaO_2);
- the amount of CO_2 in arterial blood (expressed as the partial pressure of carbon dioxide or $PaCO_2$);
- the amount of bicarbonate and bases available to buffer acids in arterial blood (expressed as mmol/L);
- arterial blood potassium levels;
- arterial haemoglobin;
- blood urea nitrogen, creatinine, and glomerular filtration rate to monitor kidney function.

Blood urea nitrogen (BUN), the measurement of creatinine, and glomerular filtration rate are very important measures of renal function and will give an indication of how efficient the patient's kidney function is. If the patient has impaired kidney function, the ability for the kidneys to act as the fourth line of action in maintaining acid-base balance is impaired and will lead to the development of metabolic acidosis (Chapter 9).

What do these values tell us?

The pH value determines the presence of acidaemia and alkalaemia.

- Acidaemia: pH <7.35 (a value below 7.35).
- Alkalaemia: pH >7.45 (a value above 7.45).

Respiratory acidosis/alkalosis

The partial pressures of oxygen and carbon dioxide give a measure of respiratory function and the presence of respiratory acidosis/alkalosis. Respiratory acidosis is caused by an acute or chronic failure of ventilation when the level of CO_2 in the blood rises. For example, respiratory obstruction, acute type II respiratory failure caused by infection and/or inflammation, and chronic respiratory failure caused by COPD.

- Chemical and clinical signs of respiratory acidosis include:
  - pH <7.35;
  - $PaCO_2$ >6.0 kPa;

- o dyspnoea/increased or decreased respiratory function;
- o headache;
- o restlessness, confusion;
- o drowsiness/unconsciousness;
- o tachycardia and arrhythmias.

Respiratory alkalosis occurs in the presence of hyperventilation and the level of CO_2 in the blood falls (see Table 3.2).

- Chemical and clinical signs of respiratory alkalosis include:
  - o pH >7.45;
  - o $PaCO_2$ <4.6 kPa;
  - o feeling light-headed;
  - o numbness and tingling in the mouth and peripheries;
  - o inability to concentrate, confusion;
  - o palpitations.

The levels of bicarbonate give a measure of metabolic function and represent either a failure to buffer hydrogen ion concentrations with bases, leading to acidosis, or a failure to buffer bicarbonate concentrations with acids, leading to an alkalosis. Base excess gives an indication of the deficit or excess of bicarbonate required to normalise pH. In metabolic acidosis the concentrations of acids (other than carbonic acid) increase, or bicarbonate concentrations in the blood fall. Causes include reduced perfusion of cells such as is caused by shock, hypoxaemia (low oxygen), renal failure, starvation, and diabetic ketoacidosis.

- Chemical and clinical signs of metabolic acidosis:
  - o pH <7.35;
  - o HCO_3 <22 mmol/L;
  - o headache;
  - o restlessness, confusion;
  - o coma;
  - o cardiac arrhythmias;
  - o Kussmaul respirations (rapid shallow)/**respiratory depression**;
  - o skin warm and flushed.

In metabolic alkalosis, the concentration of metabolic acids is reduced or the concentration of bicarbonate is increased. Causes include prolonged vomiting, gastric suctioning, and diuretic therapy leading to an increased loss of potassium and hydrogen ions, and excessive bicarbonate intake.

- Chemical and clinical signs of metabolic alkalosis:
  - o pH >7.45;
  - o HCO_3 >27 mmol/L;
  - o muscle twitching and cramps;

- feeling dizzy;
- confusion;
- lethargy;
- seizures/coma;
- nausea and vomiting.

In Table 2.4 you will find clinical examples of patients who have experienced an acid-base imbalance.

Arterial blood gas analysis	Patient examples
Respiratory acidosis: pH <7.35 $PaCO_2$ >6.0 kPa	Gladys Cabrera (62 years) suffers from COPD, and she is admitted to hospital with an acute exacerbation of her condition. She is unable to talk due to her breathlessness, rate of 40 bpm, SpO_2 is 72%, she is centrally cyanosed, and she is unable to respond to commands. The results of an arterial blood sample are pH 7.29, PaO_2 4.8 kPa, $PaCo_2$ 8.4 kPa, HCO_3 28.5 mmol/L. Following a rapid assessment of Gladys's condition, she was admitted to intensive care for respiratory support and intensive treatment for type II respiratory failure.
Respiratory alkalosis: pH >7.45 $PaCO_2$ <4.6 kPa	Joan Butcher (50 years) suffers from anxiety attacks, and these have become worse since progressing to the menopause. On this occasion she has been involved in a minor road traffic collision and she has no obvious injuries. However, when the paramedics arrived at the scene, they found her to be breathless and disorientated. She was complaining of pins and needles in her hands and arms, and she felt she couldn't get her breath. Joan was taken to accident and emergency where her ABG result following admission was pH: 7.49; $PaCO_2$: 3.2 kPa; HCO_3: 24.2 mmol/L. Joan was hyperventilating and needed to be encouraged to reduce her respiratory rate and allow her carbon dioxide levels to rise back to normal levels.
Metabolic acidosis: pH <7.35 HCO_3 <22 mmol/L	Mary Bevan (58 years) was found by her neighbour lying at the front door in a drowsy and confused state. Mary has type 2 diabetes and has recently developed a severe infection on her leg. Mary's neighbour called the emergency services and Mary was admitted to accident and emergency. Her ABG following admission was pH: 7.24; $PaCO_2$: 3.8 kPa; HCO_3: 15.1 mmol/L; BE: −13.7. Mary had Kussmaul respirations at a rate of 35 bpm and a blood glucose of 22 mmol/L. Mary had developed a metabolic acidosis secondary to infection that triggered an increase in blood glucose that necessitated management with insulin.
Metabolic alkalosis: pH >7.45 HCO_3 >26 mmol/L	Gary Smith (54 years) has been suffering from indigestion-type pain for several days. Rather than go to the GP he has been treating himself with large doses of antacids such as bicarbonate of soda. That afternoon he felt nauseated, weak, and tired and still had the persistent indigestion. He visited the GP, who decided to admit him to hospital for an assessment of his chest pain. His arterial blood gas following admission was pH: 7.49; $PaCO_2$: 5.6 kPa; HCO_3: 29.7 mmol/L; BE: +9.0.

Arterial blood gas analysis	Patient examples
Respiratory and metabolic acidosis: pH <7.35 $PaCO_2$ >6.0 kPa HCO_3 <22 mmol/L	Peter Baker (41 years) was admitted to an acute ward with a history of abdominal pain, nausea, and vomiting. Peter's condition deteriorated during the first 24 hours, and that evening he had a cardiac arrest. He was resuscitated and transferred to ICU for respiratory support and management of acute pancreatitis. His ABG following admission was pH: 7.15; $PaCO_2$: 7.6 kPa; HCO_3: 16.7 mmol/L; BE: −9.8. Peter has developed a combined acidosis because of his cardiac arrest (failed respiration) and sepsis associated with pancreatitis and lactic acidosis (see Chapter 7).

Table 2.4 Clinical examples of patients with changes in acid-base balance

Because breathlessness can result from the body's compensation in relation to the respiratory, circulatory, neuromuscular, renal, and metabolic systems, you will find breathless patients of all ages and in all clinical settings. Breathing rates change quickly in response to demands from body systems, so breathlessness is an early indicator of acute illness and should not be ignored (NICE, 2007; NPSA, 2007a). To prevent further deterioration, you need to be alert to breathless patients and undertake an initial rapid assessment using the ABCDE approach (Resuscitation Council (UK), 2015), as outlined in Chapter 1, including a detailed assessment of breathing. This needs to be combined with the clinical assessment process of 'Look: Listen: Feel: Measure', which will then enable you to respond appropriately to your patients' needs in a timely manner (Zinchenko, 2018).

As part of the ABCDE approach to organising rapid assessment, it is important to ensure that your patient's airway is patent before going on to assess breathing. On assessing your patients, you will be aware of several aspects of breathing, and noting these can be very useful in identifying risks and changes in your patients' conditions. Let's review Mr Morris's story and assess his situation by using the ABCDE and SBAR approaches described in Chapter 1 to explore the relationship between breathlessness and cardiac failure.

Breathing Assessment

Case study: Mr Morris

Situation:

Mr Morris was visited for assessment and management of chronic leg ulcers. On assessment he was found to be breathless at rest, tachycardic, hypotensive, and with leg and ankle oedema. He is tired and had experienced several episodes of paroxysmal nocturnal dyspnoea.

Background:

History of chronic heart failure secondary to hypertension. Medications include daily beta blockers and ACE inhibitors to manage blood pressure, and diuretic therapy to reduce fluid overload and support cardiac function.

(Continued)

(Continued)

Assessment:

Airway:

- Mr Morris is alert, responsive, and able to maintain airway.

Breathing:

- Respiration rapid and deep and using accessory muscles to breathe with equal chest expansion
- Rate: 32 bpm
- SpO_2: 94%
- Able to speak four or five words between breaths
- On auscultation: inspiratory crackles and a faint wheeze on expiration
- Paroxysmal nocturnal dyspnoea overnight

Circulation:

- Pale, cool, and clammy skin
- Heart rate: 115 bpm
- BP: 100/75
- Has not passed urine this morning
- Ankles and legs swollen

Disability and Exposure

- ACVPU: Alert
- No pain but tired and uncomfortable and too breathless to move
- Both legs are pale and cool to touch, with wound dressing and pyjamas tight around the legs

Mr Morris has a history of chronic heart failure, which has been managed with support and medication at home. His deterioration overnight and the following morning indicates that he is experiencing an acute exacerbation of his heart failure, which has negatively impacted on his breathing and circulation, as well as his activities of living. Heart failure can be described as inadequate pump function caused in Mr Morris's case by systemic hypertension. As his heart failed to pump effectively, there was reduced cardiac output and inadequate circulation to maintain his blood pressure and internal respiration, resulting in poor tissue oxygenation. Mr Morris's frequent episodes of breathlessness during the night (paroxysmal nocturnal dyspnoea) occurred when he awoke after slumping down in the bed. He would have experienced extreme breathlessness, with an urge to sit up to get more breath and this is an example of the body trying to compensate by improving ventilation (Hammer and McPhee, 2014). A person experiencing left ventricular failure will not be able to eject the whole volume of blood that comes from the pulmonary circulation. This means that there is an increase in pressure in the left ventricle, and a subsequent rise in pulmonary capillary pressure as fluid backs up in the pulmonary circulation. This increase in pressure causes fluid in the pulmonary capillaries to move into the interstitial spaces of the lung (pulmonary oedema) (Ashelford et al., 2019). This can also put pressure on the right side of the heart as pulmonary circulatory pressures increase, causing congestion in the venous system. Mr Morris also had swelling (oedema) of his lower legs, and this was a key indicator of venous congestion (Ashelford et al., 2019).

Activity 2.1   Critical thinking

Consider the patients in Table 2.2 and note down how many different aspects of breathing you can think of. Remember to use the 'Look: Listen: Feel: Measure: Respond' approach discussed in Chapter 1.

Table 2.6, at the end of the chapter, shows what you could identify.

Returning to Mr Morris, from his ABCDE assessment he was alert and able to maintain his airway, indicating that his brain was receiving adequate oxygenation to maintain consciousness. He was pale and his chest was rising equally on both sides. He was breathing fast and shallow (32 respirations per full minute). Mr Morris's oxygen saturations (SpO$_2$) were 94%, indicating that he was just achieving the target range of 94–98% recommended by O'Driscoll et al. (2017). He did not look distressed, but he was using his accessory muscles (pulling his shoulders up and pushing his abdomen out). He was only able to speak four or five words between breaths and, as such, it was important to use a closed questioning technique to preserve Mr Morris's energy. Breathing looked hard work for him and his nostrils were flaring slightly on inspiration. Based on his medical history there was early evidence of dyspnoea associated with acute heart failure. Further investigation through auscultation of the lungs was required. The position and sequencing of stethoscope placement is identified in Figure 2.1.

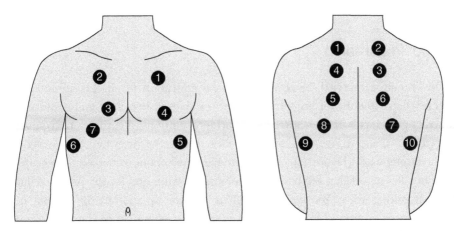

Figure 2.1   Position and sequence for stethoscope placement when listening to breathing sounds as shown by numbered dots

Auscultation of Mr Morris's lungs identified that there were crackles all over his chest at the end of inspiration and a faint wheeze on expiration. This suggested that he had fluid accumulating in the tissues of his lungs (pulmonary oedema), which would obstruct external respiration.

Activity 2.2   Evidence-based practice and research

Visit the 3M Library (www.3m.com/healthcare/littmann/mmm-library.html) to listen to different breath and heart sounds. After gaining consent, practise the 'Look: Listen: Feel: Measure' approach to perform a respiratory assessment on a well person and on your patients with breathlessness.

Practise using your stethoscope to listen to the areas of the chest identified on Figure 2.1. Make notes and compare your findings.

As this answer is based on your own observations, there is no outline answer at the end of the chapter.

Assessment of Mr Morris's circulation confirmed signs of inadequate circulation and perfusion of tissues. He was cool and clammy, experiencing tachycardia, hypotension, and had been unable to pass urine since the previous evening, and there was evidence of fluid overload consistent with an acute exacerbation of heart failure (Innes and Tiernan, 2018). An emergency referral to the General Practitioner using the SBAR approach led to rapid further assessment and treatment. Mr Morris was admitted to the local medical admissions unit for management of his heart failure.

Why is oxygen important?

Scenario: Pneumonia

Siobhan French, a married, 38-year-old physical education teacher, is admitted to the emergency department with breathing difficulties, pain in her chest and confusion. The paramedics give details of their assessment and interventions: due to her **tachypnoea**, respiratory distress, and oxygen saturations of 90%, they have given high-flow oxygen via a non-rebreathing mask (Figure 2.2) and inserted an intravenous cannula into her left hand. The paramedics report that she has had influenza-like symptoms for the past four days and feels she is getting worse. You see that Siobhan is sitting up and talking, but she appears weak and unable to support herself. You have difficulty getting her to concentrate on what you are telling her and asking her to do. Your mentor asks you to do her observations while she goes to get the doctor, and you find that Siobhan's respiratory rate is 38 bpm. She is still wearing the non-rebreathing oxygen mask that the paramedics gave her and this is delivering oxygen to her at around 70%. Siobhan's oxygen saturations are now 92%. Her pulse rate is 122 bpm and her blood pressure is 105/48 mmHg (normal adult blood pressure 100–140 mmHg systolic, 60–90 mmHg diastolic). She has a temperature of 38.6 °C.

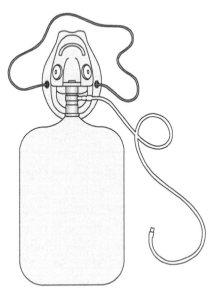

Figure 2.2 A non-rebreathing mask with reservoir bag. The reservoir fills with oxygen and the mask delivers up to 70% oxygen. These masks are used for patients who are in severe respiratory distress.

The main concern for Siobhan is that her SpO_2 levels are too low and have improved only marginally from 90% to 92% since receiving high-flow oxygen at about 70% via the non-rebreathing mask. These levels are worrying because the target saturations for an adult are 94–98% without supplementary oxygen (O'Driscoll et al., 2017). It is worth considering the accuracy of the reading, but in relation to ABCDE assessment Siobhan is dyspnoeic, tachypnoeic, tachycardic, and confused. These are signs of low blood oxygen levels (hypoxaemia). The rapid assessment and NEWS2 score of 15 indicate that her situation is critical and she has a high risk of further deterioration. Siobhan also has four Red Flags for sepsis in the presence of a possible respiratory infection and this should be communicated to the emergency team and Sepsis Six initiated (see Chapter 7) (NICE, 2017a; Nutbeam and Daniels, 2021). The RCP (2017) recommends that any patient with a NEWS2 score above 7 must prompt an emergency assessment by the critical care outreach team and senior physicians. Continuous monitoring and management of Siobhan while waiting for the team's arrival is critical to ensuring her safety.

Siobhan is already receiving high-flow oxygen and you must consider other ways of improving her oxygenation because she has not responded sufficiently; she needs more oxygen delivered to her body cells and you cannot increase the oxygen further by face mask. Despite her blood pressure being borderline low, it is important for her to sit as upright as possible to maximise her pulmonary ventilation (Table 2.2). Gravity helps to increase lung compliance (elasticity) and lung volume by allowing her accessory muscles to work more easily, thus enabling larger breaths for less effort (Katz et al., 2018). Breath size is important as not all inspired air reaches the alveoli. No gas exchange takes place in the nasal passages, trachea, bronchi, and bronchioles, known as anatomical dead space, and these constitute approximately 150 ml of inhaled air. It is more effective for Siobhan to increase her breath size, known as tidal volume (the volume of air inhaled and exhaled at each breath), than her respiratory rate (the number of breaths taken within a set amount of time, typically 60 seconds); she is already breathing very fast and is getting tired. She needs to get more oxygen into her blood to cope with the demands of her body cells (Woodrow, 2019). The medical team needs to perform further investigations to give an indication of how this might be achieved. These should include a chest X-ray to give a picture of lung inflation, and blood tests for full blood count (FBC), urea and electrolytes (U&E), liver function tests (LFT), arterial blood gas analysis (ABG), and blood cultures. Together these will give indications of blood oxygen-carrying capacity (haemoglobin from FBC), renal function (U&E levels), hydration (U&E levels plus haematocrit from FBC), presence of and response to infection (blood cultures and white cell count from FBC), and Siobhan's ability to exchange inspired oxygen for carbon dioxide (ABG). ABG analysis will also indicate the acidity of Siobhan's arterial blood and whether she has progressed to anaerobic metabolism due to reduced oxygenation, by measuring her arterial or venous lactate level.

What does Siobhan's ABG result tell us about her condition?

By using the step-by-step guide illustrated in Table 2.5, an analysis of Siobhan's ABG results and general condition indicate the following.

- Step 1: Assess oxygenation

PaO_2 – 7.8 kPa: there is evidence of hypoxaemia (SpO_2 91%) with supplemental oxygen of 70%.

- Step 2: Assess pH level

pH – 7.37: there is no evidence of acidosis or alkalosis.

- Step 3: Assess respiratory component

$PaCO_2$ – 5.2 kPa: this measure is within the normal range.

- Step 4: Assess the metabolic component

HCO_3 – 21 mmol/L: this indicates that Siobhan's HCO_3 is slightly below the normal range but not sufficient to indicate metabolic acidosis as the pH is still within the normal range.

- Step 5: Combine your findings

Siobhan is hypoxaemic (PaO_2 <8 kPa) with normocapnia (normal carbon dioxide levels: $PaCO_2$ <6 kPa).

- Step 6: Clinical interpretation and recommendation

Siobhan presented with type 1 respiratory failure (O'Driscoll et al., 2017) with evidence of new confusion, tachypnoea, tachycardia, hypotension, and elevated lactate. Things happened very quickly from that point. The anaesthetist reviewed Siobhan and recommended her transfer to the high dependency unit with a diagnosis of type I respiratory failure secondary to community-acquired pneumonia. She needed respiratory support to improve her oxygenation, pain management, and close monitoring of her ABGs, breathing, and consciousness.

Always risk assess	Look: Listen: Feel: Measure
ABG: Step 1 Assess oxygenation Normal: PaO_2 11.5–13.5 kPa	Is there evidence of hypoxaemia? Is there evidence of high levels of oxygenation? Is the patient receiving supplemental oxygen?
ABG: Step 2 Assess pH level Normal: 7.35–7.45	Is there evidence of acidosis? pH <7.35 Is there evidence of alkalosis? pH >7.45
ABG: Step 3 Assess the respiratory component Normal $PaCO_2$: 4.6–6.0 kPa	Is the $PaCO_2$ <4.5 kPa? Is the $PaCO_2$ >6.0 kPa?

ABG: Step 4
Assess the metabolic component
  Normal HCO_3–: 22–27 mmol/L
  BE +/− 1
	Is the HCO_3 <22 mmol/L?
	Is the HCO_3 >27 mmol/L?
	The base excess level (BE) is the quantity of acid or base required to restore the pH to 7.4. Base excess will mirror the bicarbonate level and simply reinforces evidence of a metabolic component (Higgins, 2013).

ABG: Step 5 Combine your findings	Combine your findings from steps 2/3/4 and identify if there is evidence of: • respiratory acidosis; • respiratory alkalosis; • metabolic acidosis; • metabolic alkalosis;

(Continued)

Table 2.5   (Continued)

Always risk assess	Look: Listen: Feel: Measure
	• signs that the respiratory system has compensated for a metabolic acidosis by increasing the respiratory rate and reducing the CO_2 level; • signs that the renal system has compensated for chronic respiratory acidosis by increasing the level of HCO_3-.
ABG: Step 6 Clinical interpretation and recommendation	Interpret the ABGs in the context of all available patient data.

Table 2.5   A step-by-step approach to assessing ABG results

How did Siobhan become so ill so quickly when she is so young and usually very fit? Siobhan has been suffering with influenza-like symptoms, most probably from a virulent infection of her upper airways. Bacteria have been aspirated into her lungs during breathing, where they have caused inflammation of the bronchioles and alveoli. The air spaces have filled with exudate (escaping fluid containing cell debris and pus), which in turn filled with white blood cells and fibrin to create a solid mass known as consolidation (Brashers and Huether, 2019). This blocks inhaled oxygen from contact with the alveolar surface, thus restricting external respiration.

Siobhan reports localised, sharp chest pain known as pleuritic pain, which results from inflammation spreading to the pleura. The pain restricts her ability to take deep breaths and, combined with the inefficient external respiration, she has quickly become hypoxaemic and breathless. Despite her young age and usual health, Siobhan's defence mechanisms are failing to cope with the virulence of the infection. Without intervention to control the infection, clear secretions, and correct her poor oxygenation, Siobhan is at serious risk of death from pneumonia and respiratory failure. The British Thoracic Society (BTS, 2015) recommend the CURB65 score to ascertain risk from community-acquired pneumonia. One point is awarded for each symptom.

- C – confusion of new onset.
- U – urea level >7 mmol/litre.
- R – respiratory rate >30 bpm.
- B – blood pressure: systolic <90 mmHg or diastolic <60 mmHg.
- 65 years of age or more.

A score of 2 or more indicates moderate to high risk of death and the need for treatment in hospital with a minimum of 12-hourly medical review, while intensive care assessment should be considered for patients scoring 3 or more (NICE, 2014a [updated 2019]). From the nursing assessment we can see that Siobhan scores 4, confirming the need for level 2 care.

Types of respiratory failure

Type 1 respiratory failure is characterised by:

- PaO_2 less than 8 kPa;
- low or normal $PaCO_2$.

It is also known as hypoxaemic respiratory failure and can progress to type II respiratory failure if not treated.

Type II respiratory failure is characterised by:

- PaO_2 less than 8 kPa;
- $PaCO_2$ more than 6.0 kPa (hypercarbia);
- respiratory acidosis.

Type II respiratory failure is also known as ventilatory respiratory failure.

Type I respiratory failure

Siobhan has type I respiratory failure indicated by hypoxaemia. This must be treated to prevent progression to type II respiratory failure and the risk of tissue hypoxia, whereby insufficient oxygen is available for cell metabolism. Without adequate levels of oxygen for aerobic cell metabolism, anaerobic metabolism begins, thus producing lactic acid. Anaerobic metabolism is less efficient and, if prolonged, cells begin to swell and cell death can occur (White and Tait, 2019).

Siobhan is already trying to compensate by breathing faster and trying to increase her pulmonary ventilation. She is receiving as much oxygen as can be given to her via oxygen mask and her SpO_2 readings of 92% and her confusion tell us that her body is failing to compensate. NICE (2014 [updated 2019]) recommend that she needs dual antibiotic treatment for the infection. Because she is so unwell, the antibiotics will need to be given intravenously and she needs additional interventions such as humidification and nebulisers to loosen the viscous secretions that are blocking external respiration (O'Driscoll et al., 2017). If her cough is too weak to expectorate the thick sputum, Siobhan may need chest physiotherapy, and consideration should be given to controlling her pain to facilitate this. If her condition does not improve and she becomes more tired, she may need respiratory support by non-invasive **ventilation** (NIV), which will help her to take bigger breaths with less effort. This system uses a very tight-fitting face mask so that extra air and oxygen can be pushed into the lungs via a series of pipes. The larger breaths help to improve gaseous exchange at the alveoli, while Siobhan's demand for oxygen should be reduced due to not needing to work so hard. Similarly, if Siobhan's ability to sustain spontaneous breathing is further reduced, she may need invasive positive pressure ventilation (IPPV) in the intensive care unit. In this instance Siobhan will need to have an endotracheal tube inserted to have her breathing totally controlled by a ventilator (see Chapter 3). Both invasive and non-invasive respiratory support carry risks so, for this reason, it is important to continually monitor Siobhan using the 'Look: Listen: Feel: Measure: Respond' approach. Her respiratory rate, SpO$_2$ against inspired oxygen, pulse, blood pressure, mental state, and temperature should be closely observed and recorded (Gibson, 2015). Any changes should be reported immediately to prompt a timely response.

You must ensure that measurements recorded are accurate to facilitate administration of the most appropriate treatment and care for Siobhan. Accurate monitoring of SpO$_2$ requires good peripheral perfusion, which can be assessed by measuring capillary refill. This is the time taken in seconds for colour to return after compressing a fingernail bed (you could practise this on your own fingernail). Capillary refill should be used as part of holistic assessment, although its value is sometimes questioned. In altered pathophysiology states, such as peripheral vascular disease, results can mislead interpretation (Creed and Spiers, 2010). Reliability of oxygen saturations can be affected by poor peripheral perfusion, anaemia, hypothermia, false or painted nails, bright environmental lights, or incorrect probe positioning (Creed et al., 2010).

Because Siobhan is acutely ill, her peripheral perfusion may be compromised, affecting the accuracy of her SpO$_2$ reading. The reading is most significant when considered against the inspired oxygen percentage. A low reading recorded on breathing room air is less worrying than a low reading on high-flow oxygen. As Siobhan is receiving high-flow oxygen, it is important to check her ABGs again to evaluate the effectiveness of any treatment and care. Results should be considered alongside other findings from clinical assessment.

Activity 2.3   Evidence-based practice and research

In clinical practice where an oxygen saturation monitor, with finger probe, is available, ask your practice supervisor/assessor if you and a fellow student can experiment to test the accuracy of oxygen saturations measurement on a healthy person (each other). If you ask your teacher, you may also be able to do this in your university clinical skills laboratory. Apply the following variances.

- Apply a blood pressure cuff.
- Hold the arm up in the air for a few minutes.
- Apply nail polish.
- Shine a bright light close to the probe.

Note the variations in results of these actions and consider how these things apply to your patients.

As this answer is based on your own observations, there is no outline answer at the end of the chapter.

Type II respiratory failure

The scenario below gives you an opportunity to understand a clinical example of type II respiratory failure.

Case study: Chronic obstructive pulmonary disease

Pav, a student nurse, was asked to look after 64-year-old Brian Carter, who was known to have COPD and previous type II respiratory failure. He was well known on the ward, having been an inpatient on several previous occasions. Three days ago, he was admitted with an infected exacerbation of COPD. Following medical review, Brian was prescribed care including intravenous antibiotics, nebulisers, steroid therapy, and oxygen at 24% via a venturi device (Figure 2.3) to keep his oxygen saturations between 88 and 92% (NICE, 2018 [updated 2019]).

Pav went to do Brian's observations and found that he looked quite uncomfortable. On further ABCDE assessment he found Brian's respiratory rate was 36 bpm and his oxygen saturations were reading 88% on his ear probe. His pulse rate was 127 bpm and his blood pressure was 98/52 mmHg. Pav noticed that Brian's fingers were slightly blue, and his nose and lips were also rather dusky coloured. Pav tried to comfort Brian and asked how he was feeling, but his answers were difficult to hear because he seemed so short of breath and sounded wheezy. Brian looked as if he was working hard to breathe, pulling his chest up by his shoulders and breathing through pursed lips while his oxygen mask hung around his neck. He looked frightened and his hand was shaking as he reached out for a glass of water.

From Pav's assessment based upon 'Look: Listen: Feel: Measure: Respond', we can deduce that Brian is in respiratory distress. This is a serious situation with risk of further deterioration if appropriate action is not taken. Brian is struggling to get air into his lungs and his oxygen saturation levels are too low, suggesting hypoxaemia and respiratory failure. Without ABG analysis to indicate Brian's $PaCO_2$ levels we do not know whether Brian is in type I or type II respiratory failure. Brian is, however, showing signs that he is in type II respiratory failure. We know this because Pav noticed the tachycardia under circulation assessment and, under exposure, should find dilation of Brian's peripheral veins and hand tremor, which are because of hypercarbia on the vascular system and central nervous system (Woodrow, 2019). Pav now needs to organise his findings using SBAR and ABCDE, to enable him to prioritise his response to reduce the risk of Brian deteriorating further.

As a student nurse, it is important that he gets help to deal with this situation, but Pav should not leave Brian alone. He can summon his mentor by use of the bedside emergency call bell. The aim is to make breathing easier for Brian, thus improving his oxygenation and reducing his carbon dioxide levels. Considering the different phases

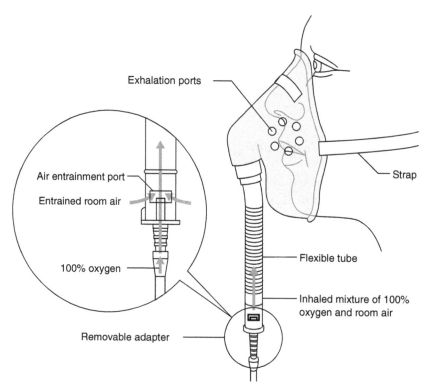

Exhalation ports

Air entrainment port

Entrained room air

100% oxygen

Removable adapter

Strap

Flexible tube

Inhaled mixture of 100% oxygen and room air

Figure 2.3 Venturi device used to administer controlled oxygen. The inhaled mixture of oxygen and room air comprises varied percentages of oxygen, depending upon the size of the air entrainment port.

of respiration, Pav is able to help with pulmonary ventilation and the supply of oxygen but is unable to control other respiratory processes.

Case study

Pav explained to Brian what he was going to do and summoned his mentor. He sat Brian more upright by using the profiling action of the bed. He helped Brian to take some sips of water and made sure that the oxygen was flowing through the mask correctly, then replaced it over Brian's nose and mouth. He checked the accuracy of the oxygen saturations probe by repositioning it and continued to observe Brian's breathing effort, rate, and depth. When his mentor arrived, Pav asked if he should increase the oxygen in view of Brian's breathlessness and low oxygen saturation readings, but he was advised not to. Instead, he assisted his practice supervisor to give two litres of oxygen via nasal cannulae while giving Brian an air-driven nebuliser. The mentor asked Pav to stay with Brian to reassure him and to make sure that he breathed in all the nebulised liquid. Pav's mentor also adjusted the bed so that it formed a chair shape. She asked Pav to call her when the nebuliser started to splutter.

After some time and two further nebulisers, Brian's breathing slowed down, and he looked more comfortable. The physiotherapist helped him to have a good cough. He expectorated large amounts of thick green-yellow sputum.

Why did Pav's mentor insist on these interventions for Brian? Sitting Brian upright would immediately make a difference to his pulmonary ventilation (see Table 2.2) by enabling larger breaths for less effort. Lowering his legs and making the bed into a chair shape reduces intra-abdominal pressure, thus allowing more space for chest expansion. As with Siobhan, it is more effective for Brian to increase his breath size than his respiratory rate, thus promoting better intake of oxygen and allowing exhalation of carbon dioxide. Brian may have felt anxious and acutely aware of the effort required to breathe, so it was important that Pav stayed to help and reassure him. The simple act of helping Brian take sips of water relieved the stress of discomfort from a dry mouth, caused by mouth breathing and the use of oxygen.

Once Pav had improved Brian's pulmonary ventilation, quickly checking and replacing Brian's oxygen mask over his nose and mouth would ensure that Brian was receiving the prescribed level of oxygen. Pav could not know how long Brian had been without the extra oxygen, and so it was sensible to check and reposition the oxygen saturations probe to ensure a good pulse was sensed, thus ensuring accuracy of the reading. Pav could then also check that the displayed pulse rate corresponded to Brian's palpated pulse rate.

Even though Brian's oxygen saturations were low at 88%, Pav's mentor was correct to advise him not to increase the oxygen, but to give two litres per minute via nasal cannulae while also giving an air-driven nebuliser via a face mask. Inpatients with COPD and risk of hypercarbic respiratory failure should aim for oxygen saturations of 88–92% using only 24% oxygen via a venturi mask until ABG analysis is available (O'Driscoll et al., 2017). Brian's COPD was longstanding, and whereas hydrogen ions resulting from synthesis of carbon dioxide would normally be a major stimulus for breathing, people such as Brian, with long-term increased carbon dioxide levels, cease to respond to this stimulus. Instead, they depend on stimulation provided by a sensed reduction in oxygen levels (Grossman and Porth, 2013). By increasing the percentage of oxygen, particularly in people with severe COPD, there is an increased risk of oxygen-induced hypercapnoea (Abdo and Heunks, 2012). British Thoracic Society guidance (O'Driscoll et al., 2017) recommends that oxygen titrated to achieve oxygen saturations of 88–92% avoids hypoxaemia and reduces the risk of oxygen-induced hypercapnoea.

Brian's hypoxaemia required continued low-level oxygen therapy to correct it, but it was equally important to reduce his carbon dioxide level. Nebulising prescribed drugs, such as salbutamol and ipratropium bromide to treat bronchoconstriction and reduce air trapping, helps to reduce the feeling of breathlessness and aid smoother air flow through the airways (Merritt, 2009). NICE (2018 [updated 2019]) recommends increasing the frequency of nebulisers in exacerbations of COPD and to drive them with air in patients at risk of hypercarbic respiratory failure. Pav's mentor gave him accurate instructions and observed guidelines that the nebuliser is ineffective once it starts to splutter (Kelly and Lynes, 2011).

Brian's inability to exhale sufficient carbon dioxide (CO_2 retention) was probably caused by sputum retention, although poor posture and air trapping could also contribute. Physiotherapy can help with clearing sputum by helping to shake it loose, precipitating coughing. Brian was able to do as the physiotherapist asked, cough and expectorate sputum, but had he been unable to do so, insertion of a naso-pharyngeal airway, through which secretions can be removed by suctioning, should be considered. Because Brian was already receiving antibiotic therapy for his exacerbation of COPD, it would be necessary to review its effectiveness in relation to available sputum culture results, which would indicate the antibiotic sensitivity.

Pav was quick to respond to Brian's respiratory distress by immediate ABCDE assessment using the 'Look: Listen: Feel: Measure: Respond' approach. He responded by asking for help, sitting Brian up, ensuring correct oxygen delivery and continually monitoring Brian while he received nebuliser therapy. Pav's interventions under his mentor's guidance were instrumental in preventing deterioration that could have led to the need for NIV (Chapter 3).

Monitoring to prevent breathlessness

Scenario: Asthma

You are working alongside the hospital respiratory nurse specialist, and you are asked to gather initial information from patients as they arrive for asthma clinic appointments. You meet 24-year-old Liz Gardiner, who appears anxious, wheezy, and a little out of breath. She tells you she has been rushing and that she will be fine in a few minutes.

It is important that you observe Liz as she waits to see the respiratory nurse. She may be well enough to walk into the department and be convincing in her story, but she has an appointment time lasting only a few minutes and then she will leave again. You have very little time to determine whether Liz has health needs that require immediate attention by way of investigation, intervention, or education. Anything that is not attended to now may have to wait six months, and during that time Liz may be at risk of severe respiratory problems leading to hypoxia and associated with uncontrolled asthma, infection, or allergy. Any of these may require hospital admission, which would put her more at risk.

Activity 2.4   Critical thinking

Make a list of the possible causes of Liz's symptoms and try to prioritise them in order of significance from very important to not important. Give reasons for your answer.

A list of symptoms and significance is given at the end of the chapter.

Liz already has a diagnosis of asthma: a chronic inflammatory lung disorder that causes obstruction of airflow. The fact that she attends hospital appointments suggests that she has had problems in the past with control of her asthma or acute, life-threatening episodes (BTS and SIGN, 2019). Liz's breathlessness and wheeze on arrival are significant and warrant further exploration. After allowing her to rest for a few minutes, you should note her degree of recovery and inform the respiratory nurse. She will want to know what triggers Liz's wheeze and dyspnoea, the frequency that Liz has been experiencing symptoms such as breathlessness, wheeze, chest tightness or a cough, how she deals with them, and how long they last (BTS and SIGN, 2019).

The respiratory nurse should review Liz's use of any asthma medication, such as inhalers for prevention or treatment of symptoms. She should check that Liz uses the correct techniques when using her inhalers, to ensure that medication is effectively administered. Inhaler technique has important clinical consequences and while 98% of people think they use their inhalers correctly, only 8% of people do (BTS and SIGN, 2019). Liz may well need some additional advice to improve her technique. Any psychosocial factors that could contribute to exacerbating Liz's asthma should be considered, and it would be useful for Liz to use a peak flow meter to monitor and keep a diary of her peak expiratory flow rate (PEFR). Peak flow measurements give an indication of airway resistance by measuring the force of expiration in litres per minute (Wheeldon, 2013). Normal values of PEFR vary depending upon age, sex, and height of the individual, and recordings of 70% of expected value or less indicate airway obstruction (BTS and SIGN, 2019). Peak flow trends are more useful than single values recorded, as they highlight deviations from normal for individual patients. These can serve to warn of potential instability in response to infection or other asthma triggers, thus allowing the patient to take appropriate preventative action. More information on peak flows can be obtained from the peak flow website listed at the end of the chapter.

Identifying the lowest level of treatment to maintain control for Liz's asthma and preventing life-threatening episodes depends upon her understanding her condition, being involved in monitoring, and her honesty and concordance with prescribed therapy and health promotion advice, such as inhaler technique. For this reason, the relationship that you develop with Liz on your first encounter could have implications for her lifelong respiratory health.

Activity 2.5 Practical health promotion skills

Visit the Asthma UK website on the link below to see demonstrations of how techniques vary for different kinds of inhalers.

https://www.asthma.org.uk/advice/inhalers-medicines-treatments/using-inhalers/

Chapter summary

Within this chapter we have used examples of patient situations to demonstrate why patients become breathless, how we can specifically assess breathing and the most appropriate interventions for some common clinical situations. We have considered patients in a variety of healthcare settings to demonstrate how acute situations can arise and how your response can have a significant impact upon patient outcomes.

Activities: brief outline answers

Activity 2.1: Critical thinking (page 55)

Assessment method	Making note of	Significance
Look	Rate of breaths – how many per minute. Rhythm. Depth. Symmetry. Smoothness. Effort used.	Breathing should be effortless 10–20 breaths per minute. Bradypnea (<10 bpm) could be a sign of central nervous system depression. Tachypnoea (>20 bpm) could indicate hypoxia but is normal after exercise. Both sides of chest should rise equally and evenly.
	Facial expression – pursed lips, nasal flaring, grimace with pain. Skin colour. Use of accessory muscles. Ratio I : E (inspiration time : expiration time). General distress.	Asymmetrical inflation could signify injury, pneumonectomy, or pneumothorax. Mucous membranes should be pink and moist; pale mucous membranes could indicate low oxygen saturations or low haemoglobin content. Skin – should be pink and warm. Breathing should not be painful – pain could indicate infection of lungs, airways, or inflammation of pleura. Distress, use of accessory muscles, and facial expressions are evidence of hypoxia and need for patient to take bigger breaths.
Listen (with and without stethoscope)	Is breathing noisy or quiet? Where does the sound come from: throat,	Is normally quiet in clear airways and is quieter on expiration than inspiration. Different noises can indicate

Assessment method	Making note of	Significance
	upper or lower airways? What type of sound? At what stage of the breath does the sound occur – inspiration or expiration? Beginning or end? Equality/symmetry. Front and back. Sound of each breath in and out. Airflow noise. Quality of breath sounds. Ability to speak – how many words?	bronchospasm (intermittent closing of the airways), blockage, sputum retention, pulmonary oedema. Visit the following website to listen to different breathing sounds. www.3m.com/healthcare/littmann/mmm-library.html When using a stethoscope, you will hear better quality sounds than without. Inability to complete sentences in one breath indicates hypoxia.
Feel	Breath/air movement on hand. Chest expansion – rise and fall. Sensations on chest movement. Skin temperature. Movement.	Feeling for air movement can augment other methods of assessment to confirm what you see or hear, especially if breathing is shallow or you are in a noisy environment. Different sensations can indicate sputum retention (rattles), surgical emphysema (like crepe paper), or pulmonary oedema (boggy). Skin should be warm and dry to touch – cold clammy skin can indicate hypoxia.
Measure	Number of breaths per minute. Size of breaths in millilitres. Force of breaths in millilitres per second. Oxygen saturations. Acid-base balance results from ABG analysis. Number of words spoken between breaths.	Respiratory rate (RR), number of complete breaths (in and out) per minute, also known as respiration rate, respiratory frequency (R_f), ventilation rate (VR), ventilation frequency (V_f), breathing frequency (B_f), or pulmonary ventilation rate. These abbreviations may be seen on respiratory support equipment. The size in millilitres of a normal exhaled breath (without force) is known as (expiratory) tidal volume. This can only be effectively measured through a tracheostomy or endotracheal tube. Peak flow measures force of breaths and is useful to establish effects of therapy. Oxygen saturations in conjunction with therapy response: 98–100% in normal. 94–98% aim in acute. 88–92% in risk of hypercapnic respiratory failure (HRF). Levels of oxygen in peripheral circulation and carbon dioxide in blood = type of respiratory failure. Gives an indication of degree of improvement or deterioration in breathing efficiency.

Table 2.6 Answer to Activity 2.1: different aspects of breathing that can be assessed

Activity 2.4: Critical thinking (page 67)

The possible reasons why Liz is anxious, wheezy, and out of breath are given in order of importance.

1. She may have a chest infection: secretions and inflammation within the airways as a result of chest infection will narrow her airways and make Liz more prone to bronchospasm, which creates the wheeze. If the wheeze is audible without a stethoscope, it is significant. Wheeze indicates constriction of the airways, thus airflow is restricted and Liz will find it harder to breathe in the oxygen she needs, particularly if she is rushing and using more energy. This is the priority problem as it needs to be treated with antibiotics and Liz will need to temporarily increase the use of her inhalers, making sure that she takes both the preventer and reliever. She will also need to monitor her peak flows to make sure that her asthma symptoms are being adequately controlled. If Liz does not get early treatment for a chest infection, she could have severe respiratory difficulties, leading to hospitalisation and intensive care (BTS and SIGN, 2019).

2. Liz's asthma may not be as well controlled as she says it is. If she is becoming anxious prior to her appointment and this is triggering wheeziness and shortness of breath, it is important to ascertain what Liz understands about her asthma symptoms and the medication she takes, how often she takes it, what time of day she takes it, and her technique. She may need to increase her medication, she may need to be taught better inhaler techniques, or she may not be taking her medication as prescribed. Liz may need some information to help her decision making. She may also need information about peak flow monitoring so that she can see clearly when her asthma is not well controlled. It would be useful to find out what triggers Liz's symptoms and to reiterate when Liz needs to seek help from her doctor or respiratory nurse. Giving Liz good health promotion advice can help to prevent her asthma getting severely out of control and necessitating hospital admission.

3. Liz may have been subjected to an allergen that triggers her asthma symptoms while on her journey. Much of the educational and health promotion information detailed in Answer 2 still applies as it is important that Liz responds quickly when her asthma is triggered.

4. She may just have been rushing and may have had a stressful journey. However, she is clearly showing symptoms of asthma, which should ideally be better controlled. Good health promotion advice is needed as in Answer 2.

Further reading

Higginson, R and Jones, B (2009) Respiratory assessment in critically ill patients: airway and breathing. *British Journal of Nursing*, 18(8): 456–61.

This article gives a good overview of respiratory assessment and the skills needed by ward nurses as well as critical care nurses. There is clear advice about use of oxygen masks.

Rolfe, S (2019) The importance of respiratory rate monitoring. *British Journal of Nursing*, 28(8): 504–08.

The article focuses on the importance of respiratory rate as a key element of breathing assessment and why a detailed assessment of breathing is essential in the recognition of clinical deterioration.

O'Driscoll, BR, et al. (2017) *Guidelines for Emergency Oxygen Use in Adult Patients.* London: British Thoracic Society. Accessed at: www.brit-thoracic.org.uk/quality-improvement/guidelines/emergency-oxygen/

These are the guidelines for oxygen use that should be applied nationally.

Elliott, M and Baird, J (2019) Pulse oximetry and the enduring neglect of respiratory rate assessment: a commentary on patient surveillance. *British Journal of Nursing*, 28(19): 1256–59.

Useful websites

www.asthma.org.uk/index.html

The Asthma UK website gives a lot of information about asthma, including inhalers and nebulisers. There is useful information for both professionals and patients.

www.brit-thoracic.org.uk/quality-improvement/guidelines/

The British Thoracic Society quality improvement guidelines offer the most up-to-date evidence to support the management of asthma, COPD, emergency use of oxygen, pneumonia, and other clinical conditions that impact on respiratory function.

Chapter 3 — The patient who needs respiratory support

Desiree Tait

NMC Future Nurse: Standards of Proficiency for Registered Nurses

This chapter will address the following platforms and proficiencies:

Platform 3: Assessing needs and planning care

Registered nurses prioritise the needs of people when assessing and reviewing their mental, physical, cognitive, behavioural, social and spiritual needs. They use information obtained during assessments to identify the priorities and requirements for person-centred and evidence-based nursing interventions and support. They work in partnership with people to develop person-centred care plans that take into account their circumstances, characteristics and preferences.

At the point of registration, the registered nurse will be able to:

3.2 demonstrate and apply knowledge of body systems and homeostasis, human anatomy and physiology, biology, genomics, pharmacology, and social and behavioural sciences when undertaking full and accurate person-centred nursing assessments and developing appropriate care plans.

3.3 demonstrate and apply knowledge of all commonly encountered mental, physical, behavioural and cognitive health conditions, medication usage and treatments when undertaking full and accurate assessments of nursing care needs and when developing, prioritising and reviewing person-centred care plans.

3.5 demonstrate the ability to accurately process all information gathered during the assessment process to identify needs for individualised nursing care and develop person-centred evidence-based plans for nursing interventions with agreed goals.

Platform 4: Providing and evaluating care

Registered nurses take the lead in providing evidence-based, compassionate and safe nursing interventions. They ensure that care they provide and delegate is person-centred and of a consistently high standard. They support people of all ages in a range of care settings.

They work in partnership with people, families and carers to evaluate whether care is effective and the goals of care have been met in line with their wishes, preferences and desired outcomes.

At the point of registration, the registered nurse will be able to:

4.10 demonstrate the knowledge and ability to respond proactively and promptly to signs of deterioration or distress in mental, physical, cognitive and behavioural health and use this knowledge to make sound clinical decisions.

4.12 demonstrate the ability to manage commonly encountered devices and confidently carry out related nursing procedures to meet people's needs for evidence-based, person-centred care.

Chapter aims

By the end of this chapter, you should be able to:

- identify why a person may need advanced respiratory (ventilatory) support to maintain effective respiratory function;
- describe non-invasive ventilation (NIV) and invasive mechanical ventilation (IMV) as forms of respiratory support;
- demonstrate an awareness of the factors influencing the choice of appropriate respiratory support;
- describe the fundamentals of providing a safe holistic approach to caring for patients receiving NIV and IMV following clinical deterioration.

Introduction

In Chapter 2 you were introduced to the nursing assessment and management of a person experiencing breathlessness as well as the common conditions that are associated with breathlessness. The importance of oxygen was addressed and how to recognise the signs and symptoms of acute hypoxaemic (Type I) and hypercapnic (type II) respiratory failure. The relationship between breathing and homeostasis was explored, together with the significance of ABG analysis. In this chapter you are introduced to people who require advanced respiratory support that goes beyond oxygen therapy. We continue to explore the importance of a detailed assessment, interpretation, and management of medications in this context and will explore how a holistic assessment of a person, including analysis of ABGs (introduced in Chapter 2), can inform both the prioritisation and management of a deteriorating patient. The chapter begins by introducing you to Mrs Jenny Matthews. The scenario box below provides a summary of her admission to the emergency department, and we will continue to follow her story as the chapter develops.

Scenario: Jenny Matthews

Situation

Mrs Jenny Matthews, age 43 years, married with no children.

Jenny has been admitted to the emergency department with a seven-day history of short-ness of breath and productive cough. She had previously been seen by her GP, diagnosed with a chest infection, and treated with a combination of broad spectrum antibiotics and an increased dose of salbutamol. She was progressing well at home but a sudden onset of increased shortness of breath at 2 a.m. prompted a 999 call from her husband. The paramed-ics reported that Jenny was in respiratory failure with an SpO_2 of 87% when breathing air, respirations of 38/minute and a heart rate of 130/minute. High-flow oxygen therapy was commenced at 60% to improve Jenny's SpO_2 to within the range of 94–98% (BTS and SIGN, 2019; O'Driscoll et al., 2017).

Background

Jenny has a 20-year history of acute asthma and has been admitted to hospital as an emer-gency on five occasions during the last seven years. On the previous occasion she required emergency intubation and ventilation and stayed in intensive care for 48 hours. Jenny has smoked cigarettes for 22 years and continues to smoke ten cigarettes a day every day. There is a strong family history of reactive airways disease.

Assessment in the emergency room

Airway (A): She can maintain her own airway, she is agitated and struggling to breathe but is responding to commands with no evidence of confusion.

Inspiratory and expiratory wheeze can be heard during lung auscultation

Breathing (B): Dyspnoea

Sitting upright and using her accessory muscles to breathe.

Unable to complete a full sentence when responding to questions.

Chest auscultation indicates an expiratory wheeze and bilateral crackles.

Respiration (R): 36/min.

SpO_2 91%, on 60% O_2 via a venturi mask

Arterial blood gas showed:

pH: 7.42

PaO_2: 8.7 kPa

$PaCO_2$: 3.6 kPa

HCO_3: 24 mmol/L.

PEFR (Peak Expiratory Flow Rate): 120 ml/min, 40% of her normal predicted volume (Jenny's normal PEFR: 300 ml/min).

Circulation (C): HR: 125/min.
BP: 125/72 mmHg.

Disability (D): Blood glucose: 6.8 mmol/L.
General body pain expressed at 2/10
ACVPU: Alert and agitated.

Exposure (E): Temp: 37.4 °C.
NEWS2 Score = 10

Recommendations

A NEWS2 of 10 indicates a senior review and escalation to the critical care outreach team (CCOT) in accordance with the RCP's guidance (RCP, 2017).

The medical team recommend the following according to BTS and SIGN guidance (2019):

- Humidified high-flow oxygen 60%, together with salbutamol 5 mg nebulisers continuously until improvement in PEF.
- Hydrocortisone 100 mg IV.
- Continuous monitoring and review every 15 minutes, with a review by the CCOT after 30 minutes or if there is further deterioration in Jenny's condition.

Thirty minutes later Jenny had shown no signs of improvement in her PEF or SpO_2. Repeat ABG results also showed no signs of improvement and Jenny was drowsy but responsive. The CCOT reviewed her situation and recommended an immediate transfer to ICU, with Jenny's consent, for continued monitoring and review of her treatment.

When Jenny's husband, Brendan, was informed of her transfer to ICU he became very angry and started shouting at his wife. Jenny ignored him, and Brendan Matthews was asked to leave the treatment room. The staff invited him to stay in a quiet room. He refused and instead gave the staff alternative details of next of kin, insisting that they no longer contact him.

Why did Jenny's situation deteriorate at home and lead to an emergency admission to ICU?

Less than 24 hours ago Jenny was seemingly making a good recovery from a chest infection when she experienced a sudden deterioration in her condition. Asthma is a chronic inflammatory disorder of the mucosal lining of the bronchi which is associated with bronchial hyper-responsiveness, reversible airway constriction, and variable airflow obstruction (McCance and Huether, 2019). The cause of asthma is complex and usually involves both genetic and environmental factors (Morris and Pearson, 2020). In Jenny's case non-atopic causes include evidence of a recent respiratory tract infection, high levels of emotional stress associated with her marriage, and exposure to tobacco smoke acting as a bronchial irritant. Jenny also has a strong family history of hypersensitivity reactions (atopic reactions) and is sensitive to environmental allergens including pollen and moulds.

Following seven days of antibiotic treatment, Jenny decided it was time to resume smoking, as this was her main way of coping with the stresses of life. This action triggered a long and aggressive argument with her husband that continued over the course of the evening. It was later that night that Jenny developed the acute exacerbation of asthma reported in her story. According to Polosa and Thompson (2013), cigarette smoking in asthma is associated with a higher frequency and severity of exacerbations and a higher risk of mortality than for non-smokers. There is also evidence to suggest that regular smoking leads to significantly reduced lung function when measured with FEV_1 (Jaakkola et al., 2019). According to Leander et al. (2014), smoking is often used as a coping strategy for anxiety and depression, as in Jenny's case, leading to an increased frequency of exacerbations for people living with asthma. This finding is supported by BTS and SIGN (2019) when they identify psychological factors such as severe domestic, marital stress as being associated with a higher risk of near fatal or fatal asthma. They also identify that a pattern of recent admissions to hospital associated with an acute asthmatic episode, and previous treatment with advanced respiratory support, are also associated with a higher risk of developing near fatal or fatal asthma. When the above factors are applied to Jenny's situation, she has a high risk of experiencing a near fatal or fatal asthma attack.

When Jenny was admitted to the emergency room, she was presenting signs and symptoms of the 'early response' phase. According to McCance and Huether (2019), this phase is initiated by exposure to the inhaled irritant and triggers a cascade of inflammatory events that lead to acute and chronic airway dysfunction. They go on to describe the combined impact of mast cell activation, which triggers the release of vasoactive mediators, the degranulation of inflammatory mediators, and innate immune activation. The clinical features associated with this process include the following:

- bronchial vasodilation and increased capillary permeability;
- vascular congestion;
- bronchospasm;
- increased contractile response of the bronchial smooth muscle;
- mucus secretion;
- thickening of airway walls;

- bronchial hyper-responsiveness;
- airway obstruction.

A summary of this process is illustrated in Figure 3.1.

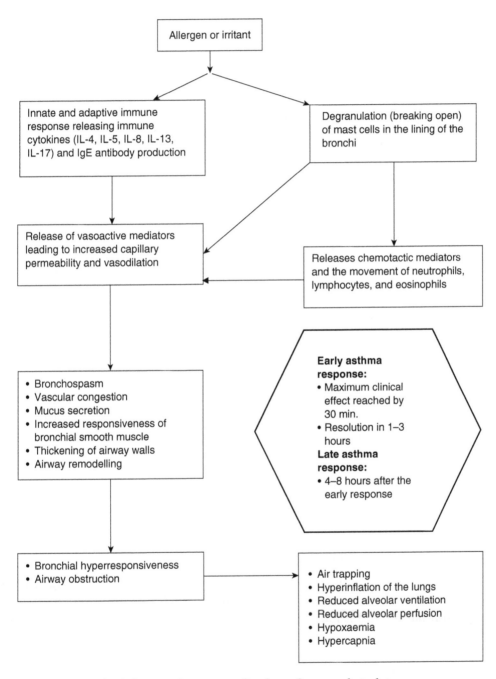

Figure 3.1 Pathophysiology and process of asthma from early to late response

Source: McCance and Huether, 2019.

For Jenny the presence of a PEFR of less than 50% of her predicted normal range, a respiratory rate of 36 breaths per minute, a pulse of 125 beats per minute and an inability to complete a sentence in one breath indicated the presence of acute severe asthma (BTS and SIGN, 2019). With oxygen saturations of 91% and signs of developing type I respiratory failure indicated by her ABG result of PaO_2 8.7 kPa (see Chapter 2), Jenny's condition was becoming life threatening and she required level 2 and potentially level 3 critical care (BTS and SIGN, 2019). We will revisit Jenny's story following her transfer to intensive care.

What does Jenny's ABG result tell us about her condition?

By using the step-by-step guide illustrated in Table 2.5, an analysis of Jenny's ABG results and general condition indicate the following.

- **Step 1: Assess oxygenation**

  PaO_2 – 8.7 kPa: there is evidence of hypoxaemia (SpO_2 91%) with supplemental oxygen of 60%.

- **Step 2: Assess pH level**

  pH – 7.42: there is no evidence of acidosis or alkalosis.

- **Step 3: Assess respiratory component**

  $PaCo_2$ – 3.6 kPa: this measure is lower than the normal range and indicates that Jenny has been hyperventilating and expiring CO_2 to cope with reduced volumes of air movement in her lungs due to bronchospasm. This is supported by her reduced PEFR of 120 ml/min (her normal PEF: 300 ml/min).

- **Step 4: Assess the metabolic component**

  HCO_3^- 24 mmol/L: this indicates that Jenny has no evidence of metabolic acidosis or alkalosis.

- **Step 5: Combine your findings**

  Jenny is not experiencing any form of acidosis or alkalosis based on these blood gas results, however, the presence of a $PaCO_2$ of 3.6 kPa indicates that Jenny's hyperventilation and a lower than normal $PaCO_2$ are correcting any potential for acidosis.

- **Step 6: Clinical interpretation and recommendation**

  Clinically Jenny is showing signs of developing type I respiratory failure (see Chapter 2), she is experiencing increased work of breathing and a reducing peak expiratory flow. There has been some improvement in her PaO_2 since the commencement of 60% humidified oxygen; however, the combination of salbutamol (bronchodilator) nebulisers and hydrocortisone has produced no improvement in her signs and symptoms. Jenny continues to be at risk of further deterioration requiring an escalation of her condition due to a secondary or late response to the initial trigger and requires close monitoring and support during this critical stage (BTS and SIGN, 2019; McCance and Huether, 2019). There are several factors that now become significant when monitoring Jenny's condition. For example, we know that:

- Jenny has now been awake and fighting for breath (in respiratory distress) since 2 a.m. and it is now 4 a.m.;
- she is emotionally distressed after her husband appears to have left her;
- she is still recovering from an acute respiratory infection and is presenting with developing type I respiratory failure and about to be transferred to intensive care.

In the next section of the case study, we rejoin Jenny in ICU.

Activity 3.1   Decision making

Read the scenario below and think about the significance of the ABG results, using Table 2.5 as a guide.

Joseph Baglio (age 68 years) has smoked 40 cigarettes a day since his twenties and has experienced angina on exertion for the last five years, although this has been managed using beta blockers and GTN. He was admitted to the medical ward six hours ago following a diagnosis of pneumonia. Following his admission, he seemed to be responding well to the oxygen therapy and intravenous antibiotics when he pressed the buzzer and fell forward clutching his chest. When the nurse arrived, she found that Joseph was unresponsive with absent respirations and pulse. A cardiac arrest call was placed and he was resuscitated successfully. His ABG results 30 minutes after his resuscitation were:

pH: 7.05

PaO_2: 8.5 kPa on 60% high-flow oxygen (SpO_2 84%)

$PaCO_2$: 14.1 kPa

HCO_3: 20.5 mmol/L

BE: −3.0

Joseph was conscious, flushed, and anxious. His vital signs were T: 38.0 °C, R: 32/min, P: 95/min, BP: 110/70 mmHg.

- Using the step-by-step guide in Table 2.5, what can you interpret from the ABG result?

One hour later Joseph was conscious but confused. His skin was cold and clammy to touch, and his vital signs were T: 38.0 °C, R: 32/min, P: 94, BP: 110/70 mmHg. He was receiving

(Continued)

(Continued)

60% humidified high-flow oxygen and diagnosed with acute coronary syndrome with evidence of ST elevation myocardial infarction (STEMI). As well as his beta blockers, he has been prescribed statins for reducing cholesterol (he had previously refused to commence statins when prescribed), clopidogrel to reduce the risk of another thrombotic event, and morphine and nitrates for chest pain. Joseph was not considered a suitable candidate for percutaneous coronary angiography because of his pneumonia and was assessed as a candidate for thrombolysis instead, but this was also decided against in light of his traumatic resuscitation. He now has two acute morbidities affecting his respiratory and cardiac system. A second ABG result was:

pH: 7.30

PaO_2: 9.4 kPa (SpO_2 89%)

$PaCO_2$: 6.70 kPa

HCO_3: 21.4 mmol/L

- Using the step-by-step guide in Table 2.5, what can you interpret from the ABG result?
- What are your priorities of care for this patient?

Outline answers to this activity are given at the end of the chapter.

As we rejoin Jenny in ICU, the clinical staff have just completed her initial assessment.

Case study: Jenny's transfer to ICU

Situation: Following her assessment in the emergency room, Jenny was a level 2 patient requiring high dependency care for assessment and monitoring of her respiratory system. She was admitted to ICU and assessed as follows:

A: Responding to commands and maintaining her airway.

B: SpO_2: 90%

60% high-flow humidified O_2

R: 36/min

Blood gases showed:

pH: 7.36

PaO_2: 8.2 kPa

$PaCO_2$: 4.5 kPa

HCO_3: 23 mmol/L

C: HR: 128/min

BP: 130/72 mmHg

D: Blood glucose: 6.7 mmol/L

Agitated and disorientated

E: Temp: 37.5 °C

Recommendations from ICU intensivist:

- Commence NIV as Continuous Positive Airways Pressure (CPAP) using a face mask and initiate inspiratory pressure at 5 cm H_2O increasing to a total inspiratory pressure of 13–15 cm H_2O as tolerated.
- Continually monitor ABCDE and specifically aim for reduced respiratory rate and improved tidal volumes as the work of breathing is supported.

According to BTS and SIGN (2019), the evidence of hypoxia in the presence of a normalising $PaCO_2$, and persistent disorientation following intensive treatment, indicates Jenny is having a life-threatening attack. She has been prescribed ipratropium bromide in conjunction with salbutamol and a once only dose of intravenous magnesium sulphate to produce further bronchodilation (BTS and SIGN, 2019). When her current situation is assessed in the context of her previous admission to ICU, the ICU specialist suggests that she meets the criteria for NIV and that commencement of CPAP could prevent her from needing tracheal intubation and invasive ventilation (Tuxen and Hew, 2019). BTS and SIGN (2019) demonstrate that there is limited evidence to support the use of NIV for managing asthma; however if there is sufficient evidence to support its use the patient should be managed in ICU and be monitored continuously by specialist practitioners (Lim et al., 2012). The plan for Jenny is to commence her on CPAP and monitor her ABCDE continuously for signs of improvement or deterioration.

Activity 3.2 Reflection

Reflect on patients you have nursed and ask yourself the following questions:

- Have I looked after patients with acute respiratory failure either in hospital or the community?
- If so, how did I assess and document the patient care?
- Did the patient need support with oxygen therapy or NIV?
- Did the patient have support from the physiotherapist, dietitian, and respiratory nurse or the critical care outreach nurse?

(Continued)

(Continued)

Hint: This reflection is meant to encourage you to think critically about assessing and managing care and should help you to identify good practice and areas for improvement.

As this answer is based on your own reflection, there is no outline answer at the end of the chapter.

What is NIV and why has it been considered as a type of respiratory support for Jenny?

Pulmonary ventilation, or breathing, is essential for life, and the purpose of NIV is to provide varying levels of positive pressure air flow through a tight-fitting mask to improve the patient's levels of PaO_2 and $PaCO_2$ by improving gaseous exchange and reducing the work of breathing. Breathing involves the inhalation of gases in air into the lungs and exhalation of gases from the lungs into the atmosphere. All gases in air collectively exert a pressure known as atmospheric pressure. The gases in the lungs also exert a pressure known as alveolar pressure. In air, gases always flow from an area of high pressure to an area of low pressure. During inspiration the thoracic space expands because of contraction of the intercostal muscles and diaphragm (see Table 2.2 in this volume and Hall (2016)). This increase in space reduces the overall alveolar pressure in the lungs and atmospheric air flows into the airways to equalise the pressure. Expiration involves relaxation of the respiratory muscles and natural elastic recoil of the lung tissue so that air is expelled back into the atmosphere. Normal breathing therefore relies on negative pressure ventilation.

For 120 years the principal method of supporting ventilation for patients with respiratory failure was based on the principle of negative pressure ventilation. For example, the **iron lung** was used successfully for patients with respiratory failure caused by neuromuscular diseases such as polio. This method was challenged in the 1950s when, during the polio epidemic in Europe, the demand for iron lungs outstripped supply and alternative methods for providing respiratory support were tried (Lassen et al., 1954). This led to the development of **invasive mechanical ventilatory** (IMV) support, which involved air being forced under pressure into patients' lungs via a tracheostomy tube or endotracheal tube at a rate of between 10 and 20 times per minute to mimic normal respiration, described as intermittent positive pressure ventilation. This dramatically reduced the mortality rate of patients suffering from respiratory failure and became the mainstay treatment for ventilatory support until towards the end of the twentieth century (Borthwick et al., 2003).

In the last 25 years, the use of NIV techniques that supply air through a tight-fitting face mask rather than an endotracheal tube have escalated, and this method is recommended by BTS and ICS (2016) and Duke and Bersten (2019), as a viable form of respiratory support in the management of people with either acute or chronic respiratory failure, and has been used to support people with:

- sleep apnoea;
- acute exacerbations of COPD;
- pulmonary oedema;
- neuromuscular disease;
- pneumonia;
- weaning from IMV.

In Jenny's case the use of NIV to manage an acute severe asthma attack does not have such a strong evidence base (Tuxen and Hew, 2019). However, BTS and SIGN (2019) recommend that it should be considered as an option to prevent the risk of intubation in patients with acute severe asthma, but should be based on a skilled clinical assessment and knowledge of the patient's condition. Jenny's respiratory function is compromised but not so impaired that she is in imminent danger of complete respiratory collapse. She can protect her own airway, has only mild disorientation and there is no evidence of a **pneumothorax** on chest X-ray (Tuxen and Hew, 2019). The types of NIV and their use are explained in Table 3.1.

Type of NIV	Benefits	Risks	Patient examples
Continuous positive airways pressure (CPAP). This method provides a continuous flow of positive pressure during the complete respiratory cycle. Some air always remains retained in the alveoli so that they never collapse. This enables oxygen exchange to continue during the whole respiratory cycle and prevents alveolar collapse (atelectasis).	• Improves oxygenation in patients with type I respiratory failure. • Reduces the risk of atelectasis (collapsed non-functioning alveoli).	• There is reduced clearance of CO_2 due to air being trapped in the alveoli. • Not suitable for patients with type II respiratory failure where there are increased levels of CO_2. • The airway is not protected so patients must be able to maintain their own airway.	Mrs Smith is admitted with severe breathlessness and is producing excessive amounts of pink frothy secretions from her airways. She is diagnosed with acute pulmonary oedema and is commenced on CPAP starting at 5 cm H_2O as part of her ongoing treatment to reduce pulmonary secretions by increasing alveolar pressure to above capillary hydrostatic pressure. Chao Chan is diagnosed with pneumonia and type I respiratory failure. His PaO_2 is 6.2 kPa and his $PaCO_2$ is 3.6 kPa. He is commenced on CPAP with an inhaled positive respiratory pressure of 5 cm and then 10 cm H_2O.

(Continued)

Table 3.1 (Continued)

Type of NIV	Benefits	Risks	Patient examples
			Bryn Jones has been diagnosed with **obstructive sleep apnoea**. He suffers from morbid obesity, snoring, and daytime fatigue. He has now been fitted with a face mask and CPAP machine for home use. The equipment delivers CPAP at 10 cm H_2O, to be used at night while sleeping.
Bilevel NIV or bilevel positive airways pressure ventilation. This method provides two alternating levels of positive pressure during respiration. During inspiration, there is an inspired pressure level (IPAP) and during expiration, an expired pressure level (EPAP).	• Improves oxygenation and CO_2 clearance in patients with type II respiratory failure. • IPAP reduces the work of breathing and conserves the use of oxygen by the body. • A lower EPAP pressure reduces air trapping but still allows continuous gas exchange during respiration while preventing atelectasis.	• The airway is not protected so patients must be able to maintain their own airway.	Henry Jones has pneumonia. His PaO_2 is 6.8 kPa and his $PaCO_2$ is 6.5 kPa. He is breathless and agitated. He is commenced on bilevel positive airways pressure with an inspiratory pressure of 10 cm H_2O and an expiratory pressure of 4 cm H_2O. Gladys Cabrera (62 years) suffers from COPD and she is admitted to hospital with an acute exacerbation of her condition. She was commenced on bilevel positive airways pressure at an inspiration pressure (IPAP) of 12 cm H_2O and an expired pressure (EPAP) of 5 cm H_2O with 40% oxygen. She didn't like the face mask but was prepared to give it a try if the nurse reminded her.

Table 3.1 Types of non-invasive ventilation and their use

Contraindications for using NIV

The success of NIV techniques in the support of respiratory function relies on effective patient selection. For Jenny, CPAP was chosen as the optimum treatment regime, but this does not mean that the use of NIV will always lead to a successful outcome for every patient. Patients need to be risk assessed for any contraindications before commencing the therapy and then risk assessed for evidence of any change or deterioration in their condition. This is illustrated in Table 3.2. The contraindications of NIV rarely exist in isolation: often patients will present with one or more of these factors. Knowing the patient and their medical history is an essential part of the rapid decision-making process required when determining a patient's suitability for NIV and relies on good communication between the recipient and all practitioners involved (Scala and Pisani, 2018). Contraindications include:

- patient unable to protect their own airway;
- life-threatening hypoxaemia;
- severe confusion/agitation/cognitive impairment;
- unconscious patient;
- airway obstruction due to vomiting or a foreign object;
- facial trauma/burns/surgery;
- pneumothorax;
- copious amounts of respiratory secretions/sputum;
- inability to fit the mask and maintain effective positive pressure;
- haemodynamic instability and/or cardiac arrhythmias;
- recent surgery in the upper gastrointestinal tract;
- severe co-morbidity;
- presence of bowel obstruction.

Table 3.2 offers a summary of the risk assessment and nursing interventions required to care for patients receiving NIV.

Risk assessment	Nursing interventions
Contraindications for use of NIV	Rapid assessment of ABCDE using 'Look: Listen: Feel: Measure' is important to measure the risk of contraindications to treatment with NIV. In particular, the risk of a spontaneous pneumothorax should be ruled out by reviewing the patient's chest X-ray following their admission.
	A patient may decide to refuse treatment.
	NIV should only be commenced following specialist medical assessment of the patient's clinical need against contraindications.
Preparation of the patient and technology	If the patient has consented and understands what is happening, ensure the equipment has been prepared and checked to ensure it is in working order.
	Sit the patient upright and, with their cooperation, attach the face mask, nasal mask, or hood. The patient will need a few minutes to get used to the mask. Often NIV is commenced at a low level of positive pressure and increased according to the clinical state of the patient (Tuxen and Hew, 2019).
	Document baseline clinical data.
	Agree and document a treatment plan for escalating and identifying a ceiling of treatment.
Airway and respirations	Monitor the patient's airway and respiratory rate, look for signs of respiratory distress and air entry as illustrated in Figure 2.1, page 55.
	Monitor SpO_2 for evidence of improvement or deterioration.
	Monitor the patient's arterial blood gas results after:
	one hour:
	if there is no change in the patient's condition or a slight improvement, then monitor again in four hours;
	one hour:
	if there is a deterioration in the patient's condition:

(Continued)

Table 3.2 (Continued)

Risk assessment	Nursing interventions
	• assess patient and check the equipment; • consider either increasing the oxygen or pressures as prescribed; • consider a change to mechanical ventilation in line with the nurse's scope of practice.
Haemodynamic state	The increase in pulmonary airway pressure from NIV can cause a rebound reduction in the patient's blood pressure, particularly with CPAP pressures above 10 cm H_2O. Monitor the patient's blood pressure every five minutes during the first 30 minutes and then at 30 minutes to hourly as the patient's blood pressure stabilises. Continuous arterial monitoring of blood pressure via an arterial catheter provides an effective way to monitor BP as well as obtaining arterial samples for blood gas analysis.
Fluid balance and gastrointestinal function	There is a risk of fluid retention triggered by the body's response to a reduction in BP (Chapter 6). Look for evidence of reduced urine output and interstitial oedema. There is a risk of increased air swallowing and gastric distension associated with the air flow. This may be reduced by inserting a nasogastric tube and may be used to support nutrition and hydration.
Mental state and level of consciousness	Monitor for signs of increased confusion or agitation. Any deterioration in level of consciousness is an indication that the NIV should be discontinued, and the treatment plan reviewed. Patients on NIV should not normally be sedated as this can compromise their airway and compliance with treatment.
Psychological distress	Patients receiving NIV experience discomfort and distress due to the tight-fitting mask and side effects of the treatment. Communication is difficult with the face mask in place, although this may be resolved for some patients by using a nasal mask. Alternative techniques for delivering the air under pressure include a mouthpiece and a hood. The role of the nurse in providing support and reassurance is essential. Frequent removal of the mask is counterproductive, and it is important to encourage the patient to keep the mask in situ for at least 30 minutes if any benefit is to be achieved. This can involve the use of a pressure relief to the bridge of the nose. If a patient is becoming very distressed, this will impact on their physiological state and is often an indication to discontinue the NIV and refer to the treatment plan (Jarvis, 2006).
Skill mix	Optimum management of patients with acute respiratory failure and NIV is achieved in ICU. However, patients can be nursed in acute respiratory wards and accident and emergency provided there is an appropriate skill mix and staff ratios of 1 or 2 patients to 1 nurse.

Table 3.2 Risk assessment and management of patients receiving NIV

Returning to Jenny's story, we find that she has consented to the use of NIV and commenced the support at a low level of positive pressure (5 cm) and this was gradually increased to 10 cm with support and encouragement from the nursing staff. There seemed to be an initial improvement with an increase in SpO_2 (94%).

Case study: Jenny's condition changes

Two hours after commencing the NIV, Jenny's condition rapidly deteriorated as illustrated in the following ABCDE assessment.

A: Difficult to rouse but still able to maintain her airway.

B: SpO_2 91% on O_2

60% high-flow humidified O_2

R: 39/min, with shallow respirations

Blood gases showed:

pH: 7.20

PaO_2: 7.9 kPa

$PaCO_2$: 7.8 kPa

HCO_3: 24 mmol/L

C: HR: 128/min

BP: 110/72 mmHg

D: Blood glucose: 6.7 mmol/L

Glasgow Coma Score (GCS) had dropped to 9 (eyes opening to pain 2, inappropriate words 3, and normal flexion to pain 4).

E: Temp: 37.5 °C

ABG analysis

- Jenny has persistent hypoxaemia.
- Her pH indicates acidosis.
- The high CO_2 indicates a respiratory acidosis.
- No sign of a metabolic acidosis.

Jenny's worsening clinical condition, including a high respiratory rate, reduction in her level of consciousness, and increasing heart rate, combined with hypoxia and respiratory acidosis, indicates severe type II respiratory failure. Immediate intervention with intubation and mechanical ventilation is now required.

On reflection, the critical care intensivist recognised that although he identified some clinical grounds for the use of NIV, in Jenny's case, any improvement was limited, and her condition had now become life threatening (see Table 3.3).

Reason for IMV	Look: Listen: Feel: Measure	Patient examples
Hypoxaemic respiratory failure, for example: • pneumonia; • lung consolidation; • atelectasis; • pulmonary oedema; • acute respiratory distress syndrome (ARDS); • **pulmonary embolism;** • **carbon monoxide poisoning**.	• Central cyanosis • Altered respiratory pattern • Agitation/irritability • Confusion • Exhaustion • Seizures • SpO_2 <90% • PaO_2 <8.0 kPa	Chao Chan is diagnosed with pneumonia and type I respiratory failure. His PaO_2 is 6.2 kPa and his $PaCO_2$ is 3.6 kPa. He was commenced on CPAP at 5 cm H_2O then 10 cm H_2O. However, after the first hour he was confused and agitated, pulling off his mask and refusing to put it back on. His ABGs were PaO_2 5.7 kPa and $PaCO_2$ 5.0 kPa. It was agreed that treatment should be escalated to IMV.
Hypercapnic respiratory failure, for example: • COPD; • asthma; • airway obstruction/anatomical; • deformity; • cervical injury above level c4 and/or damage to the brain stem; • excessive sedation; • Guillain-Barré syndrome; • cardiac arrest; • heart failure; • pulmonary embolism.	• Increased work of breathing • Use of accessory muscles • Shallow breathing • Dyspnoea • Agitation/irritability • Confusion • Exhaustion • Seizures • Cardiovascular collapse and cardiac arrest • $PaCO_2$ >6.0 kPa	Mariana Banica (27 years) has a severe scoliosis of her spine (the spine is curved from side to side in an S shape). Since childhood she has been prone to respiratory infections due to reduced and uneven lung capacity. Mariana was admitted to ICU after having collapsed at home following a flu-like illness for three days. On admission she was very confused, cyanosed and her breathing was shallow. Her ABGs were pH: 7.19; PaO_2: 12.7 kPa; $PaCO_2$: 10.7 kPa; HCO_3: 24.0 mmol/L. Mariana was intubated and commenced on Bilevel Positive Pressure ventilation at a rate of 15/min, with an IPAP of 20 cm H_2O and EPAP of 5 cm H_2O.
Impaired consciousness and/or the patient's inability to protect his/her airway. Glasgow Coma Scale (GCS) score of <8 indicates the potential for further deterioration in consciousness, reduced ventilation, and poor airway protection, for example: • severe brain injury; • prolonged effects of general anaesthetic; • traumatic injury of the face and neck.	• Inability to maintain airway. • Unconscious. • GCS <8.	Pete Williams (19 years) was assaulted on his way home from the pub. A witness said that Pete had been kicked repeatedly on the head while he lay on the floor. In ICU he was agitated and unable to communicate except with grunts. He was opening his eyes and flexing his arms to pain, GCS 7. The computerised tomography (CT) scan showed evidence of progressive brain swelling. The management plan for Pete in the first 24 hours was to intubate him with an oral endotracheal tube and provide continuous positive pressure ventilation (IPAP 30 cm H_2O) with a rate of 15/min in order to protect his airway and maintain PaO_2 >8.0 kPa and $PaCO_2$ 4.5–6.0 kPa. Pete developed ventilator-acquired pneumonia on day four and stayed on IMV for seven days.

Table 3.3 Indications for mechanical invasive ventilation in the critically ill patient

What happens when NIV is not suitable? The case for IMV

The benefits of supporting patients in respiratory failure with NIV include the following (BTS/ICS 2016):

- There is reduced risk of ventilator-acquired pneumonia.
- The patient is fully awake and an active partner in their care.
- The use of NIV may prevent the requirement for invasive respiratory support.

There are, however, several reasons why patients may require an escalation of treatment to IMV or direct intervention with IMV without NIV (Bersten, 2019). These include:

- life-threatening hypoxic (PaO_2 below 8.0 kPa) respiratory failure accompanied by patient confusion and/or exhaustion;
- life-threatening hypercarbic ($PaCO_2$ above 6.0 kPa) respiratory failure accompanied by patient confusion and/or exhaustion;
- impaired consciousness and/or the patient's inability to protect their airway.

For patients in these situations, clinical assessment, combined with medical and nursing experience, will determine when invasive support with intubation and mechanical ventilation is required. Based on Jenny's assessment following her deterioration, she met all the three criteria above for intubation and mechanical ventilation. Jenny's sudden deterioration may have been related to the combined effects of physical exhaustion and the latent release of inflammatory mediators triggered by the initial inflammatory response several hours before. This can lead to further bronchospasm, oedema, mucus secretion and obstruction of air flow, an increase in variable and uneven airway obstruction, and air trapping in the alveoli (McCance and Huether, 2019). Jenny initially presented with hypoxaemia (low oxygen in the blood) which triggered an increase in respiratory rate. This, together with the combined effects of uncontrolled inflammation and airway obstruction, led to a reduction in her tidal volumes (the volume of air in each breath) and an increase in CO_2 retention. This led to a rise in $PaCO_2$, respiratory acidosis, and progressive hypoxaemia: type II respiratory failure.

Mechanical invasive ventilation in adults can only take place when a patient is intubated with a cuffed endotracheal or tracheostomy tube. The cuff provides a seal around the tube and prevents leaks. The purpose of IMV is to push air under pressure into the patient's lungs to ensure there is effective movement of oxygen and carbon dioxide in and out of the lungs (pulmonary ventilation). There are increasing numbers of types and modes of IMV, but for the purposes of this chapter we will limit discussion to two core modes: pressure-controlled ventilation and volume-controlled ventilation (Bersten, 2019). In Table 3.4 you will find an explanation of these modes together with the advantages and disadvantages of both.

IMV mode	Risks	Benefits
Pressure-controlled ventilation: air is pushed into the lungs until a preset alveolar pressure is reached. For example: • bilevel positive airways pressure (BiPAP) (see NIV); • continuous positive airways pressure (CPAP) (see NIV).	Ineffective ventilation. Hypo ventilation and variable tidal volumes triggered by reduced lung compliance in the presence of acute lung injury, sputum, and/or bronchospasm. Compliance measures the 'ease of stretch' ability in the lungs. The more compliant the lungs are, the less pressure is required to open the airways during IMV.	Reduces the risk of ventilator-associated lung injury.
Volume-controlled ventilation: a preset volume of air is delivered to the lungs with each breath. For example: • synchronised intermittent mandatory ventilation (SIMV), where the breaths are synchronised with the patient's own breathing; • controlled mechanical ventilation (CMV) where the patient requires higher levels of sedation for effective ventilation.	Ventilator-associated lung injury: • barotrauma: over-distension of some alveoli; • volutrauma: over-distension of the alveoli caused by large tidal volumes; • biotrauma: the release of inflammatory mediators that may increase patient mortality. Increased requirement for the use of sedation to support effective ventilation, which may delay the process of weaning from respiratory support.	The machine delivers a set tidal volume with each breath, thus improving overall ventilation.
Modes that deliver a combination of both. For example: • pressure-regulated volume-controlled ventilation.		Reduces the risk of ventilator-associated lung injury. Ensures effective tidal volumes and pulmonary ventilation.

Table 3.4 A comparison of pressure-controlled and volume-controlled ventilation modes

In both pressure-controlled and volume-controlled ventilation, the patient's respiratory rate can be managed in one of three ways.

- The patient breathes spontaneously and controls their own rate.
- The patient's respiratory rate is set and controlled by the machine.
- The patient's respiratory rate is supported by a minimum respiratory rate set by the machine and supplemented by the patient's own respiratory rate.

The option of as much or as little respiratory support through IMV allows the patients to be involved in the process of respiratory support and aids their readiness to wean from IMV as they improve (Nichol et al., 2016). Other clinical examples of situations when IMV is required are included in Table 3.3.

Case study: Jenny's intubation and ventilation with IMV

Jenny now required immediate intubation and mechanical ventilation and she was induced into anaesthesia with ketamine and alfentanil (short-acting anaesthetic agents) and paralysed with suxamethonium (a fast-acting muscle relaxant) to facilitate safe tracheal intubation with an oral endotracheal tube. Because of the combination of risks related to hyperinflation of the lungs, air trapping, and increased airways resistance caused by bronchospasm, inflammation, and mucus production, it was decided that the best clinical intervention for Jenny was controlled ventilation with SIMV (Table 3.4), with an inspired tidal volume set at 400 ml and a rate of 12 breaths per minute and a plateau airways pressure of less than 30 cm. The respiratory rate was set to give Jenny a short inspiration time and a prolonged expiratory time to reduce the risks of further air trapping and barotrauma (Tuxen and Hew, 2019). Alternative methods of respiratory support, such as pressure-controlled ventilation, were also considered. To achieve this type of controlled ventilation it was necessary, in Jenny's case, to provide a deep level of sedation and paralyse with neuromuscular blockade. This was achieved using propofol (a short-acting anaesthetic) and cisatracurium (a short-acting neuromuscular blocking agent). Jenny's airway resistance was reduced by suctioning of the airways to remove secretions. A chest X-ray was performed to check the position of the endotracheal tube and for pneumothorax in the context of Jenny's clinical deterioration.

Sedation: what is the evidence base?

The aim of using drugs to sedate patients during IMV is to promote comfort, relieve distress and anxiety, facilitate effective respiratory function, and reduce the risk of ventilator-associated injury. The Intensive Care Society have maintained that most drugs used for this purpose can cause side effects. These include depression of the cardiovascular system leading to reduced BP; respiratory depression and delayed weaning from respiratory support; reduced motility of the gastrointestinal tract with delayed absorption of nutrients and poor-quality sleep (Whitehouse et al., 2014). The use of sedation assessment scales and sedation protocols has been recommended as a method for getting the balance right between the advantages and disadvantages of using sedation. The Ramsay scale, Riker Sedation Agitation scale, and Richmond Agitation and Sedation scale are examples of tools adapted for patients on IMV (Ramsay et al., 1974; Riker et al., 2001; Ely et al., 2003). There is limited evidence that such scales and protocols can improve patient outcomes, however some studies do identify that patients are achieving a more clinically effective sedation level together with reduced opioid and **benzodiazepine** use (Whitehouse et al., 2014; Kaplan et al., 2019). Some studies have tested the consistency between the various tools as well as interrater reliability and conclude that the tools have a high level of consistency and reliability (Stasevic Karlicic et al., 2016; Namigar et al., 2017). There is evidence, however, that daily sedation interruption combined with patient assessment can improve patient outcome (Chen et al., 2014) and daily sedation interruption has become an essential element of an internationally recognised ventilator bundle (see Concept summary: care bundles below) (Hellyer et al., 2016). There is also evidence that healthcare staff do not always follow sedation recommendations due to lack of awareness, lack of conceptual agreement with the guidance, poor strength of evidence in their use, and lack of clarity over who is responsible for prescribing the guidance (Sneyers et al., 2014; Miller et al., 2012). In a qualitative study of eight ICUs in Scotland, the authors found that there are several complex factors that influence both nursing and medical sedation practices, including complex clinical decision making and organisational factors (Kydonaki et al., 2019). In summary, the use of sedation protocols and daily sedation interruption, while seen to be clinically effective, continue to be areas that require further research and should always be used in the context of the patient's clinical condition and as part of the ventilator bundle to reduce the risk of ventilator-acquired pneumonia (see Table 3.5).

Risk assessment	Nursing interventions

Airway
 	
 • Risk of the endotracheal tube/tracheostomy (tube) occluding due to poor humidification, the patient biting down on the tube and/or secretions.
 	
 • Risk of airway irritation.
 	
 • Risk of the tube becoming dislodged.
 	
 • Risk of unplanned extubation.
 	
 Breathing
 	
 • Risk of airways becoming partially occluded leading to a rise in airway pressure and ineffective ventilation.
 	
 • Risk of air leak due to poor connections.
 	
 • Risk of inappropriately set alarm parameters.
 	
 • Risk of ventilator-associated lung injury and ventilator-associated pneumonia (VAP).
	• Look for evidence of distress and agitation such as coughing and biting on the tube, assess the patient's sedation score and reassure. If the patient continues to be distressed, there is a higher risk of unplanned extubation and/or trauma to the patient's airways. If necessary, increase the sedation according to the prescribed guideline until the patient is comfortable.
	
	 • Humidification of the airways can be achieved by:
	    o heat/moisture exchange (HME) filters that are attached to the ventilator circuit close to the endotracheal tube;
	    o hot water humidifiers (37 °C);
	
	 • Narrowing or occlusion of the patient's airway can be identified by an increase in the inspired airway pressure and evidence of patient agitation, rattling/bubbling on chest auscultation.
	
	 • Endotracheal suction is used to remove secretions in the trachea but should only be performed when there is evidence of the above. Endotracheal suction can be either open suctioning (where the circuit is broken to enable a suction catheter to be inserted) or closed-circuit suctioning (where the suction catheter is integrated into the ventilator circuit). Suction can be painful, distressing, and can increase the risk of infection and trauma to the airways.

Risk assessment	Nursing interventions
	• A loose connection can be identified by a reduction in inspired airway pressure, expired tidal volume, and reduction in SpO_2.
	• Assess respirations, inspired and expired tidal volumes and airway pressure, SpO_2, and ABG analysis if the patient's condition changes.
	• Set alarm limits on the ventilator to between 5 and 10 marks above and below the prescribed range and assess the patient hourly.
	• Adhere to the ventilator bundle (see Concept summary: care bundles).
Circulation • Risk of impaired circulation and cardiac function: IMV increases central venous pressure (CVP) because the right side of the heart has to pump against a higher alveolar pressure. Left ventricular cardiac output is reduced due to more blood staying in the venous circulation. Thus, the patient is at risk of hypotension and oedema. • Risk of liver dysfunction leading to clotting disorders, immunosuppression, and reduced albumin production. *Disability* • Inability to communicate verbally due to the endotracheal tube and sedation. • Risk of pain. • Risk of anxiety, delirium, and/or boredom.	• Assess the patient's vital signs for evidence of impaired circulation using continuous monitoring: heart rate and rhythm; BP; CVP; chest X-ray; signs of venous thrombosis; urine output, which should be ≥0.5 ml/kg/hr (> about 30 ml/hr). • Adhere to the ventilator bundle to reduce the risk of VAP. • Assess the patient for signs of peripheral oedema, bruising. • Assess blood results at least daily, including serum electrolytes; urea and creatinine; liver function tests; clotting. • Assess and screen for sepsis daily (Chapter 7). • When appropriate, encourage the patient to use non-verbal means of communication, such as picture cards and alphabet cards. Use eye contact and explain all procedures before they are attempted. • Assess the patient's pain using non-verbal cues and pain scores and manage appropriately with the aid of pharmacological and non-pharmacological methods. • Help the patient to be orientated to night and day and assess for signs of delirium (Chapter 8). • Encourage family-centred care and patient-focused care. • Encourage the patient to be involved in decisions and, where possible, life outside the unit. • Monitor and maintain nutrition and hydration.

(Continued)

Table 3.5 (Continued)

Risk assessment	Nursing interventions
Exposure and safe environment • Risk of poor skin integrity, dry eyes and mouth. • Risk of infection associated with the use of invasive procedures. • Risk of noise and the environment disturbing sleep and rest.	• Assess the integrity of the patient's eyes and mouth hourly and manage appropriately according to each patient's needs (RCO and ICS, 2017). • Manage pressure ulcer prevention: risk assess on admission; reassess daily: inspect skin, manage moisture on the skin, optimise nutrition and hydration, minimise pressure through positioning (Institute for Healthcare Improvement (IHI), 2009; NICE, 2014c). • Risk assess and manage the patient with due regard to the ventilator bundle and risk assessment for sepsis (IHI, 2012; NICE, 2017a). • Assess noise levels and reduce noise pollution where possible. Reorientate the patient to their environment and offer reassurance when appropriate.

Table 3.5 Risk assessment and plan of care for a ventilated patient

Why are tidal volume, respiratory rate, and airway pressure important in promoting optimum ventilation?

The tidal volume (TV) is the volume of air in each breath and can be measured as inspired (iVt) and expired (eVt) tidal volume. The respiratory rate (R) describes the total number of respirations in a minute. If a patient is on IMV this may include set ventilator breaths and the patient's own breaths. Minute volume is the total volume of air either inspired (iVm) or expired (eVm) in one minute and is equal to TV times respiratory rate (Hall, 2016). Airway pressure is the same as alveolar pressure and is the pressure required to push air into the patient's lungs during inspiration.

When assessing and monitoring a patient receiving IMV, TV, rate, minute volume, and airway pressure are some of the important indicators for measuring effective ventilation. For example, increasing iVt, R, or iVm can improve the elimination of CO_2. If, however, by doing this the inspired airway pressure (peak pressure) goes above 30–35 cm H_2O, then the patient becomes at risk of acute lung injury. It is equally important to monitor plateau pressure (airway pressure achieved when inspiration is complete) to monitor lung compliance (degree of elastic recoil of the lung). Patients such as Jenny often have high airway resistance due to narrow and inflamed bronchi, and it becomes harder to push air into the lungs. In this situation it is important to reduce the risks of barotrauma (ruptured alveoli) and pneumothorax caused by high inflation pressures.

This is achieved by balancing the controlled respiratory rate and iVt to ensure inspired peak airway pressure does not exceed 30 cm H_2O. The intensivist can utilise pressure-controlled ventilation as an alternative to volume-controlled ventilation in this case. Promoting effective patient ventilation, therefore, requires assessment, monitoring, communication, and collaboration with the patient, nurse, intensivist, and physiotherapist to promote optimum lung function, and with the dietitian to promote optimum nutrition to support the patient's metabolic requirements and promote recovery (Woodrow, 2019). A summary of the risk assessment and management of patients such as Jenny is illustrated in Table 3.5.

Concept summary: care bundles

Evidence-based practice is concerned with ensuring that the best available evidence is applied to practice. One method for achieving this is using care bundles. A care bundle is a group of evidence-based interventions that, when combined, provide the most clinically effective method for reducing risk and improving patient outcome (Horner and Bellamy, 2012). The ventilator care bundle is an example of how combining selective interventions appears to have reduced the incidence of ventilator-acquired pneumonia (Lawrence and Fullbrook, 2011; Eom et al., 2014) and has been recommended by IHI (2012) as an effective group of interventions to reduce the risk of ventilator-acquired pneumonia.

The current IHI (2012) ventilator bundle identifies five components:

1. *Elevation of the head of the bed to 30–45%* to prevent aspiration of gastric contents.
2. *Daily interruption of the patient's sedation and daily assessment of the patient's readiness for extubation.* This intervention aims to reduce the accumulation load of sedatives during mechanical ventilation and encourages readiness to wean the patient from ventilation.
3. *Peptic ulcer disease prophylaxis* when clinically relevant to balance the risk of a gastrointestinal bleed against an increased risk of aspiration pneumonia when the pH of the stomach is elevated.
4. *Venous thromboembolism prophylaxis* to reduce the risk of venous thromboembolism.
5. *Daily oral care with chlorhexidine* to promote good oral hygiene.

It should be noted however that the Intensive Care Society recommends that the evidence base for the ventilator bundle should be reviewed regarding the use of chlorhexidine for oral decontamination and gastrointestinal stress ulcer prophylaxis (Hellyer et al., 2016).

In Jenny's story, she continued to be ventilated, sedated, and paralysed for a further 12 hours until her clinical condition improved, allowing the neuromuscular blocking agent to be discontinued, followed by a gradual reduction in sedation. We join Jenny as her sedation was stopped.

Case study: Jenny's ventilation with IMV

Jenny's sedation was ceased, and she was assessed:

A: Airway maintained through an oral endotracheal tube.

   Drowsy, responds to normal verbal stimuli

B: SpO_2: 95%

   O_2 60%

   Ventilation mode: SIMV

   iTV: 400 ml, eTV 400 ml

   Controlled R: 16/min

Blood gases showed:

   pH: 7.34

   PaO_2: 11 kPa

   $PaCO_2$: 6.0 kPa

   HCO_3: 24 mmol/L

C: HR: 120/min

   BP: 110/70 mmHg

D: Blood glucose: 6.7 mmol/L

   Sedated with reducing levels of propofol according to protocol, drowsy, responds to normal verbal stimuli: Ramsay scale 3

E: Temp: 37.5 °C

ABG analysis

- Jenny's oxygen levels have improved and are now within the accepted safe range.
- She is slightly acidotic but considerably improved from her results prior to IMV.
- The high CO_2 indicates the upper limit of normal.
- No sign of a metabolic acidosis.
- Jenny no longer has hypoxia or hypercapnia.

Her clinical condition has improved, and she no longer has evidence of respiratory failure. The recommendation is to continue to reduce her sedation and encourage her to trigger her own breaths while reducing the preset ventilator rate. Once she is breathing without the help of the IMV the plan is to extubate her and monitor her condition.

Chapter summary

In this chapter you have been introduced to patients who need advanced respiratory support. The technology and assessment strategies for patients in these situations are often complex and the patient's condition can change suddenly. We have seen how Jenny's condition initially deteriorated, but continuous assessment of her condition alerted staff to changes in her condition and she received intensive care. Within 24 hours Jenny's condition had improved sufficiently for her to be transferred to level 2 care and then a general ward. She was discharged from hospital five days later. Jenny agreed to separate from her husband and a year later has managed to give up smoking and make a new life for herself. She can still remember her time in the intensive care unit and is determined to improve how she manages her asthma to reduce the risk of another admission with the support of the respiratory nurse specialists, physiotherapy, her GP, and her family.

The important messages to gain from this chapter are as follows.

- Always begin by assessing the patient's airway, breathing and circulation, disability, and environment, and you will always be able to prioritise care and communicate your concerns using SBAR.
- Interpretation of the patient's condition through blood gas analysis means much more if the results are assessed in the context of the patient's whole situation.

Activities: brief outline answers

Activity 3.1: Decision making (page 79)

Using the step-by-step guide in Table 2.5, what can you interpret from the ABG result?

These are the first set of ABG results.

- Joseph was showing signs of hypoxaemia on 60% oxygen.
- pH 7.07: shows evidence of acidosis.
- $PaCO_2$ 14.1 kPa: shows evidence of respiratory acidosis.
- HCO_3 20.5 mmol/L: shows evidence of metabolic acidosis also.
- Joseph shows signs of both a respiratory and metabolic acidosis.
- This result in the context of his clinical situation is consistent with a period of inadequate oxygenation and tissue perfusion related to his cardiac arrest. Re-establishment and maintenance of Joseph's respiration and circulation will provide an opportunity for acid-base balance to be restored.

Using the step-by-step guide in Table 2.5, what can you interpret from Joseph's second ABG result?

- Joseph's oxygen levels had improved; however his PaO_2 and SpO_2 are still below the accepted levels.
- His pH of 7.20 is still showing signs of acidaemia.
- $PaCO_2$ 6.70 kPa: still shows evidence of respiratory acidosis but has improved from his previous results.

- HCO$_3$ 22.5 mmol/L: shows evidence of a resolving metabolic acidosis compared to the previous result.
- Joseph still shows signs of both a respiratory and metabolic acidosis; however, this is not as severe as his post cardiac arrest results.
- Joseph's ABGs still indicate evidence of type II respiratory failure, which has now been complicated by a diagnosis of a STEMI.

What are your priorities of care for this patient?

- Joseph needs to receive support for his respiratory failure and should be assessed to determine the most suitable treatment plan. This may be a combination of nebulised short-acting **beta agonist**, short-acting **muscarinic antagonist**, and intravenous antibiotics. He should be encouraged to sit up in the most comfortable breathing position and be assessed for NIV. Following an assessment from the CCOT, Joseph was transferred to ICU for NIV and was commenced on bilevel positive airways pressure.
- Your role is to risk assess the patient and reassure him and, if he is commenced on NIV, to support him to promote his comfort.
- Joseph will require continuous assessment of his respiratory and cardiac function with a view to reducing the NIV support over the next few hours if his condition continues to improve.
- He will need continued support and reassurance to maximise the effect of the respiratory support, and his cardiovascular status should be monitored to assess for signs of deterioration following his cardiac event.

Further reading

Adam, S, Osborne, S and Welch, J (2017) *Critical Care Nursing Science and Practice.* Third edition. Oxford: Oxford University Press.

This book offers more detail about working in a critical care environment.

Moore, T and Woodrow, P (2009) *High Dependency Nursing Care: Observation, Intervention and Support for Level 2 Patients.* Second edition. London: Routledge.

This book offers practical help with learning how to use the technology when involved in the care of level 2 patients.

Useful websites

www.ics.ac.uk/ICS/GuidelinesStandards/ICS/GuidelinesAndStandards/
StandardsAndGuidelines.aspx?hkey=4ed20a1c-1ff8-46e0-b48e-732f1f4a90e2

The Intensive Care Society site provides access to relevant innovations and standards that relate to the care of patients who are critically ill. The website is multidisciplinary and offers information to patients and relatives in user-friendly guides. A revised edition of sedation guidance is now available on this website.

www.hqinstitute.org/post/icu-sedation-guidelines-care

The documents accessed here give you a helpful introduction to some of the drugs used to promote safety and pain relief for patients receiving mechanical ventilation. It also gives you examples of some of the assessment tools available for monitoring pain and sedation for both adults and children.

www.ihi.org

The Institute for Healthcare Improvement website offers evidence-based and practical ways in which to provide safe and effective care for patients with acute and critical care needs. Registration is free.

Chapter 4

The patient with chest pain

Thomas C. Barton, David Barton and Desiree Tait

NMC Future Nurse: Standards of Proficiency for Registered Nurses

This chapter will address the following platforms and proficiencies:

Platform 3: Assessing needs and planning care

Registered nurses prioritise the needs of people when assessing and reviewing their mental, physical, cognitive, behavioural, social and spiritual needs. They use information obtained during assessments to identify the priorities and requirements for person-centred and evidence-based nursing interventions and support. They work in partnership with people to develop person-centred care plans that take into account their circumstances, characteristics and preferences.

At the point of registration, the registered nurse will be able to:

3.2   demonstrate and apply knowledge of body systems and homeostasis, human anatomy and physiology, biology, genomics, pharmacology and social and behavioural sciences when undertaking full and accurate person-centred nursing assessments and developing appropriate care plans.

3.3   demonstrate and apply knowledge of all commonly encountered mental, physical, behavioural and cognitive health conditions, medication usage and treatments when undertaking full and accurate assessments of nursing care needs and when developing, prioritising and reviewing person-centred care plans.

3.5   demonstrate the ability to accurately process all information gathered during the assessment process to identify needs for individualised nursing care and develop person-centred evidence-based plans for nursing interventions with agreed goals.

Annexe B: Nursing procedures

2.7   undertake a whole-body systems assessment including respiratory, circulatory, neurological, musculoskeletal, cardiovascular, and skin status

(Continued)

(Continued)

3.1 observe and assess comfort and pain levels and rest and sleep patterns

3.5 take appropriate action to reduce or minimise pain or discomfort

Chapter aims

By the end of this chapter, you should be able to:

- identify common causes of chest pain;
- identify and explain the different causes of chest pain;
- critically examine vital signs and understand other related investigations when assessing chest pain;
- identify and prioritise the most appropriate clinical nursing interventions for the management of chest pain;
- undertake a person-centred approach to assessing and managing a person experiencing chest pain.

Introduction

As a nurse, you will often work with patients who present with chest pain. Despite being a common symptom, it is also one of the most alarming for the patient and their family because most people associate chest pain with having a heart attack or a cardiac event. The heart is the most vital of organs: we can feel it beating and hear its activity, and we all know that if it stops, this will quickly lead to death. Not all chest pain is cardiac in origin and this chapter aims to introduce you to the common causes of chest pain including cardiovascular, musculoskeletal, gastric, or respiratory. This chapter also explores the crucial part that the nurse and multidisciplinary team play in assessing, prioritising, and managing interventions and care that enable recovery and rehabilitation, or palliative care.

We will examine four patient scenarios that are typical of chest pain presentations. While the scenarios are condition based, you can follow the logical prioritisation of nursing interventions that are vital in assessing and managing such presentations. To do this, you will need to develop and apply your knowledge of undertaking a person-centred nursing assessment informed by biopsychosocial aspects of the person, pathophysiology, and your ability to identify clinical signs, prioritise, plan, and evaluate care.

The nature of acute care is that often complete patient notes are not immediately available or patients themselves give incomplete or varying histories. As you work through each scenario you will note that we have not necessarily given comprehensive information on every aspect of the patient's needs, or all the information that may have been gleaned by the nursing assessments. We hope that you will pick up on these omissions, as there are activities where you will be able to reflect on this. It will be you (the nurse) who should be seeking out and identifying these 'wider' concerns that extend beyond the patient's immediate presenting symptoms. Each of the scenarios is divided into three sections:

- the person's situation and background;
- the ABCDE assessment and interpretation of findings;
- prioritisation of immediate and ongoing care.

Possible causes of chest pain

According to Mills et al. (2018), the most common causes of chest pain are:

- cardiovascular disease (ischaemic coronary artery disease, conduction and rhythm disorders, congenital disorder, dissecting aortic aneurism);
- respiratory disease (COPD, infection, asthma, cancer, pneumothorax, and pulmonary embolism);
- musculoskeletal disorder or injury (mechanical injury, trauma, arthritis, osteoporosis, and other congenital or degenerative diseases that affect the thoracic skeleton);
- gastrointestinal disease (gastritis, infection, herniation, pancreatitis, and gall bladder disease);
- psychological causation (emotional distress/disturbance, mental health disorder).

How do you assess and prioritise care for patients with chest pain?

A person experiencing chest pain has the potential to deteriorate rapidly and suddenly, particularly if the underlying cause is cardio-circulatory or respiratory. A rapid assessment of the patient experiencing chest pain, and the crucial information that arises from this, is vital in enabling the nurse to prioritise nursing interventions. Regardless of location a potentially deteriorating patient should be assessed using the ABCDE approach advocated by the Resuscitation Council UK (2015) and the findings communicated using the SBAR approach explained in Chapter 1 and illustrated in Table 1.10. It is important to remember that information may be gained from several sources: from the patient and their family and from other members of the care team such as doctors, nurses, healthcare assistants, and physiotherapists. What is crucial is that all this information is properly collated and acted on in an appropriate way by all members of that multidisciplinary team (MDT).

This assessment, illustrated in Table 4.1, will enable you to prioritise the most immediate acute presentation of chest pain. Significant interventions will almost always include ongoing monitoring of ABCDE, undertaking electrocardiographs (ECGs), administering prescribed medication, and preparing the patient for percutaneous coronary intervention (PCI) if diagnosed with acute coronary syndrome (ACS) (unstable angina, non-ST elevation myocardial infarction (NSTEMI), or ST elevation myocardial infarction (STEMI), has been diagnosed).

ABCDE	Factors to assess and prioritise for a person with chest pain	Interpretation and decision making
Airway	Is the person able to respond and are they breathing? Is there evidence of airway obstruction, accompanied by stridor or wheezing on expiration?	If the answer is no: pull the emergency buzzer and phone 2222. The person is needing immediate resuscitation. Evidence of partial airway obstruction may be associated with inflammation or infection of the upper airways, asthma, or an acute exacerbation of COPD. Identify the patient as having risks to the airway and alert the medical team using SBAR and NEWS2 criteria identified in Chapter 1.
Breathing	Is the patient breathless? Is there evidence of increased work of breathing, including use of accessory muscles? Is there thoracic pain associated with deep breaths or a cough? What is the pattern, rate, and depth of respiration? What is the SpO$_2$?	A combination of chest pain associated with breathlessness may indicate the following: • Sudden onset of sharp pleuritic pain suggests pulmonary embolus and you need to check for evidence of haemoptysis and a swollen, inflamed leg (deep vein thrombosis). Assess the need for oxygen according to BTS (O'Driscoll et al., 2017) guidance. • Sudden crushing central chest pain and breathlessness is suggestive of myocardial infarction (MI) and pulmonary oedema, angina, aortic dissecting aneurysm. Assess the need for oxygen according to BTS (2017) guidance. • Progressive breathlessness associated with some chest pain may be associated with pneumonia. Assess the need for oxygen according to BTS (2017) guidance. • Chest pain associated with an altered pattern or depth of breathing may be associated with a thoracic musculoskeletal injury. • Thoracic pain on inspiration or during coughing, together with pyrexia, may be associated with either pericarditis (inflammation of the cardiac pericardium) or inflammation of the pleural layer of the thorax.

ABCDE	Factors to assess and prioritise for a person with chest pain	Interpretation and decision making

Circulation	Does the person with chest pain show signs of shock (pale, cold, mottled skin, capillary refill time >2 secs)? (See Chapter 6)
	
	Is there other evidence of reduced perfusion: systolic BP below 90 mmHg, tachycardia above 90/min, reduced urine out below 0.5 ml/kg/hr?
	
	Is there evidence of changes in cardiac rhythm or signs of ST elevation or depression?
	
	Is there evidence of weight gain, peripheral oedema?
	
	Is there evidence of nausea and/or vomiting?
		Chest pain associated with evidence of shock and or tachy- or brady-arrhythmias can be associated with:
		
		• MI and cardiogenic shock
		
		• trauma in the thoracic region such as a stab wound or rib fractures
		
		• pneumothorax
		
		• thoracic discitis (infection/abscess between thoracic discs)
		
		• sepsis secondary to lung infection – risk assess for sepsis
		
		• continuous cardiac monitoring for life-threatening arrhythmias such as:
		
		  o ventricular fibrillation
		
		  o ventricular tachycardia
		
		  o atrial tachycardia
		
		  o complete heart block
		
		  o severe bradycardia/asystole.
		
		• Evidence of peripheral oedema and weight gain is suggestive of progressive heart failure and/or acute kidney injury. Monitor fluid intake and output according to NICE CG174 (2017b).

Disability	Is there evidence of new confusion? Is there a deterioration in level of consciousness? What are the pain characteristics? Site, Onset, Character, Radiation, Associated features, Timing, Exacerbating/relieving factors, Severity (SOCRATES) Blood glucose?	Chest pain when associated with reduced perfusion and new confusion may be caused by cardiogenic shock, sepsis, or heart failure. Retrosternal pain can be caused by angina, MI, aortic aneurysm, pericarditis, oesophageal pain. Onset of pain is usually sudden for all the above causes. Character of cardiac pain is described as constricting and heavy. For a person experiencing an aortic aneurysm, the pain is described as tearing or ripping, tight and stabbing for pericarditis and gripping or burning for oesophageal pain. This is a surgical emergency. Cardiac pain is described as radiating to the arms, neck and sometimes the jaw. Aortic pain radiates through to the back, between the shoulders, pericardial pain can radiate to the left shoulder while oesophageal pain can radiate through to the back. Pain associated with angina is intermittent, lasting for up to 10 minutes and is triggered by stress, exercise, and the cold. It is relieved by rest or glyceryl trinitrate (GTN). MI pain is severe and is not relieved by rest or GTN and has a prolonged duration.

(Continued)

Table 4.1 (Continued)

ABCDE	Factors to assess and prioritise for a person with chest pain	Interpretation and decision making
		Pain from an aortic dissection is acute, severe, and prolonged. Oesophageal pain can be very similar to cardiac pain and is not usually relieved by rest or GTN.
		Blood glucose may be elevated as part of the stress response.
Exposure	Are there signs of physical trauma, blood loss or severe injury? Is there evidence of surgical emphysema (air or gas located in the subcutaneous tissue layer)?	Look for signs of possible causes of the chest pain caused by trauma such as injury to the thoracic cavity, localised bruising indicative of a previous injury. This may indicate severe asthma with evidence of leakage of air under pressure from the alveoli to interstitial tissues, or trauma from rib fractures.

Table 4.1 A summary of factors to assess and interpret chest pain, guided by Innes et al. (2018) and Zinchenko (2018)

When assessing the person's situation and background, the primary nursing assessment is always 'Look: Listen: Feel: Measure' as an integral part of the ABCDE assessment. Establishing the situation and the immediate priorities for assessment and management can give an early indication of possible cause as well as the potential for deterioration. You may receive this information from the patient and family, paramedics who initially assessed the patient, or as part of a ward handover. This information may include:

- a recent history of the problem causing concern;
- the timeline of events leading to the problem;
- related factors such as biological, medical, pharmacological, psychological, and social history.

For a person presenting with chest pain a summary of the person's pain experience can be structured using a model for rapid pain assessment such as the mnemonic SOCRATES (Gregory, 2019; Mills et al., 2018), which guides practitioners to ask the following questions:

- *Site:* Where is the site or focus of pain?
- *Onset:* What were they doing at the time of onset? Was it gradual or sudden and is the pain progressive or regressive?
- *Character:* What is the pain like? Is it sharp, aching, burning, crushing, or stabbing?
- *Radiation:* Does the pain radiate anywhere?
- *Associations:* Are there any other symptoms associated with the pain (i.e. nausea)?
- *Time course:* Does the pain follow any pattern?
- *Exacerbating/relieving factors:* Does anything change the pain?
- *Severity:* How bad is the pain?

When the situation has been established, a full ABCDE assessment should follow.

ABCDE assessment for a person with chest pain

A summary of the ABCDE assessment, together with normal and abnormal ranges, can be found in Chapter 1 and illustrated in Tables 1.3 to 1.9. Table 4.1 identifies key factors to assess and manage for people who present with chest pain.

The ABCDE assessment is *not* a one-off activity and the plan for further assessment will depend on the patient's condition, NEWS2 (RCP, 2017) guidance on escalation of care, and, in specialist clinical areas, the expert judgement of the medical and senior nursing staff.

Chest pain of acute onset of suspected cardiac origin

While there are many different causes of chest pain, many people readily associate chest pain, particularly if the pain is severe and sudden in onset, with a cardiac cause. There is a widespread fear of cardiac events being associated with a high mortality even though other causes of chest pain such as asthma, pneumothorax, or gastrointestinal bleeding can also be potentially deadly. Crucially, however, these can often be entirely reversible or curable when assessed and managed in a timely manner; acute asthma can be reversed, pneumothorax and gastrointestinal bleeds can be resolved. Cardiac causes of chest pain can vary in clinical severity but in many cases can be alarming for the patient. Whether the cause is angina or myocardial infarction (MI), the key factor, as above, is to assess and manage the situation in a rapid and timely manner to improve patient outcome.

Conversely, from a healthcare professional's point of view, it is entirely appropriate to be concerned about cardiac causes of pain, not just because they can be fatal, but also because, if survived, there is a distinct possibility of later significant morbidity. Cardiac muscle cells (myocytes) can function within ischaemic (reduced blood flow and oxygen availability) conditions for approximately 20 minutes before cell death and tissue necrosis take place (Brashers, 2019). When a person has an MI, structural and functional change can occur. This includes myocardial stunning, a temporary loss of contractile function associated with ischaemic damage and an imbalance of energy-dependent electrolyte pumps which maintain the balance of calcium, sodium, and potassium, increasing the risk of heart failure, cardiac arrhythmias and reduced cardiac output (Brashers, 2019). Heart failure arising from myocardial muscle ischaemia and subsequent scarring of the myocardium can result in poor cardiac muscle function and/or cardiac remodelling, leaving the heart vulnerable to decompensation. Myocardial remodelling, initiated as part of the inflammatory response to ischaemia and cell damage, causes an increased growth in myocardial cells (myocytes) and myocardial scarring. The damaged and scarred myocardium loses contractile function, and these factors can lead to a poor ejection fraction (the percentage of blood expelled from a ventricle during systole). This may be compounded further if the papillary muscles are affected by the myocardial ischaemia. This can cause dysfunction of the tricuspid and/or mitral valves (depending on the site of the ischaemia).

Pathophysiological changes that occur with heart failure are complex and occur as the body tries to compensate for the reduction in cardiac output (systolic dysfunction) and/or decreased filling capacity of the ventricles (diastolic dysfunction). A summary of these changes can be seen in Table 4.2. Failure to initiate appropriate treatments, or failure of treatments to fully resolve cardiac ischaemic events, is likely to result in ischaemic heart disease. Resolution can be achieved by rapid restoration of coronary blood flow and the use of ACE inhibitors to reduce ventricular remodelling and the use of beta blockers and statins to stabilise myocardial function (Brashers, 2019; NICE, 2020a). Early rehabilitation and secondary prevention should occur following ACS to maximise the potential for recovery and reduce the risk of further ischaemic events (NICE, 2020a).

Pathophysiological changes	Compensatory physiologic actions	Findings on clinical assessment
Haemodynamic changes • Decreased cardiac output/stroke volume (systolic dysfunction) • Decreased filling (diastolic dysfunction) caused by decreased relaxation of cardiac muscle, reduced elastic recoil, increased ventricular stiffness)	Reduction on stroke volume triggers: • Increased venous return to the heart (preload) and a subsequent increase in the force of contraction (increased ventricular volume results in enhanced contraction – Frank-Starling Relationship). This will be impaired in the presence of diastolic dysfunction. • Increased release of catecholamines (dopamine, norepinephrine (noradrenaline), and epinephrine (adrenaline)) to improve rate and force of contraction and peripheral vascular resistance (afterload). • Ventricular hypertrophy and an increase in ventricular volume. These mechanisms can maintain cardiac output temporarily but without urgent diagnosis and management of the cause, the heart will fail.	• > respiratory rate • > heart rate • Temporary > BP • > peripheral vascular resistance, PVR (peripheral shutdown)

Neuro-hormonal changes
 	
• Activation of the sympathetic nervous system (SNS)
 	
• Activation of the renin-angiotensin-aldosterone system and vasopressin release (RAAS)
	• Initially the activation of the SNS and RAAS will provide a compensatory response that will maintain perfusion of blood to the vital organs.
	
	• However, the increased preload and afterload that occur increases the workload of the heart leading to increased risk of further damage and release of inflammatory mediators, leading to myocyte hypertrophy and controlled cell death.
		• Initial compensatory changes will continue to promote:
		  o > respiratory rate
		  o > heart rate
		  o > BP
		  o > PVR
		• Reduced glomerular filtration rate and < urine output

Pathophysiological changes	Compensatory physiologic actions	Findings on clinical assessment

Cytokine release (interleukins and tumour necrosis factor)		• However, a vicious circle of hyperactivity of RAAS will cause further cardiac pump failure and lead to:
		
		  ○ < cardiac output
		  ○ < BP
		  ○ < urine output
		  ○ > PVR

Cellular changes: • Inefficient use of calcium ions (Ca^{2+}) and the force of myocyte contraction • Adrenergic desensitisation • Muscle (myocyte) hypertrophy • Programmed cell death • Fibrosis	• Ca^{2+} is necessary for efficient cardiac contraction. Loss of Ca^{2+} function leads to reduced rate and force of contraction. • Heart muscle becomes less responsive to increased levels of catecholamines. • Myocyte hypertrophy leads to increased demand for oxygen due to increased workload, cell damage leads to controlled cell death and increase in interstitial fibrosis and ventricular stiffness.	• < cardiac output • < BP • < urine output • Fluid overload leading to either pulmonary oedema with left-sided heart failure, peripheral oedema with right-sided failure, or both in progressive heart failure • Progressive heart failure and mortality

Table 4.2 A summary of the pathophysiological changes related to heart failure
Source: Hammer and McPhee, 2014.

With so much at stake, the importance of early recognition, diagnosis, and treatment for patients with chest pain that may be cardiac in origin cannot be overestimated. NICE (2020a) has produced guidance on treating ischaemic heart conditions. While the guidance is extensive and cannot be reproduced in this chapter, the following crucial points are highlighted.

- Chest pain recognised as angina should be differentiated as either stable or unstable angina. Factors to consider include whether the pain is brought on by exercise and relieved by rest (stable) or if pain develops at rest (unstable). If the pain is stable, the patient should be treated for stable angina as advised by the NICE pathway for stable angina (NICE, 2020a). If the pain is unstable, it is an ACS (NICE, 2020a) and requires further investigation and treatment urgently.
- If the onset of pain was within the last 12 hours, the person still has pain, and their ECG is abnormal or unavailable, emergency admission to hospital is needed following the treatment pathway (reperfusion therapy) identified (NICE, 2020a).
- If onset of the pain was between 12 and 72 hours ago and ACS is suspected, the patient requires urgent same-day referral for review in hospital.
- If onset of the pain was more than 72 hours ago and has completely resolved but there are signs of complications such as pulmonary oedema, medical management

is recommended and should follow the guidance offered by NICE (2020a). If there are no complications, ECG and blood troponin levels (troponin T is a cardiac enzyme released during damage to the myocardium; it can be used to assess for MI/ACS) should be tested and a cardiology assessment offered.

With ACS, 300 mg of aspirin should be given at the earliest opportunity if available, and so long as there is no clear evidence the patient is allergic to it. Written documentation should be sent with the patient that aspirin has been given. Oxygen saturations should be maintained between 94 and 98% (or 88–92% if the patient has a background of COPD at risk of hypercapnic respiratory failure) with supplementary oxygen if required (O'Driscoll et al., 2017). If a 12-lead ECG is available this should also be done at the earliest opportunity. Once an ECG is obtained and interpreted as an MI, there are essentially two possible conclusions: either an ST elevation myocardial infarction (STEMI) or a non-ST elevation myocardial infarction (NSTEMI).

The acronym MONA can be applied to support decision making regarding medications management for this client group, but this approach can be challenged based on current evidence (Alencar Neto, 2018) and a more comprehensive approach to pharmacological management is now recommended, as illustrated below:

- M: The assessment of pain and administration of morphine. While morphine continues to be the drug of choice for pain relief for cardiac pain, there is some evidence from clinical trials that morphine is associated with delayed activity of anti-platelet drugs in patients presenting with STEMI (Hobl et al., 2014).
- O: The assessment of requirement for oxygen maintained between 94 and 98% (or 88–92% for COPD) is critical to reduce the risk of further injury to the myocardium (Alencar Neto, 2018). The American Heart Association recommend the use of supplemental oxygen for NSTEMI and STEMI only when the saturation falls below 90% (Amsterdam et al., 2014).
- N: Assessment for the use of nitrates to reduce preload and afterload when symptoms indicate. There is a lack of sufficient evidence to argue that the standard use of nitrates, unless symptom specific, provides benefit (Alencar Neto, 2018).
- A: Assessment and management of anti-platelet medication and anticoagulants according to NICE NG185 (2020a) and dual anti-platelet therapy should be initiated and continue for up to 12 months.
- Other drugs found to improve patient outcome include:
  - Beta blockers prescribed within 24 hours of a cardiac event is associated with a lower incidence of re-infarction (Alencar Neto, 2018; NICE, 2020a).
  - ACE inhibitors should continue indefinitely to reduce morbidity and mortality (NICE, 2020a).
  - Statin therapy to reduce the risk of recurrent angina and MI (NICE, 2020a).

For patients experiencing a STEMI there is elevation of the **ST segment** of the patient's ECG. A blood test to assess the level of troponin will also be undertaken. A troponin test assesses the levels of either Troponin T or Troponin I proteins in the blood.

These proteins are released into the circulation when heart muscle becomes damaged and can be used as a biomedical marker for the diagnosis of MI (Sharma et al., 2004). In this situation, the next step depends on the time of onset of pain and the services available at the hospital or nearby hospitals. If the hospital has a cardiac angiography service, the preferred treatment is cardiac angiography with follow-on primary PCI to revascularise the ischaemic myocardium (NICE, 2020a). Angiography is a non-surgical technique using an inflatable balloon to widen the coronary arteries; a stent can then also be placed if required.

If a PCI cannot be offered then fibrinolysis using a thrombolytic, 'clot busting', drug can be prescribed as an alternative. Administering such a drug will render a patient completely incapable of making clots and, as a result, they will be at high risk of bleeding. Certain patients will not be eligible for this treatment due to other health problems (recent surgery, for example) and careful assessment of the risks versus benefit of administering the drugs must take place by the specialist healthcare team involved. Early assessment can be initiated by the paramedics or specialist cardiac nurses or the medical team, depending on the patient's circumstances. Certain drugs can only be given once, specifically streptokinase (BNF, 2021), so if the patient has had this before, it is accepted UK practice that they cannot have it again and they will be asked to carry a medical alert card indicating when the drug was administered. A thrombolised patient requires close monitoring in hospital and referral to a specialist cardiologist who may consider follow-up angiography and PCI.

In the absence of the more obvious ST segment elevation, diagnosis of MI is more difficult. ECG should be interpreted by an expert who will look for patterns that may indicate myocardial ischaemia. Blood tests such as troponin T may give an indication of the extent of myocardial damage. If the result is extremely high this, combined with any ECG findings, may lead to a diagnosis of NSTEMI. More subtle findings or results may result in a diagnosis of unstable angina. The management of both conditions is essentially the same (NICE, 2020a).

Initially these patients will all be treated with aspirin, with a loading dose of 300 mg if not given at an earlier point in their care. They will also be anticoagulated using a low molecular weight heparin such as fondaparinux if angiography is likely within 24 hours. Within the following six months, all patients should be risk assessed as part of a thorough clinical assessment, and will be judged as being at a certain level of risk of mortality and risk of adverse cardiac events from their myocardial ischaemia. Patients at lowest or low risk should be offered conservative management, have ischaemia testing and assessment of their left ventricular function by echocardiogram (ECHO). These patients can be discharged home if well prior to outpatient follow-up and possible coronary angiography. Patients with intermediate or higher risks require more urgent assessment and intervention. New generation cardiac computerised tomography (CT) scanners can offer more information on the extent of a patient's cardiac ischaemia and need for **revascularisation**, but ultimately angiography or CT assessment of ischaemia is indicated within 96 hours of admission so long as there are no contraindications such as bleeding. The results of these investigations will then allow the cardiologists to decide, with the patient, whether PCI or coronary artery bypass grafting (CABG) is the best option for the patient (NICE, 2020a).

Finally, NICE (2020a) guidance crucially advises that patients suffering from ACS/MI should have discharge and follow-up arrangements, a course of cardiac rehabilitation, management of risk factors and secondary prevention measures, i.e., high cholesterol, high blood pressure, aspirin, statins, and advice on lifestyle changes such as smoking cessation, diet, and exercise.

Cardiopulmonary arrest

With severe cardiac and respiratory causes of chest pain such as cardiac ischaemia or other conditions causing respiratory distress, there is always the possibility that a patient will become so unwell that their breathing or circulation fails to provide adequate oxygenation and perfusion to the body, and they collapse. Generally, such an event will lead swiftly to unconsciousness, and without immediate life-sustaining care and treatment of the underlying condition the patient will die. Nurses should receive at least emergency life support teaching as part of their ongoing mandatory training and some nurses may undertake intermediate or even advanced life support training depending on where they work. The Resuscitation Council provides up-to-date, evidence-based treatment algorithms of care for healthcare professionals to follow at their respective levels of training, which is too extensive to reproduce in this chapter. However, being a nurse involved in the care of a patient in cardiopulmonary arrest, be it in a community setting with no immediate clinical support or in a critical care unit, is an alarming and challenging experience both professionally and personally (emotionally). It is recommended that nurses follow the advice of the Resuscitation Council to debrief any cardiac arrests either as part of a team, with senior colleagues/line managers or even with your organisation's resuscitation officers. It is essential that nurses recognise the tremendous impact that these events can have on their own wellbeing and that they develop mechanisms of routine support and reflective practice, and access further support if required.

It is worth noting the messages of the Resuscitation Council regarding professionals' concerns about doing harm when undertaking cardiopulmonary resuscitation in circumstances where they are uncomfortable (such as in the community). A patient who you have established to be in cardiopulmonary arrest is not alive, you cannot make the situation worse and any help you can provide without putting yourself at risk can only offer help to that person (NMC, 2018c). Remember the mnemonic DRSABCD (St John Ambulance, 2021):

- **D** – Danger: always assess the situation around the patient for danger to you or other bystanders. Do not put yourself at risk.
- **R** – Response: is the person conscious? Call to them, shake their shoulder.
- **S** – Send for help: ensure there is help on its way, if you are alone, make this call yourself, otherwise you can delegate this to a bystander or colleague but be sure

that they return to confirm that help is coming. If you are in a community setting with no phone signal, you should leave the patient and return knowing help is coming rather than indefinitely performing CPR.

- **A** – Airway: check the patient's airway for soft or hard obstruction. Clear foreign bodies if able to do so as per ELS training. Use a head tilt, chin lift technique when assessing or maintaining the airway.
- **B** – Breathing: Assess if the patient is breathing. Use a head tilt, chin lift technique, place your cheek close to their mouth and watch the chest for signs of breathing for ten seconds. If you are trained to do so, you can also check the carotid pulse at the same time. If the person is breathing but unconscious, put the patient into a recovery position and monitor them until help arrives. In hospital settings, an oropharyngeal airway can be used to help maintain an airway and oxygen applied via a face mask until clinicians arrive.
- **C** – CPR: If a patient is unconscious and not breathing, ensure once again that help is coming and commence CPR as per the latest resuscitation guidelines and your life support training. Be sure to work with those around you to take turns in delivering CPR as it is a physically demanding activity, and you can become exhausted quickly. The quality of CPR deteriorates as people tire.
- **D** – Defibrillator: In a hospital setting, defibrillators are standard equipment in many healthcare facilities and as a nurse responding to a patient in cardiopulmonary arrest you should call 2222. Stay with the patient and ask a colleague to fetch the cardiac arrest trolley (containing the resuscitation equipment and defibrillator). In community settings, there are now increasing numbers of automated external defibrillators (AEDs) located in local communities. 999 operators can direct callers to an AED if they are near the incident.

Cardiac chest pain leading to acute heart failure and cardiogenic shock

In the scenario below you are introduced to Harry Smith, a 58-year-old retired manager. He is married and a grandfather. He was diagnosed with type 2 diabetes when he was 48 years old and takes metformin (see Chapter 12) twice a day. Harry also suffers from hypertension and **hyperlipidaemia** and has been prescribed an ACE inhibitor to reduce his blood pressure, statins to reduce his blood cholesterol, and aspirin to reduce the risk of clot formation. Harry began smoking when he was 15 years old and only gave up smoking 40 cigarettes a day when he was diagnosed with diabetes. He had given up completely by the age of 50. Harry is known to be at high risk of developing acute cardiovascular disease (NICE, 2020a). Harry generally does not enjoy physical exercise, but he does enjoy gardening, and on the morning of his admission he had decided to start the first grass cut of the spring. Halfway through the job he developed central chest pain and he rested until the pain subsided. Not willing to leave a job half done, Harry went back outside to finish the grass. Later that afternoon Harry's wife came home to find him collapsed in the chair with severe central crushing chest pain.

Case study: Harry Smith

Following an urgent admission by ambulance to A&E, Harry was immediately seen by A&E nurses and doctors and diagnosed with a primary MI due to occlusion of a coronary artery. The ECG revealed evidence of ST elevation indicating an antero-lateral MI and Harry's troponin levels were elevated above the accepted reference limit.

The A&E nurses quickly assessed Harry's condition on admission. They found the following.

- Respirations: 22 bpm.
- Pulse: 110 bpm, sinus tachycardia.
- BP: 110/80 mmHg.
- Temperature: 37.5 °C.
- SpO_2: 96%.
- He was pale and anxious.
- He had central chest pain and a 'heavy' left arm.

Activity 4.1   Critical thinking

Are these observations normal? What do you make of these observations?

An outline answer to this activity is given at the end of the chapter.

Reviewing Harry's condition

Harry was compensating for the loss of cardiac output by increasing his heart rate and respirations. A major nursing priority was to relieve his pain, which subsequently would alleviate ongoing stress on the heart. Pain assessment using a pain scale is a nursing priority. Harry was prescribed diamorphine to relieve the chest pain; this was administered by the nurses with measurable good effect. He was also prescribed aspirin to prevent further platelet aggregation and oxygen therapy to support an SpO_2 between 94/min and 98%. He was booked for immediate angiography and PCI within 90 minutes of admission to A&E (Karkabi et al., 2021; ICSI, 2009).

Monitoring fluid balance is a crucial nursing intervention in the patient with compromised cardiac function, and it was noted that Harry had not yet passed urine. Following a bladder scan to exclude urinary obstruction, the nurses inserted a urinary catheter, which drained 90 ml of urine. He had last passed urine while at home before the onset of his symptoms. Renal function is reliant on adequate perfusion of the kidneys (see Chapter 9). They are therefore sensitive to low blood pressure or poor perfusion resulting from compromised cardiac function, and monitoring urine output can give an indication of how well the patient's organs are being perfused. This is crucial information as the other major organ most sensitive to damage from poor perfusion is the brain. Identifying poor perfusion is the first and most important step in being able to enact interventions to protect the patient from further organ damage.

Remember

Always 'Look: Listen: Feel: Measure'.

Harry's ongoing management

Just prior to transfer for angiography, the A&E nurses reassessed Harry and found the following.

- SpO$_2$: 85%
- HR: 120/min
- BP: 83/55 mmHg
- His skin was cold and clammy.
- He had central cyanosis.
- He was nauseated.
- He was confused.

Activity 4.2 Critical thinking

Are these observations normal? What do you make of these observations?

An outline answer to this activity is given at the end of the chapter.

Harry was presenting with the clinical features of uncompensated and progressive **cardiogenic shock**. Cardiogenic shock or cardiac shock is a clinical state where the cardiac output (volume of blood ejected from the left ventricle) is reduced, leading to inadequate perfusion of blood to the tissues, triggering the shock response (Martin et al., 2019). This can also be described as pump failure.

The most common cause of cardiogenic shock is MI, when 40% of the heart muscle in the left ventricle has been damaged and the ventricle fails (Gowda et al., 2008). Other causes include severe contusion or bruising to the myocardium or a ventricular septal defect that reduces the efficiency of the left ventricular chamber as a pump. Cardiogenic shock can also occur in patients who develop septic shock, and this is discussed in Chapter 7.

Regardless of the cause, the onset of cardiogenic shock triggers a cycle of events that lead to a continuing decline in cardiac function. Patients who develop cardiogenic shock often present with dramatic and distinctive features including:

- having increased respiratory rate, tachycardia, and hypotension;
- being pale and cyanosed;
- feeling cold and clammy to touch;
- being confused and disorientated.

Treatment and care planning

It is a priority that the nurses caring for Harry continue with a full systematic regime of ongoing regular assessment from the outset. The rationale for this is that patients such as Harry may be admitted to A&E with clinical features already present, but in many cases the cardiogenic shock may develop between five to seven hours after the onset of chest pain and the initial MI (Babaev et al., 2005).

Harry's presentation and past medical history highlight several factors that increase the risk of patients developing cardiogenic shock.

- He has a history of diabetes.
- He has had a large anterior-lateral MI.
- He has an elevated troponin level.

The extent of ST elevation suggests that the damaged area involves both the front (anterior) and side (lateral) sections of his left ventricular myocardium and could involve 40% of his left ventricle.

Harry should remain in the resuscitation unit of A&E until they are ready to receive him in the cardiac catheter suite and/or operating department. He will need to be closely monitored every 15–30 minutes for a change in his condition. Following PCI or additional cardiac surgery, Harry will require support in the coronary care or cardiac intensive care unit. Here nurses will provide continuous highly specialist support.

Further treatments and care planning

For Harry, the large area of ischaemia and inflammation to his heart muscle (myocardium) in the left ventricle caused by the coronary occlusion has led to reduced blood pressure and cardiac output. This has happened because the reduction in blood flow and oxygen available to the heart has led to a reduction in the energy available to support cardiac contraction. Consequently, Harry has reduced perfusion of vital organs and tissues.

The physiological response to shock in Harry's case would involve the triggering of the flight/fight response, including nervous and hormonal responses. This includes stimulation of the sympathetic nervous system to increase heart rate and peripheral vasoconstriction and the release of epinephrine (adrenaline) and norepinephrine (noradrenaline). However, due to the damage to Harry's heart, his body is unable to compensate for the reduction in cardiac output, and despite an increase in heart and respiratory rate, his blood pressure is below the level required to achieve adequate tissue perfusion (see Table 4.2). With no intervention the progressive reduction in blood pressure will continue, leading to the progressive stages of shock, including a further reduction in cardiac output, metabolic acidosis, further myocardial depression, loss of consciousness, and reduced urine output.

The initial clinical priorities of care for patients in Harry's situation are the same as for ACS and that is to restore tissue perfusion to stabilise and facilitate recovery of the damaged myocardium. For Harry, restoring the circulation to the muscle damaged by the coronary occlusion will prevent the continual cycle of deterioration into cardiogenic shock.

Heart muscle will begin to die through the process of necrosis and form scar tissue in the absence of reperfusion therapy within 120 minutes (Greulich et al., 2019). The primary treatment for patients in cardiogenic shock, therefore, is PCI and restoration of blood flow. This has been demonstrated to improve the long-term survival rates of patients such as Harry when compared to medical stabilisation alone (Vahdatpour et al., 2019).

To safely transfer Harry to the operating department, medical stabilisation is first required. The nursing priorities for this will include:

- providing oxygen therapy to restore SpO_2 to 98%;
- instituting and monitoring of prescribed fluid resuscitation to improve vascular circulation;
- administration and monitoring of intravenous drugs to improve cardiac function (**inotropic therapy**) such as **dobutamine, dopamine** and milrinone (see Chapter 7).

If Harry's condition does not respond to PCI, or if he is unsuitable for reperfusion therapy with thrombolytic drugs (dissolving the blood clot) or coronary artery bypass surgery, medical support will be the most effective option (Vahdatpour et al., 2019). In this case Harry may need the support of NIV (see Chapter 3) and intra-aortic counterpulsation. The nursing management of such complex procedures will be undertaken within high dependency areas.

The provision of intra-aortic counterpulsation involves the insertion of a catheter into the aorta. The catheter has a balloon at the distal end and during cardiac diastole (ventricular relaxation) the balloon will inflate. This creates a back pressure during ventricular relaxation that will improve the blood supply to the coronary arteries that branch off the aorta above the catheter tip. During cardiac systole the balloon deflates and creates a reduction in peripheral resistance, thus reducing the workload of the left ventricle and improving cardiac output.

Harry was commenced on oxygen therapy and received fluid resuscitation. An intravenous anti-emetic was prescribed and administered by the nurses to relieve the nausea. He was transferred immediately to the cardiac catheter suite and underwent PCI with the insertion of two stents to the left anterior descending artery. A stent is a 'stainless' tube that, when inserted and guided into place with a cardiac catheter, expands and pushes against the inner (endothelial) layer of the coronary artery, expanding the diameter of the artery and improving blood flow to the ischaemic myocardium.

The key interventions responsible for Harry's recovery were:

- timely assessment and diagnosis;
- fast and efficient communication;
- the work of the paramedical staff that transferred him to A&E;
- efficient and thorough nursing and medical assessment in A&E, and early recognition and reporting of his deterioration to the cardiology team;
- cardiology intervention;
- critical care support – specialist nursing care.

Activity 4.3   Reflection

With appropriate intervention, Harry will be able to return home. What do you think are the main issues that the nurses should consider in enabling the 'journey' to recovery when Harry goes home?

An outline answer to this activity is given at the end of the chapter.

A person with a respiratory cause of chest pain

In Mr Adams's case study, we will explore a person's experience of chest pain related to a respiratory condition.

Case study: Mr Adams

Mr Adams, a 57-year-old man who has retired early, has attended his local GP surgery as he has become increasingly short of breath during a summer heatwave. His wife insisted that he go to see his GP. He tells the receptionist that he is feeling very unwell, that he has chest tightness and a generalised dull pain in his chest. He is asked to wait and told that a doctor will see him very soon. Shortly afterwards, following a spasmodic episode of coughing, he collapses in the waiting room. The receptionist reports to the attending practice nurse that Mr Adams became suddenly very short of breath and was wheezing and that he had attempted to use an inhaler prior to collapsing on his chair.

The practice nurse makes an immediate initial visual and verbal assessment of Mr Adams and finds him to be conscious but clearly in distress. He appears flushed and sweaty, is breathing noticeably quickly and has an audible wheeze. He can speak in short sentences only, but with assistance he can be helped to a wheelchair and moved to another room to be assessed. This immediate assessment informs appropriate interventions and the urgency of the presenting condition.

In a quiet room, Mr Adams manages to take his inhaler himself and appears to settle slightly. The practice nurse records his clinical observations – an important baseline – and they are as follows.

- Respiratory rate: 28 bpm (audible wheezing)
- SpO_2: 94%
- Pulse: 100 bpm (regular, bounding)
- Blood pressure: 140/78 mmHg
- Temperature: 37 °C.

Activity 4.4   Critical thinking

Are these observations normal? What do you make of these observations?

An outline answer to this activity is given at the end of the chapter.

The practice nurse undertakes a more detailed assessment of Mr Adams's recent health history – this is important in developing a more detailed picture of the patient. Mr Adams reports that he has chronic bronchitis, having previously been a heavy smoker, and that he has been short of breath and coughing more than normal for a couple of days. He feels the hot weather is making his shortness of breath worse and this in turn is making his chest very tight. He has had to use his inhalers more frequently over the past couple of days. He is also treated for hypertension and high cholesterol, and he is overweight. In recent years, his chronic bronchitis has become more severe and led to long periods off work before he retired. He is well known to the GP. Due to the collapse of Mr Adams, and his distressed state, the practice nurse makes the decision that he is an immediate priority and that he requires constant observation. She stays with him, monitoring his respiratory status and offering him reassurance.

One of the surgery's GPs arrives and takes a full medical history and performs an examination of Mr Adams. This reveals that, in addition to the practice nurse's observations, Mr Adams has also been coughing up green sputum for the past two days (it is normally a light creamy colour).

The details of the GP's examination and ABCDE assessment of Mr Adams are that:

- he is breathless at rest;
- he is using his accessory muscles to breathe;
- he has poor chest expansion;
- he is peripherally warm;
- he is peripherally cyanosed;
- when auscultated, he has quiet breath sounds with a wheeze throughout his lung fields. He also has some basal crackles, which are worse on the right.

Activity 4.5   Critical thinking

Given this information, at this point what do you think is causing Mr Adams's chest pain?

An outline answer to this activity is given at the end of the chapter.

Management of the presenting condition

The GP diagnoses Mr Adams with infective exacerbation of his chronic bronchitis. The immediate action necessary is urgent admission to hospital. Because of his collapse and the severity of his presentation, the GP wants Mr Adams to be admitted to hospital as a priority for initial investigation and treatment of acute exacerbation of chronic bronchitis.

Following admission to hospital, a first nursing priority is to ensure that he remains closely monitored given that he has collapsed because of his significant respiratory difficulties. The other clinical findings (green sputum) suggest he may have an infection, and his history suggests it is getting worse – he requires further and immediate investigations (Bridges and Dukes, 2005). The hospital nurses will need to ensure that the interventions listed below are quickly organised and undertaken so that appropriate therapeutic interventions can be commenced as soon as possible. The further investigations needed are:

- chest X-ray;
- sputum sample for culture and sensitivity;
- blood tests – FBC to identify evidence of a raised white cell count, haematocrit, and haemoglobin level; U&E to identify evidence of dehydration and renal function; and C-reactive protein to identify evidence of inflammation.

These investigations will indicate the location of his infection (chest X-ray), the type of infection (sputum), and the severity of the infection (bloods). They may also highlight any other developing problems or otherwise undiagnosed issues. A next priority for nursing care is to initiate and provide the treatments prescribed, to monitor their effects and to oversee the patient's care pathway. The nursing responsibilities related to supporting a person's respiratory function can be found in Chapters 2 and 3.

Treatment and care planning

- Antibiotics, broad spectrum as per local health provider policy, which should be reviewed when a positive sputum culture is available.
- Bronchodilators, which will improve the patient's symptom of shortness of breath and wheeziness and hopefully reduce care requirements by allowing independence.
- Corticosteroids, which may be useful in COPD patients whose symptoms are not controlled by bronchodilators but should be stopped if there is no significant clinical improvement.
- Humidified oxygen if clinically required to maintain SpO_2 between 88% and 92% according to medical prescription (RCP, 2017) – and only in small concentrations as higher concentrations can disrupt the patients who have reverse drive respiratory effort and worsen their condition. If they remain unwell or are deteriorating with low concentration oxygen, then specialist respiratory medicine opinion should be sought.
- Discharge when improving.

Activity 4.6   Critical thinking and group working

While Mr Adams was awaiting admission from the GP surgery to hospital, what other wider concerns should the practice nurse be considering?

Write down a list of points, then compare notes with one or more friends or colleagues. Did you think of the same ones or were there differences?

An outline answer to this activity is given at the end of the chapter.

A person experiencing musculoskeletal causes of chest pain

Case study: Mr Knight

Mr Knight, a frail 82-year-old widower, has been admitted to a clinical decision unit (CDU) for 24 hours' observation and monitoring of chest pain, having fallen at home tripping

(Continued)

(Continued)

over his cat. He has fallen onto the left side of his chest and has had excruciating pain since. He was referred to hospital by his GP following a home visit; the GP was subsequently concerned when he noted that Mr Knight was on warfarin.

In CDU the nurses admit and undertake a primary assessment, quickly followed by a full nursing assessment including situation, background, and ABCDE assessment. The assessment reveals that Mr Knight takes warfarin, bisoprolol, simvastatin, and calcium tablets. Mr Knight tells the nurses that he is worried he is having a heart attack because of the fright, and he is clearly very anxious. In addition, it is noted that Mr Knight is lying on a bed wincing with pain and guarding the left side of his chest. It is painful for him to move, and he feels better when he is lying still. He is an articulate man, talking in full sentences, and he does not appear to be having problems breathing. He says he has awful pain in the left of his chest; it is constant and sharp, throbbing in nature and made worse on deep inspiration. The nurses noted baseline vital signs. His observations are as follows.

- Respiratory rate: 18 bpm
- Oxygen saturation: 98%
- Pulse: 90 bpm (irregular)
- Blood pressure: 120/54 mmHg
- Temperature: 36.7 °C

Activity 4.7   Critical thinking

Are these observations normal? At this point, what do you make of these observations?

An outline answer to this activity is given at the end of the chapter.

Mr Knight tells the nurses that he knows he has had an irregular heartbeat for some time, and this is why he takes warfarin as his GP tells him he could have a stroke.

An on-call junior doctor takes a full medical history and examines Mr Knight. It is ascertained that he has fallen quite accidentally and has not felt dizzy, faint, blacked out, had palpitations, or otherwise lost consciousness before or during his fall. He has pain that is isolated to the left side of his chest – it does not radiate anywhere, and he does not feel short of breath. He does find it painful to take deep breaths. The medical examination finds that:

- he is a thin, frail man;
- he is pale;
- he has very extensive bruising and some swelling to the left side of his chest;

- the left side of his chest is painful when palpated;
- there is reduced chest expansion on the left.

Activity 4.8   Critical thinking

With the information gained from the initial nursing assessment and with this information from the medical assessment, what do you now think is causing his chest pain?

An outline answer to this activity is given at the end of the chapter.

Management of the presenting condition

The doctor diagnoses Mr Knight with a haematoma and suspects possible rib fractures.

The immediate action taken is to:

- give analgesia;
- gain intravenous access;
- oxygen is prescribed should his oxygen saturations fall below 94%.

Now that Mr Knight has been assessed, it is a priority for the nurses to administer suitably strong prescribed analgesia, such as morphine or another opiate-based medication, for his pain before he goes on to have further necessary investigations. The nurses fully assess his pain both before and after administration of analgesia using a pain scale, but also with regard for any effect on respiratory effort (SOCRATES). In addition, with evidence of bleeding and anaemia, it would be prudent to gain intravenous access early and the nurses should ensure that cannulation is undertaken as soon as possible.

The further investigations undertaken are:

- blood tests –FBC, U&E, international normalised ratio (INR), coagulation screen (COAG) to identify clotting irregularities;
- chest X-ray to assess for evidence of trauma;
- 12-lead ECG to rule out the pain being cardiac in origin.

These investigations will identify with certainty whether Mr Knight is anaemic because of his haematoma, or by an as yet unidentified internal bleed (FBC). The COAG and INR tests will identify how thin his blood is and the clinicians may decide to actively reverse the effects of his warfarin. The blood tests may also identify evidence of underlying infection (often a precipitating factor of falls in the elderly). The chest X-ray will either confirm or exclude rib fractures, haemothorax or pneumothorax, and may demonstrate the extent of haematoma in the soft tissues of his chest if large. The nurses will need to perform a 12-lead ECG; this is to rule out myocardial injury that may be masked by his musculoskeletal injury symptoms.

Treatments and care planning

- Treatment will depend on the extent of bleeding. If severely anaemic, Mr Knight may require a transfusion of blood; if less anaemic, a course of iron supplements may be prescribed. A mild anaemia may be tolerated with a plan to review him in a few weeks once he is recovered. Further blood tests may be taken to identify any vitamin or iron deficiencies.
- Prompt administration (if required) of drugs such as vitamin K and beriplex (BNF, 2021) will be required to reverse the effects of the warfarin and help stop bleeding.
- Rib fractures tend to be treated conservatively with analgesia and rest.

The CDU nurses will now need to ensure that Mr Knight is admitted to a ward bed as soon as possible, where a full care pathway will be instigated. Key parts of that will include close monitoring of vital signs, pain management, and appropriate mobilisation to preserve as much of the gentleman's usual physical function as possible. A significant rationale for this is the potential for stroke, a major risk in elderly patients with atrial fibrillation, and this will be exacerbated by the necessity of stopping warfarin in the light of his bleeding. It is crucial that the nurses note that his risk of stroke is high, and that it is therefore important that he is closely monitored (see Chapter 11). Once his bleeding has stopped and he is stable, the patient's clinicians will need to decide on whether to restart his warfarin dependent on his thromboembolic and bleeding risks. Tools such as CHA_2DS_2-VASc stroke risk assessment and HAS-BLED bleeding risk tool (Lane and Lip, 2012) can assist in this decision by giving one-year risk scores of strokes versus bleed. For example, if the bleeding risk is greater than the stroke risk score, it is safer not to anticoagulate the patient. Patients who are receiving warfarin do have a higher risk of intracranial bleeding should they sustain a head injury as the result of a fall, and the patient should be fully investigated regarding the cause of their falls, as current evidence suggests that all but the most prolifically falling patients should be maintained on warfarin as instance of stroke often outweighs that of intracranial haemorrhage.

Mr Knight presents a complex case for nursing management throughout, given his frailty, polypharmacy, and multiple underlying health problems. Prioritising nursing interventions will be a pivotal part of Mr Knight's care pathway – with a central aim of enabling his eventual discharge. Full and ongoing nursing assessment, coupled with input from the MDT, will ascertain the best time for discharge. Given his age and frailty, he may require temporary support at home, and the nurses will need to be sure that a package of care (perhaps from an intermediate care team) is ready for implementation on discharge home if he requires the help.

Activity 4.9 Critical thinking

Consider what other social and community issues the nurses may have had to think of.

An outline answer to this activity is given at the end of the chapter.

A person with gastric/abdominal causes of chest pain

Case study: Mrs Thompson

Situation and background:

Mrs Thompson is an 81-year-old lady with dementia who lives in a nursing home. She complained of 'very bad' indigestion after her Sunday meal. Although forgetful and unable to live on her own as a result, Mrs Thompson is generally able to express herself well, and she told the nursing staff at the nursing home that she had severe pain in her chest. She is on regular antacid for persistent 'heartburn'. The nursing home staff called an ambulance to take her to A&E as they were concerned that she might be having a heart attack.

Assessment:

On admission, the A&E nurses assist Mrs Thompson to a trolley in the general waiting area of the emergency department. They carry out an immediate primary nursing assessment and note that she is clearly uncomfortable, sitting upright and burping a lot. She says she feels nauseous and that she has a very uncomfortable spasmodic burning-type chest pain. This pain is not radiating elsewhere. Her vital signs are as follows.

- Respiratory rate: 22 bpm
- Oxygen saturation: 95%
- Pulse: 110 bpm (regular)
- Blood pressure: 155/100 mmHg
- Temperature: 36.2 °C

Activity 4.10   Critical thinking

- Are these observations normal?
- At this stage, what do you make of these observations?

An outline answer to this activity is given at the end of the chapter.

The A&E nurses note that Mrs Thompson is cooperative. She can mobilise with nursing assistance. A full nursing assessment using the ABCDE approach is undertaken, coupled with an A&E doctor's physical examination and history. These reveal:

Airway and Breathing

- Able to maintain her airway and respond to questioning.

- She has a clear chest with normal heart sounds.
- R: 22/min
- SpO$_2$: 96%

Circulation

- HR: 102/min
- The ECG reveals sinus tachycardia.
- BP: 155/98
- She is pale, but sweaty.
- She has had mild diarrhoea for two days.

Disability

- She is an elderly frail woman with mild to moderate cognition deficits.

Exposure

- Her abdomen is tender on palpation, but no abnormal masses are identified.

> ## Activity 4.11   Evidence-based practice and research
>
> With this information, what do you think is causing her chest pain? (You might want to look up some of the web resources given on page 128.)
>
> *An outline answer to this activity is given at the end of the chapter.*

Management of Mrs Thompson

Mrs Thompson is experiencing an acute exacerbation of her chronic gastritis. The medical treatment of gastritis and the related prioritisation of nursing intervention will depend on what the underlying cause is: diet, infection, other medications such as **non-steroidal anti-inflammatory drugs (NSAIDs)**, steroids. However, a first nursing priority for Mrs Thompson is to alleviate the symptoms; this is undertaken via administration of antacids and H$_2$ antagonists (BNF, 2021) as prescribed. It is important that the nurses monitor and record the effects of these. Correction of electrolyte and hydration deficits will also be important, and a resultant nursing intervention will focus on administration of prescribed fluids and careful fluid balance monitoring.

Treatments and care planning

As Mrs Thompson is elderly and frail, she will be admitted briefly for some investigations to explore possible underlying abnormalities that could be leading to her symptoms. The nursing teams will need to ensure that these investigations are planned and undertaken as soon as possible, and these will include:

- blood tests: blood cell count, presence of *H. pylori*, liver, kidney, gall bladder, and pancreas functions;
- urinalysis;
- stool sample, to look for blood in the stool or infections such as *Clostridium difficile*;
- chest and abdominal X-rays;
- repeat 12-lead ECGs.

Activity 4.12   Reflection

Reflect on Mrs Thompson's situation and what you might do if she were your patient. What other wider concerns should the nurses caring for Mrs Thompson be thinking of relating to her total care and return to her nursing home?

An outline answer to this activity is given at the end of the chapter.

Chapter summary

This chapter has presented four clinical scenarios that have highlighted different causes of chest pain. Key points that must arise from this are:

- the need for rapid and full systematic nursing assessment using the ABCDE approach;
- the need for prioritisation of initial nursing interventions;
- the need for nurses to take immediate and regular ongoing vital signs guided by evidence-based practice;
- the need to keep an open mind on the cause of 'chest pain';
- the need for holistic nursing assessment throughout the patient journey.

We hope that you take from this chapter, if nothing else, the knowledge that there may be many causes of chest pain, and many means of assessing and intervention.

Activities: brief outline answers

Activity 4.1: Critical thinking (page 112)

The respiratory rate is significantly high; the pulse is elevated – tachycardia at rest; the blood pressure is low, even for a known and treated hypertensive; the temperature is above the normal range; the SpO_2 is acceptable.

Central chest pain radiating to the left arm accompanied with pallor is typically suggestive of MI, although this could only be confirmed in the light of other investigations.

The observations point to a physiological state of compensating shock.

Activity 4.2: Critical thinking (page 113)

The blood pressure is significantly low from the previous baseline; the SpO$_2$ is significantly low; this clinical profile points to a developing physiological state of decompensating shock.

Activity 4.3: Reflection (page 116)

Harry was commenced on a rehabilitation programme while still an inpatient and will continue that programme following discharge home. The key elements to cardiac rehabilitation programmes focus on improving diet, exercise, and appropriate medication management. Support and compliance with all of these will help to reduce the risk of further cardiac problems.

Activity 4.4: Critical thinking (page 117)

The respiratory rate is very high for a man of this age at rest, but the SpO$_2$ is within the normal range; the pulse is slightly elevated; the blood pressure is within a normal range for a man of this age; the temperature is on the border of elevation above normal. Consider medical history as part of his background assessment.

Activity 4.5: Critical thinking (page 118)

This symptom complex is highly suggestive of a chest infection that is exacerbating ongoing lung disease.

Activity 4.6: Critical thinking and group working (pages 119)

Mr Adams's wife will need to be contacted and given information regarding his prospective admission, and an opportunity to ask questions or attend the surgery to be with her husband. The nurse should be responsive to her expected concern and anxiety. In addition, the nurse should be able to provide information as to where Mr Adams will be first admitted – most likely to a medical admissions unit.

Activity 4.7: Critical thinking (page 120)

The respiratory rate is slightly elevated; his pulse would not be considered abnormal in a man of his age – later investigation revealed underlying atrial fibrillation treated with bisoprolol and warfarin; blood pressure is slightly low for a man of his age and review of his bisoprolol dose should be considered; temperature is within a normal range; oxygen saturation is normal.

Activity 4.8: Critical thinking (page 121)

With a history of a fall, this information is highly suggestive of trauma – a potential haematoma – and could point to rib fractures. The nurse should be aware of the potential for pneumothorax and monitor respiratory function closely.

Activity 4.9: Critical thinking (page 122)

You should have picked up on two key issues – the first leading you to the second. First, Mr Knight tripped over his cat: who would be available to care for the cat while he was in hospital? Second, the scenario does not provide any information on his social status. Does he live alone? Does he have family? How accessible is his accommodation for the shops? Does he have friendly neighbours? What is his financial situation? Does his accommodation need modification to make it safer for him? Will there be a requirement for community nursing or community healthcare support? Your reflection on Mr Knight should have taken in these wider holistic concerns.

Activity 4.10: Critical thinking (page 123)

The respiratory rate is elevated; the pulse is elevated – tachycardia; the blood pressure is moderately high – particularly the diastolic; the temperature is normal; the oxygen saturation is acceptable for the patient's age.

It would be difficult in isolation to make any conclusion from these readings. However, in conjunction with other findings they would evidence a patient experiencing pain.

Activity 4.11: Evidence-based practice and research (page 124)

These findings are highly suggestive of acute or chronic gastritis – and further enquiry would reveal that Mrs Thompson has a history of persistent heartburn.

Activity 4.12: Reflection (page 125)

A significant issue for this woman is her dementia. The scenario presents her as very cooperative – but as increasingly forgetful. There is also a real possibility that dementia may worsen in future. An important issue that arises from nurses planning discharge to the nursing home will be ensuring that the nursing home understands her problems. Dietary advice will need to be given to minimise episodes of gastritis, this coupled with a carefully monitored regime of H_2 antagonists and antacids.

Further reading

Albarran, J (2002) The language of chest pain. *Nursing Times*, 98(4): 38–40.

An interesting and easy read on chest pain, nursing assessment, and how patients express their pain.

Blanchard, JF and Murnaghan, DA (2010) Nursing patients with acute chest pain: practice guided by the Prince Edward Island conceptual model for nursing. *Nurse Education in Practice*, 10(1): 48–51.

An interesting paper that considers chest pain in relation to nursing models and nursing theory.

O'Shea, L (2010) Differential diagnosis of chest pain. *Practice Nurse*, 40(6): 13.

An informative review of chest pain and related physical examination and patient history taking.

Pope, BB (2006) What's causing your patient's chest pain? *Nursing Management: Critical Care Insider*, Suppl. 21–4.

An informative review of chest pain and its management in a critical care nursing environment.

White, AK and Johnson, M (2000) Men making sense of their chest pain – niggles, doubts and denials. *Journal of Clinical Nursing*, 9(4): 534–41.

An interesting paper that suggests that men's self-concept as 'healthy' may inhibit a speedy response to the signs and symptoms of acute coronary pain.

Useful websites

www.patient.co.uk/doctor/Chest-Pain.htm

Patient.co.uk offers comprehensive health information provided by GPs and nurses to patients during consultations. This PatientPlus article is written for healthcare professionals.

www.netdoctor.co.uk/diseases/facts/angina.htm

NetDoctor.co.uk is a collaboration between doctors, healthcare professionals, information specialists, and patients. It is a comprehensive web resource. This article is a useful review of angina.

www.familydoctor.org/familydoctor/en/health-tools/search-by-symptom/chest-pain-acute.html

This website is operated by the American Academy of Family Physicians (AAFP), a national medical organisation representing more than 100,300 family physicians, family practice residents, and medical students. The page presents a useful algorithm in chest pain diagnosis.

www.nice.org.uk/guidance/ng185

The National Institute for Health and Care Excellence website offers guidance, advice, quality standards, and information services for health, public health, and social care. Also contains resources to help maximise use of evidence and guidance. The guidance NG185 focuses on the management of ACS.

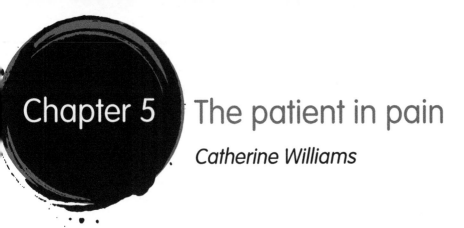

Chapter 5 · The patient in pain

Catherine Williams

NMC Future Nurse: Standards of Proficiency for Registered Nurses

This chapter will address the following platforms and proficiencies:

Platform 4: Providing and evaluating care

Registered nurses take the lead in providing evidence-based, compassionate and safe nursing interventions. They ensure that the care they provide and delegate is person-centred and of a consistently high standard. They support people of all ages in a range of care settings. They work in partnership with people, families and carers to evaluate whether care is effective, and the goals of care have been met in line with their wishes, preferences, and desired outcomes.

Outcomes: The proficiencies identified below will equip the newly registered nurse with the underpinning knowledge and skills required for their role in providing and evaluating person-centred care.

At the point of registration, the registered nurse will be able to:

4.8 demonstrate the knowledge and skills required to identify and initiate appropriate interventions to support people with commonly encountered symptoms including anxiety, confusion, discomfort, and pain.

4.14 understand the principles of safe and effective administration and optimisation of medicines in accordance with local and national policies and demonstrate proficiency and accuracy when calculating dosages of prescribed medicines.

4.15 demonstrate knowledge of pharmacology and the ability to recognise the effects of medicines, allergies, drug sensitivities, side effects, contraindications, incompatibilities, adverse reactions, prescribing errors, and the impact of polypharmacy and over the counter medication usage.

(Continued)

(Continued)

Annexe A: Communication and relationship management skills

Annexe B: Nursing procedures Part 2: Procedures for the planning, provision, and management of person-centred nursing care.

At the point of registration, the registered nurse will be able to safely demonstrate the following procedures:

Procedural competencies required for best practice, evidence-based medicines administration and optimisation

11.1 carry out initial and continued assessments of people receiving care and their ability to self-administer their own medications.

11.2 recognise the various procedural routes under which medicines can be prescribed, supplied, dispensed, and administered; and the laws, policies, regulations, and guidance that underpin them.

11.3 use the principles of safe remote prescribing and directions to administer medicines.

11.4 undertake accurate drug calculations for a range of medications.

11.5 undertake accurate checks, including transcription and titration, of any direction to supply or administer a medicinal product.

11.6 exercise professional accountability in ensuring the safe administration of medicines to those receiving care.

11.7 administer injections using intramuscular, subcutaneous, intradermal, and intravenous routes and manage injection equipment.

11.8 administer medications using a range of routes.

11.9 administer and monitor medications using vascular access devices and enteral equipment.

11.10 recognise and respond to adverse or abnormal reactions to medications.

11.11 undertake safe storage, transportation, and disposal of medicinal products.

Chapter aims

By the end of this chapter, you should be able to:

- build upon knowledge and skill to reflect what the NMC Future nurse standards (2018) will require of a newly qualified registered nurse;
- discuss the anatomy and physiology of pain transmission;
- define acute and chronic pain;
- effectively assess pain using a variety of assessment tools, interpreting findings and determine the most appropriate pain management strategy;
- reflect on clinical examples in the chapter and apply this to your own clinical situation.

Introduction

Pain assessment and management is an important aspect of the role of the registered nurse as we are the ones who are mostly involved in ongoing pain assessment and the implementation of the pain management plan.

This chapter will first discuss the aetiology of pain. We will then look at the different types of pain patients can experience and go on to explain how to perform an accurate pain assessment. The chapter will explain the importance of monitoring patients using clinical assessment skills and procedures and the use of pharmacological and non-pharmacological interventions in treating acute and chronic pain.

Pain assessment should form an integral component of your nursing assessment. If we can learn to assess a patient's pain as routinely as we take their pulse, blood pressure, temperature, respiration, and oxygen saturations, then we will have taken a huge step toward managing it.

Pain can have harmful physiological, psychological, and emotional effects on your patient. Many patients in the clinical environment experience pain, which is usually related to surgery, trauma, or some form of organ disease. Katie's story illustrates how a team approach to clinical decision making can support pain management.

Case study: Kate's story

Maddie, a student nurse, is on a placement in the burns unit and is working with her mentor on admissions. One evening a patient called Kate is transferred for assessment to the burns unit. She has sustained a 13% scald to both legs. She is still in a great deal of discomfort despite receiving a total dose of 30 mg of intravenous morphine (in increments of 10 mg) and paracetamol 1 g intravenously prior to transfer from A&E. The medical staff on call is reluctant to give further opiates at present as she is concerned that this will increase the risk of respiratory depression. However, Kate is asked to assess her pain level on a scale of 0–10 and rates the pain as 11. Maddie's mentor explains that the patient's nerve endings have been left exposed to the air by her injury and that the uncovering of the wound for assessment is contributing to Kate's discomfort. The mentor also explains that the wound will have to be cleaned and debrided prior to dressings being applied and that this is likely to make the pain worse, albeit temporarily. The mentor then becomes an advocate for the patient and suggests to the medical staff that she might benefit from using **nitrous oxide** for pain relief until the wound can be covered. Checks are made with the patient and there are no contraindications for her to receive this form of analgesia. The mentor sets about explaining to Kate how to use the nitrous oxide inhalation system; they are able to proceed with the wound assessment and types of dressings. When the wounds are properly dressed and no longer exposed to the air, Kate's discomfort abates, and she can breathe normally and no longer requires the nitrous oxide.

The aetiology of pain

Wilson (2007) describes acute pain as being a physiological response that warns us of a threat or danger to the body. Because of the increase in hormone production and sympathetic output in the body from injury or illness, your patient, when in pain, will experience an increase in heart rate and blood pressure, which increases cardiac work and oxygen consumption. Patients who are not appropriately managed for acute pain are at higher risk of developing chronic pain syndrome. Chronic or persistent pain is pain that carries on for longer than 12 weeks despite medication or treatment (Stamenkovic et al., 2019).

This physiological response comes from the nervous system that directs and manages the functions of all the cells and tissues in our body. Nociceptors are sensory receptors of the peripheral nervous system. They are located at the end of nerve cells that originate in the dorsal root ganglion and trigeminal ganglion and are responsible for sending signals to the spinal cord and the brain when damaging stimuli are detected in the skin, mucous membranes, muscles, joints, and organs. They are also known as pain receptors because they produce the sensation of pain.

For example, if you burn your finger, the tissue damage activates the nociceptors, which in turn transmit impulses to the brain via the spinal cord, causing you to experience **nociceptive pain**. Other forms of nociceptive pain arise from arthritis, sickle cell crisis, and post-operative pain.

Another type of pain stimulus is known as **somatic pain**, which is a type of nociceptive pain. The nerves that detect somatic pain are located in the skin and deep tissues and they send impulses to the brain when they detect tissue damage; for example, if you cut your finger, stretch a muscle too far, or exercise for a long period of time. The pain experienced will be sharp due to the tissues being rich in the A delta (A) fibres sending rapid signals to the brain, and this is why you are able to clearly locate the origin of the pain and it usually causes distress.

Pain from deeper tissues is known as **visceral pain**. Visceral pain, defined as pain originating from the internal organs, is a hallmark feature of multiple diseases, including inflammatory bowel disease, pancreatitis, irritable bowel syndrome (IBS), and functional dyspepsia (Zhuo-Ying et al., 2019). Like somatic pain, the nociceptors send signals to the spinal cord and brain when damage is detected. Visceral pain is often associated with marked autonomic phenomena, including pallor, profuse sweating, nausea, GI disturbances and changes in body temperature, blood pressure, and heart rate.

For example, if you suffer from IBS or bladder disorders, you will experience visceral pain. The generalised aching or squeezing felt is caused by or stretching of the abdominal cavity. Visceral pain can radiate to other areas in the body, which is why pinpointing its exact location can be difficult.

Activity 5.1 asks you to research nociceptive, visceral, and somatic pain in more depth.

Activity 5.1   Evidence-based practice and research

(a) In order to research nociceptive, visceral, and somatic pain in more depth, try to identify the specific areas of the body that may be affected, what type of injury may cause them in a patient, and how the pain for each area may be experienced. As a nurse why is it important to identify the types of pain our patients experience?

There is no outline answer provided for this part of the activity.

(b) Nitrous oxide and oxygen are an effective analgesic for the relief of procedural pain and can safely be used by nurses working in a range of settings, but what are the associated risks and contraindications for the use of nitrous oxide?

An outline answer to this question is given at the end of the chapter.

Having researched the sources of pain in Activity 5.1 we will now review the types of pain patients can experience.

Types of pain

When treating patients, you always need to consider the type of pain that they are suffering so that you can use the appropriate strategy to alleviate it.

Pain is classified as acute or chronic (Dougherty and Lister, 2020). **Acute pain** is normally of sudden onset, usually occurring because of tissue damage, injury, or disease, and it tends to resolve over time as tissues heal. **Chronic pain** begins with an episode of acute pain, but unlike acute pain, chronic pain does not resolve over time. The most common causes of chronic pain are degenerative conditions such as osteoarthritis or diabetic complications such as neuropathy. Table 5.1 shows some common examples of chronic and acute pain.

Chronic pain	Acute pain
Diabetic neuropathy	Migraine/headache
Back pain	Burns
Osteoarthritis/rheumatoid arthritis	Fractures
Multiple sclerosis	Lacerations
Cancer	Abdominal pain
Neuralgia	Toothache
Post-surgical pain	Post-surgical pain

Table 5.1   Examples of chronic and acute pain

Mixed pain is a combination of nociceptive and neuropathic pain. In the case of mixed pain syndromes, healthcare professionals are likely to hear elements of both neuropathic and nociceptive pain described by the patient (Ritchie, 2011). Mixed pain is likely to need a poly-pharmaceutical approach to manage the different types of pain. Low back pain is often classified as mixed pain, associated with both neuropathic and nociceptive pain components.

The way in which we experience pain is very complex. All sorts of factors influence our experience, including our thoughts and feelings. You need to be aware that some patients can suffer from both forms of pain (chronic and acute), and a number of nursing interventions that you routinely perform on your patient, such as suctioning, line insertion, repositioning, and physiotherapy, can cause additional pain and discomfort. One way to understand what is happening is what is called the **gate control theory** of pain (Melzack and Wall, 1965; Melzack, 1996).

In 1965, Ronald Melzack and Patrick Wall published the gate control theory of pain. The theory combined previous notions of pain and attempted to answer questions on why we may perceive pain to different degrees. The theory simply stated, in an elegant and succinct way, that the transmission of pain from the peripheral nerve through the spinal cord was subject to modulation by both intrinsic neurones and controls emanating from the brain.

Melzack and Wall (1965) suggested that before information is transmitted to the brain, pain messages encounter the 'nerve gates' which ascertain whether these pain signals are to be transmitted up to the brain. Pain impulses travel into the spinal cord along small fibres known as A delta and C fibres to the dorsal horn substantia gelatinosa, where the fibres impede the inhibitory interneurons, allowing pain information to travel up the spinal cord to the brain. Increasing activity of the transmission cells results in increased perceived pain. Conversely, decreasing activity of transmission cells reduces perceived pain. In the gate control theory, an open 'gate' describes when input to transmission cells is permitted, therefore allowing the sensation of pain, and a closed 'gate' describes when input to transmission cells is blocked, therefore reducing the sensation of pain.

Providing comfort to your patient who is in pain is a vital role of the nurse, and implementing supportive measures will minimise the overall pain and anxiety in your patient. Communication, reassurance, touch, and explanations are important skills that you need to incorporate into your practice. In addition to evidence-based analgesic management, simple measures such as reducing noise levels and light and relieving prolonged pressure or limb placement by turning pillows over may help relieve positioning discomfort in your patient and decrease anxiety levels. Activity 5.2 now asks you to consider the types of pain patients experience and how you can help in managing this.

Activity 5.2   Decision making

Think about the case study: Kate's story. What type of pain do you think Kate is suffering from and how are these factors stimulating the pain gate? What is your reasoning for deciding this? What interventions could you introduce to close the pain gate?

An outline answer to this activity is given at the end of the chapter.

Pain assessment

Having considered types of pain that a patient might experience, we will now look more closely at pain and methods of assessment.

Assessment of pain is an important aspect of your role that requires several skills, including observation, interpretation, and communication skills. Other interventions that can be used as management strategies include:

- analgesic administration;
- emotional support;
- cognitive techniques;
- comfort measures.

Assessing and managing pain are essential components of nursing practice. Pain is often categorised as acute or chronic, but it is a complex physical, psychological, and social phenomenon that is uniquely subjective. Pain traverses all clinical settings and the age spectrum (RCN, 2015) and the patient's response to pain can be affected by a multitude of variables such as age or culture, not just the type of pain and its duration.

Activity 5.3 focuses on your own experience on practice in supporting a patient in pain.

Activity 5.3   Reflection

Think of three or four patients you have cared for who were in considerable pain or whose pain needed careful management. How did they express pain? Did they express their pain in the same way as other patients? If not, what were the differences?

As this answer is based on your own reflection, there is no outline answer at the end of the chapter.

Having reflected on your own practice of pain assessment, the next section will review what needs to be covered when completing a comprehensive pain assessment.

What should be covered in your pain assessment?

Your initial assessment of the patient's pain assessment should include:

- the underlying condition;
- whether the pain is acute or chronic or mixed;
- pain history;
- location of pain;

- intensity of pain;
- cognitive development and understanding of pain;
- whether any medical treatment is being given;
- related symptoms such as vomiting and breathlessness;
- meaning or significance of the pain for the patient;
- an assessment of the influence of psychological, social, and spiritual factors on the person's experience of pain.

A pain assessment tool can be invaluable as it can aid the patient to communicate his or her pain and pain assessment and control should be a priority within nursing, yet pain may often be underassessed and unrelieved and the reasons for this are complex and varied. It is pointed out by many that for the planning of effective nursing interventions for pain, individual assessment is essential, and thus assessment tools are necessary.

Quality care for patients presenting with acute pain begins with the use of an appropriate pain assessment tool. A variety of pain assessment tools have been developed and used in clinical settings with subsequent improvements in assessment. They each have specific attributes, and their place in clinical practice is considered.

Many assessment tools are available, although the most used pain scale in the healthcare setting is the numerical rating scale. The numerical scale offers the individual in pain an opportunity to rate their pain score. The user rates their scale from zero to the higher number when asked or places a mark on a line indicating their level of pain. The lowest figure indicates the absence of pain, and the highest figure represents the most intense pain possible.

An advantage of the numerical scale assessment is that it follows the WHO analgesic ladder (WHO, 2006). Although developed and validated for cancer pain, the WHO analgesic ladder is widely used to guide the basic treatment of acute and chronic pain; while there is little evidence to support its use in chronic pain it may provide an analgesic strategy for non-specialists. While pain assessment is a prerequisite for appropriate management of acute pain, there are some concerns about the use of pain intensity scoring systems. It has been shown that pain is subjective. This suggests that self-reporting of pain is variable and a host of factors such as language, culture, and psychological factors could all influence the perception of pain (Garcia et al., 2007; Narayan, 2010). Individual responses to analgesia vary considerably, both in terms of efficacy and side effects. This provides challenges with assessment and management in routine clinical practice. If an individual either fails to tolerate, or has an inadequate response to a drug, then it is worthwhile considering a different agent from the same class (NICE, 2021b).

Medicines management and the administration of medicines is a key part of the nurse's role. As a registered nurse, it is your responsibility to work collaboratively and to address medicines-related problems, optimising the use of medicines by providing advice on prescribing, medication monitoring, and management of repeat prescribing systems. Further information is available at **nice.org.uk**

The standards for the administration of medicines have been withdrawn from the NMC from January 2019 and the NMC have worked collaboratively with the Royal Pharmaceutical Society (RPS) to produce guidance for all healthcare professionals covering areas such as the storage, transportation, and disposal of medicines (RPS, 2018).

The administration of medicines in a healthcare setting must be done in accordance with a prescription, Patient Specific Direction, Patient Group Direction, or other relevant exemption specified in the Human Medicines Regulations 2012 (Schedules 17 and 19, as amended). A nurse administering a medicine must have an overall understanding of the medicine being administered and seek advice, if necessary, from a prescriber or a pharmacist.

Activity 5.4 focuses on your own reflections of using pain assessment tools.

Activity 5.4   Reflection

Reflecting on these new standards, investigate the pain relief analgesic ladder devised by the WHO. Reflect on a patient you have cared for who benefited from having their medication linked to the principles of the ladder.

As this activity is based on your own reflections, there is no outline answer at the end of the chapter.

Another pain assessment method that is easy to remember is the PQRST mnemonic, which stands for Provokes, Quality, Radiates, Severity, and Time (Skaer, 1998), shown in the box 'Pain recognition and assessment'. This method has five simple characteristics to help you in the questioning of the patient's pain assessment, but remember that you must let the patient describe the pain, as sometimes they say what they think you would like to hear. We now go on to think of simple ways of remembering the cues to help you in assessing the patient's pain.

Pain recognition and assessment

P = Provokes

- What causes pain?
- What makes it better?
- What makes it worse?

Q = Quality

- What does it feel like? Can you describe the pain? Is it:

- sharp?
- dull?
- stabbing?
- burning?
- crushing?

R = Radiates

- Where does the pain radiate?
- Is it in one place?
- Does it move around?
- Did it start elsewhere and is now localised to one spot?

S = Severity

- How severe is the pain on a scale of 1–10? This can be a difficult one as the rating will differ from patient to patient.

T = Time

- Time pain started.
- How long did it last?
- Is it constant or does it come and go?

Because of the subjective nature of pain, the most effective method for establishing if a patient is in pain is to ask them about their pain experience.

One framework often used by healthcare professionals is the SOCRATES mnemonic, which provides a structured and systematic approach to assessment of the physical aspects of pain.

S – Site

O – Onset

C – Character

R – Radiation or referred pain

A – Associate symptoms

T – Timing

E – Exacerbating factor

S – Severity of intensity

The SOCRATES mnemonic focuses on the physical or sensory aspects of pain and does not consider the emotional effects of the pain on an individual, for example fear, anxiety, and depression. These emotional effects will influence how an individual copes with their experience of pain (Snow et al., 2004).

Pain assessment tools that are more holistic than the SOCRATES mnemonic include the McGill Pain Questionnaire (Melzack, 1975), which also asks how the pain affects an individual emotionally, and the Brief Pain Inventory (Cleeland and Ryan, 1994), which includes assessment of how the pain affects the individual's ability to undertake activities and their quality of life.

When using a pain scale, the patient needs to be able to communicate and describe their pain experience, and to understand the questions and pain scale that is used. Some patients may find communication challenging for various reasons, including language barriers, hearing impairment, cognitive impairment, learning disability, and dementia and this needs to be taken into consideration when undertaking a pain assessment and using an appropriate tool to undertake the assessment.

The following are a number of observational pain assessment tools that are seen in clinical practice. They include: the Abbey pain scale (Abbey et al., 2004), the Pain Assessment in Advanced Dementia (PAINAD) scale (Warden et al., 2003), the Doloplus-2 (Hølen et al., 2007), and the Bolton Pain Assessment Tool (BPAT) (Gregory, 2012).

It can be hard to recognise if some people with learning disabilities are in pain. People with learning disabilities may not say they are in pain. They may not act in a way that you would expect people in pain to act. It is particularly difficult to know if someone is in pain if they do not communicate verbally. People who have additional health needs, especially those who are immobile or wheelchair dependent, are likely to suffer from long-term pain. People with learning disabilities, like non-disabled people, will have individual and different responses to pain.

The Disability Distress Assessment Tool4 (DisDAT) is based on the idea that each person has their own 'vocabulary' of distress signs and behaviours. The tool builds on the ability of family and supporters to identify different signs of distress in individuals. It can be used to record the signs and behaviours of the person when they are content or distressed. There is an 18-item checklist called Non-Communicating Adults Pain Checklist5 (NCAPC). This can help assess chronic pain in non-communicating adults and has demonstrated validity and reliability for people with learning disabilities (Lotan et al., 2009).

It is vital that you regard the patient's pain as an assessment priority. Unless pain is assessed regularly and effectively, your patient will continue to suffer unnecessarily.

Assessment in the very young, the cognitively impaired (such as the sedated patient or those with dementia), and those with communication problems can pose problems, but there are suitable pain assessment tools such as verbal rating, visual analogue, body diagrams, questionnaires, and pain diaries.

Effective pain assessment is a fundamental part of your nursing care, and the accountability of pain assessment lies firmly within the domain of nursing. To enable you to do this effectively, keep in mind the following:

- Seek to establish a relationship with your patient.
- Use open questions.
- Observe your patient for clues regarding pain.
- Adopt the most appropriate pain assessment tool.
- Avoid making a subjective assessment and jumping to conclusions.

Activity 5.5 asks you to think about the pain assessment tools discussed above and which one would be most beneficial for Kate's pain assessment.

Activity 5.5   Critical thinking

Here we will look at critical thinking and decision-making skills using our case study patient Kate. Of the assessment scales that have been discussed, which one do you think would be most appropriate for her, and why? What other factors will you observe in your assessment?

An outline answer to this activity is given at the end of the chapter.

Managing your patient's pain

A key aspect of your role as a registered nurse is managing your patient's pain safely and effectively. The choice of drug used to alleviate your patient's pain depends upon the nature and severity of the pain, and many other factors that the doctor will consider.

The three main classes of drugs that are commonly used within the hospital care environment are:

- non-opioids;
- opioids;
- anti-emetics should ideally accompany an opioid prescription. Remember that anti-emetics by the oral route are ineffective in a nauseated or vomiting patient.

Non-opioids

The non-opioid drugs, paracetamol and aspirin (and other NSAIDs), are particularly suitable for pain in musculoskeletal conditions, whereas the opioid analgesics are more suitable for moderate to severe pain, particularly of visceral origin. **Non-steroidal anti-inflammatory analgesics** (NSAIDs) are particularly useful for the treatment of patients with chronic disease accompanied by pain and inflammation. Some of them are also used in the short-term treatment of mild to moderate pain including transient musculoskeletal pain.

The route of administration will depend on your patient's condition. Take care to bear in mind your patient's renal clearance, as nephrotoxic medication increases the risk of kidney failure.

Opioids

Opioid analgesics can be divided into those used for mild to moderate pain, such as codeine phosphate, and those used for moderate to severe pain, such as morphine or oxycodone hydrochloride.

Opioids should only be considered in carefully selected individuals for the short- to medium-term treatment of chronic non-malignant pain, when other therapies have been insufficient; the benefits should outweigh the risks of serious harms (such as addiction, overdose, and death). They should not be used in cases of acute respiratory depression; comatose patients; head injury (opioid analgesics interfere with pupillary responses vital for neurological assessment); raised intracranial pressure (opioid analgesics interfere with pupillary responses vital for neurological assessment); risk of paralytic ileus.

With continuous longer-term use of opioids, tolerance and dependence compromise both safety and efficacy. Potentially lethal side effects such as respiratory depression and changes in consciousness level mean that they must be appropriately selected, prescribed, administered, and monitored as they can further exacerbate conditions of an already compromised patient.

Opioids can be administered via multiple routes but have many side effects such as respiratory depression, cough suppression, constipation, urinary retention, and nausea and vomiting, with the additional potential to depress the gag reflex, causing aspiration. Hence, close observation and documentation are vital to prevent complications occurring.

New safety recommendations have been issued following a review of the risks of dependence and addiction associated with prolonged use (longer than three months) of opioids for non-malignant pain (Gov.UK, 2020).

For further information and guidance on the pharmacology and therapeutics of this group of drugs, please refer to the *British National Formulary* (**www.bnf.org**) and NICE Clinical Knowledge Summaries (CKS) on analgesia.

Many strong opioids can cause the patient to feel nauseous and managing this is an essential element of pain management. You can buy some anti-emetics that help relieve nausea and vomiting over the counter without a doctor's prescription, but generally anti-emetics are prescription-only drugs. There are many different types of drugs that are used to control nausea and vomiting. Some affect brain function by preventing the stimulation of the vomiting centre, which in turn relieves nausea by promoting gastric emptying. The most used anti-emetics such as ondansetron, prochlorperazine, and cyclizine, affect the vomiting centre, whereas metoclopramide increases gut motility. The patient's symptoms will affect the choice of anti-emetic.

For further information and guidance on the pharmacology and therapeutics of this group of drugs, please refer to the *British National Formulary* (**www.bnf.org**).

Epidurals

This next section provides an overview of other types of analgesia you will come across and how they work. There is a lot of confusion surrounding epidural and spinal anaesthesia and whether they are the same. They are not, and each has its own unique procedures and benefits.

The main difference between spinal and epidural anaesthesia is that **spinal anaesthesia** involves injecting the drug to the **cerebrospinal fluid,** whereas **epidural anaesthesia** involves passing the medication into the epidural space through a catheter.

An epidural anaesthetic works by blocking the nerve roots and can be inserted at different levels of the spine depending on the area that needs pain relief. The nerve roots are located in a space near the spinal cord called the epidural space. The epidural space extends from the base of the skull to the sacrum and the space is identified by feeling for bony landmarks on the spine and pelvis. A fine-bore catheter is inserted into the epidural space and is secured to the patient's back and then attached to the infusion device.

The area of analgesic effect is dependent on the site of insertion in relation to the surgery. Epidural location sites are:

- T6–T9 abdominal surgery – exploratory laparotomy.
- T7–T10 upper abdominal surgery – repair of abdominal aortic aneurysm.
- T9–L1 lower abdominal surgery – repair of inguinal hernias.
- L1–L4 hip and knee surgery (Dougherty and Lister, 2020).

The drugs most used for epidural analgesia are opioids such as fentanyl and bupivacaine. Bupivacaine is a medication used to decrease feeling in a specific area. In nerve blocks, it is injected around a nerve that supplies the area, or into the spinal canal's epidural space. Bupivacaine can be used on its own (usually for a bolus dose) and dosage will depend on the size of the catheter and the duration of surgery. Remember that epidural analgesia is contraindicated in patients who have:

- local or systemic infection;
- known neurological disease;
- coagulation disorders or who are undergoing anticoagulant therapy;
- spinal arthritis/spinal deformities;
- hypotension;
- marked hypertension (Hastings, 2009).

Activity 5.6 will assess what you have learned from the section above through a series of questions and answers.

Activity 5.6 Critical thinking

What is epidural analgesia? Where is it administered? What do you think might be the specific nursing care associated with administering drugs via this route?

An outline answer to this activity is given at the end of the chapter.

Good practice advises the duration of catheter placement should be determined after weighing up the associated risks and benefits. Epidural catheters should not remain in situ for longer than clinically necessary and should be removed as soon as it is safe to do so and after checking the patient's anti-coagulation status.

Dose, timings, and therapeutic effect of all anti-coagulation should be considered both when inserting and removing an epidural catheter, and while the epidural is in situ. This is to reduce the risk of bleeding into the epidural space. Please refer to your local guidance for further information on good practice. Further advice may need to be sought from a haematologist if your patient has a co-morbidity that would adversely affect coagulation or the length of action of the anticoagulant – such as impaired renal function (RPS, 2020).

As with all controlled drugs you must prepare, administer, and document the drugs according to your hospital's policy. For further information and guidance regarding pharmacology and therapeutics, please refer to the *British National Formulary* (**www.bnf.org**).

Patient-controlled analgesia

Patient-controlled analgesia (PCA) is widely used for the treatment of pain in the ICU environment. The PCA offers on-demand, intermittent, IV administration of opioids under patient control (with or without a continuous background infusion). This technique is based on the use of a sophisticated microprocessor-controlled infusion pump that delivers a pre-programmed dose of opioid when the patient pushes a demand button; lock-out controls are set to prevent excessive administration or overdose.

Activity 5.7 Critical thinking

This activity requires undertaking further research activities, this time focusing upon PCA. First, what is PCA? What are the main advantages and disadvantages of its use in patients experiencing pain in hospital or in the community?

There is no answer to this activity at the end of the chapter. The issues are discussed below.

Using a PCA system allows your patient more immediate relief of incidental (break-through) pain and can provide a greater sense of personal control over pain. It can be reassuring to your patient to know that an analgesic is quickly available and that they are in control of the administration.

As the opioid analgesia is not administered unless the patient presses the control, it is important that they are able to operate it properly. The PCA system will be unsuitable for a patient who does not have the cognitive ability to understand how to use the PCA device, or who is unable or unwilling to operate the handset.

Because a strong opioid is being administered, you will need to have a clear under-standing of the contraindications and therapeutics of the drug and its side effects. Hourly checks of the following must be completed and documented:

- heart rate;
- blood pressure;
- respiratory rate;
- oxygen saturations;
- pain score;
- sedation score;
- nausea/vomiting;
- dose used.

In addition to your patient checks, pump checks need to be completed to enable con-tinuing assessment. Pump checks include:

- programme check;
- amount delivered;
- successful attempts;
- unsuccessful attempts – this will indicate that analgesic needs are not being met and the regime needs to be urgently reviewed;
- lock-out time – the lock-out interval is designed to prevent overdose. Ideally, it should be long enough for the patient to experience the maximal effect of one dose before another is permitted.

A PCA is usually needed for a few days after surgery/medical interventions, and many ICUs have specific step-down analgesia protocols to prevent premature discontinuation and ensure patients remain pain free during the step down from intravenous to oral medication. Any concern you may have about the PCA infusion should be discussed immediately with the pain team or the anaesthetist.

As with all controlled drugs, you must prepare, administer, and document the drugs according to your local policy. For further information and guidance regarding pharmacology and therapeutics, please refer to the *British National Formulary* (**www. bnf.org**).

Recognising deterioration in your patient

Every nurse is accountable for their actions when it comes to care delivery and recognising a deteriorating patient is a fundamental assessment skill every nurse needs to be able to undertake safely. When you have a critically ill patient who has difficulty communicating their pain due to altered levels of consciousness or endotracheal intubation, you must report any changes in your patient's pain or overall condition. You will need to make frequent observations and assessments so that you spot any change in their condition or adverse effects caused by treatment. Be aware of patients receiving any medication and sedation for post-operative pain as they could be at risk of respiratory depression. You will need to assess pain and sedation hourly. When caring for a patient in pain, it is useful to remember the following:

- Always report any new sources for pain identified by your patient – this could be a sign of surgical and/or medical complications.
- Opioids have strong side effects. Your patient will require specific and close monitoring and you may need to administer other drugs to overcome the side effects.
- Never focus solely on the one aspect of your patient's pain – consider all possible factors that may be affecting their pain management.

Non-pharmacological pain management

There are other ways to manage a patient's pain other than pharmacological intervention. Non-pharmacological approaches may contribute to effective analgesia, are often well accepted by patients, and are a useful adjunct in managing pain. The role of non-pharmacological approaches to pain management is evolving and it is likely that some non-pharmacological and complementary therapies may make an important contribution to holistic patient care. The goals of non-pharmacological interventions are to:

- minimise fear and distress;
- make pain tolerable;
- give the patient a sense of control over the situation and their behaviour;
- teach and enhance coping strategies.

Common non-pharmacological pain-control methods widely used in hospitals and in the community are distraction, music therapy, hypnosis, cold and heat application, transcutaneous electrical nerve stimulators (TENS), and massage therapy. You need to be familiar with each of these methods. It is also important that you develop a therapeutic nurse–patient relationship and pay attention to comfort measures, as these will aid pain control in your patient. Fear and anxiety make pain worse, so your nursing care should aim to alleviate these feelings.

Scenario

Kate is now at home recovering from her burns and being visited by Seeta, who is the community nurse responsible for her continuing care. Seeta is accompanied by Jaimie, who is on clinical experience in the community.

Jaimie has been learning about pain management and is interested to see how Seeta will be approaching the problem in Kate's case.

Seeta asks Kate how she is coping with the pain and, rather to Jaimie's surprise, asks whether she finds listening to music helpful. Seeta explores with Kate whether adjusting the lighting in her room might help and discusses with her how best to make her as comfortable as possible. She then suggests playing some of Kate's favourite CDs in a relaxed atmosphere.

Seeta goes on to suggest to Kate that she might benefit from one or more of the following: music therapy, hypnosis, or cognitive behavioural therapy (CBT). She has leaflets about all of these, which she is able to leave with Kate.

Seeta then gives Kate a leaflet about transcutaneous electrical nerve stimulators and explains how this works. She explains to Kate how she might access any of these therapies.

As they leave Kate's house, Jaimie realises her understanding of how pain can be managed has been broadened by watching and listening to Seeta at work.

Chapter summary

Looking back over this chapter and the scenarios, we hope you take from it several key messages including that all patients have differing needs and thus require nurses to approach pain assessment and management in an innovative proactive manner. Pain can be triggered by many medical conditions, including ischaemia, infections, inflammation, oedema, distension, immobilisation, incisions, and wounds. The use of invasive and non-invasive medical devices can also cause pain in your patient. In addition, many commonly performed nursing procedures, such as suctioning, turning, dressing changes, and the insertion and removal of catheters, may be a source of pain for your patient, and these need to be taken into consideration when assessing pain.

Preventing pain will improve your patient's physiological and psychological outcomes, enabling earlier discharge. Remember that pain is individual to each patient (McCaffery and Pasero, 1999) and will always require regular individual assessment. Pain is usually a symptom of a problem, and even though analgesia will be provided, the cause of your patient's pain will still need to be investigated. Unless pain is assessed regularly and effectively, the patient will continue to suffer unnecessarily.

Pain management must be one of your top nursing priorities and you must continue to monitor outcomes related to pain management. Some patients may be able to verbally or non-verbally communicate their pain-control needs; the critically ill intubated patient may not be able to communicate their level of pain adequately, and this needs to be recognised in the care plan. To fulfil the above you will need to have a thorough understanding of the actions of analgesics, their side effects, dosages, and differing methods of administration and appropriate use within the ICU setting to ensure a positive outcome for your patient.

Activities: brief outline answers

Activity 5.1: Evidence-based practice and research (page 133)

(b) Nitrous oxide is a small inorganic chemical molecule and may also be known as dinitrogen oxide or dinitrogen monoxide. Overall, nitrous oxide is a very safe drug with few absolute contraindications but it is clearly contraindicated in patients with significant respiratory complications. This includes patients with pneumothorax, pulmonary blebs, air embolism, bowel obstruction, those undergoing surgery of the middle ear, and patients who have had eye surgery that uses an intraocular gas.

Nitrous oxide is known to interfere with vitamin B12 and folate metabolism. In patients with these pre-existing conditions, nitrous oxide should only be used with full precautionary consideration and close monitoring. Precautions should be taken in paediatric patients with underlying vitamin B12 deficiency and is relatively contraindicated in pregnancy, as it's known to have potential teratogenic and fetal toxic effect.

Activity 5.2: Decision making (page 134)

Kate is suffering from acute pain. Burn pain is one of the most difficult forms of acute pain to treat. The type of tissue damage with a burn injury is likely to generate unusually high levels of pain. The gate is opened by the activity in the small-diameter nerve fibres being exposed by the burn injury. Interventions used to close the gate can include relaxation/mental factors/activity and other physical factors.

Activity 5.5: Critical thinking (page 140)

Assessment tools are essential to the diagnosis of underlying burn pain syndromes and the effectiveness of their treatment. The better tool to use with this patient is one of the verbal self-report instruments that measure pain intensity, such as the '0–10' numeric rating scale. This is the most appropriate tool because assessing pain in the burn-injured patient is complex and, as she is able to communicate well, this assessment tool will give you a clear picture of her pain status.

Activity 5.6: Critical thinking (page 143)

An epidural is a form of regional analgesia involving an infusion of drugs through a catheter placed into the epidural space. Epidural analgesia may be administered either as a continuous infusion, as patient-controlled epidural analgesia (PCEA), or as a combination of the two. The injection can cause both a loss of sensation and a loss of pain by blocking the transmission of signals through nerves in or near the spinal cord. A comprehensive assessment should include vital signs, pain and sedation levels, level of consciousness, ability to void, sensation and motor function, presence of potential adverse side effects and complications, and evaluation of insertion site.

Your patient will require vital signs monitoring throughout its use for signs of hypotension (due to **vasodilation** of the vessels) and respiratory depression (due to opioid analgesia). Most clinical areas advocate an hourly protocol check of:

- heart rate;
- blood pressure – hypertension should not be managed by tilting the patient's head down as this will allow the drug to travel up to T4 and cause paralysis of the respiratory muscles;
- respiratory rate;
- oxygen saturations;
- pain score;
- dose delivered;
- sedation score;
- nausea/vomiting – if your patient is complaining of a headache and nausea/vomiting, this may be a sign of a dural puncture;
- level of sensory/motor block – the block should be high enough to provide effective analgesia but not to paralyse the respiratory muscles. If this occurs, you must stop the infusion immediately.
- the dressing.

Further reading

Caudill, M (2016) *Managing Pain Before It Manages You.* 4th edition. New York: Guilford Press.

This book continues to be the gold standard for the self-management of pain. It is informative and easy to read, focusing on what people can do on their own to manage persistent pain.

Herndon, DN (2017) *Total Burn Care.* Fifth edition. London: W B Saunders.

This book will give you a comprehensive overview of the assessment and management of a patient with moderate and severe thermal burns.

Macintyre, PE and Schug, SA (2015) *Acute Pain Management: A Practical Guide.* Fifth edition. CRC Press.

With a focus on practical acute pain management in adults in the hospital setting, this book provides health professionals with simple and practical information to help them manage patients with acute pain safely and effectively, and includes evidence-based information about management of acute pain in some specific patient groups.

Mann, E and Carr, E (2006) *Pain Management: Essential Clinical Skills for Nurses.* London: Blackwell Publishing.

Pain Management is a practical guide to current best practice, providing students and newly qualified nurses with the knowledge and skills required to care for a person experiencing, or at risk of experiencing, pain.

Useful websites

www.bnf.org

https://bnf.nice.org.uk/

BNF. Compiled with the advice of clinical experts, this essential reference provides up-to-date guidance on prescribing, dispensing, and administering medicines.

www.rpharms.com/

The Royal Pharmaceutical Society (RPharmS or RPS) is the body responsible for the leadership and support of the pharmacy profession within England, Scotland, and Wales and is internationally renowned as a publisher of medicines information.

https://about.medicinescomplete.com/

Medicines Complete, from the RPS, is the definitive online resource for drug and healthcare information and a useful tool for students and new registrants.

www.britishpainsociety.org

The British Pain Society. This is a useful website for current information on all matters relating to pain.

www.nice.org.uk

Website of the National Institute for Health and Care Excellence. This website allows you to access a series of national clinical guidelines to secure consistent, high-quality, evidence-based care for patients using the NHS.

Medicines and Healthcare Products Regulatory Agency (**www.gov.uk**)

The Medicines and Healthcare Products Regulatory Agency (MHRA) is an executive agency of the Department of Health and Social Care in the United Kingdom which is responsible for ensuring that medicines and medical devices work and are acceptably safe.

www.nice.org.uk/

The National Institute for Health and Care Excellence (NICE) is an executive non-departmental public body of the Department of Health in England, which publishes guidelines in four countries in the UK. The site provides practitioners with a readily accessible summary of the current evidence base and practical guidance on best practice.

Pain | Subject Guide | Royal College of Nursing (**rcn.org.uk**)

RCN subject guides are a useful and easy to navigate resources to find current evidence-based practice.

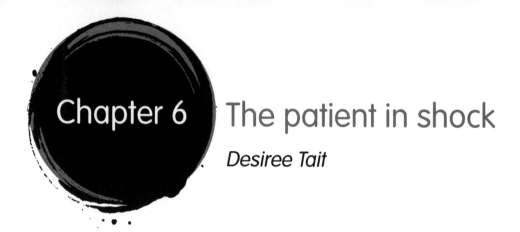

Chapter 6   The patient in shock

Desiree Tait

NMC Future Nurse: Standards of Proficiency for Registered Nurses

This chapter will address the following platforms and proficiencies:

Platform 3: Assessing needs and planning care

Registered nurses prioritise the needs of people when assessing and reviewing their mental, physical, cognitive, behavioural, social, and spiritual needs. They use information obtained during assessments to identify the priorities and requirements for person-centred and evidence-based nursing interventions and support. They work in partnership with people to develop person-centred care plans that take into account their circumstances, characteristics and preferences.

At the point of registration, the registered nurse will be able to:

3.2   demonstrate and apply knowledge of body systems and homeostasis, human anatomy and physiology, biology, genomics, pharmacology and social and behavioural sciences when undertaking full and accurate person-centred nursing assessments and developing appropriate care plans.

3.9   recognise and assess people at risk of harm and the situations that may put them at risk, ensuring prompt action is taken to safeguard those who are vulnerable.

Chapter aims

By the end of this chapter, you should be able to:

- describe and identify clinical situations that lead to the syndrome of shock;
- describe the clinical features of hypovolaemic, distributive, cardiogenic, and obstructive shock;

- differentiate between and diagnose possible causes of patient deterioration as it relates to the four types of shock;
- demonstrate how to assess, record, and respond to patients at risk of hypovolaemic shock using a person-centred approach;
- reflect on clinical examples illustrated in the chapter and apply this to your own clinical situation.

Introduction

Shock can be described as any situation that leads to a failure of the circulatory system to perfuse organs, tissues, and cells in the body; a situation where there is a mismatch between the supply and demand of oxygen. If this situation continues without intervention the person will die. Rapid assessment and recognition of a deteriorating patient, assessment of possible cause, and interventions to support oxygen supply and circulation are vital. This chapter provides an overview of the general causes and clinical manifestations of shock syndromes and examines in detail the care of a patient with **hypovolaemic shock**. The underlying physiology, social psychology, and ethical implications of the patient's care will be discussed in the context of risk assessment and collaborative management of care. The chapter proceeds with an overview of the knowledge and skills required to assess, differentiate, and manage the care of patients who present with shock. The assessment and management of patients with cardiogenic shock are discussed in Chapter 4, and patients with distributive shock, including sepsis and **septic shock**, are discussed in detail in Chapter 7.

What is shock and why does it occur?

Shock can be defined as any situation that leads to a failure of the circulatory system to perfuse organs, tissues, and cells in the body. Reduced tissue perfusion means that oxygen and nutrients are not reaching the tissues to meet demand and consequently cells, tissues, and organs begin to fail. Reduced tissue perfusion regardless of cause can result in shock, organ failure, and death (Martin et al., 2019; Standl et al., 2018).

For example, if a patient has a haemorrhage and loses 30% of their total blood volume, they will have reduced levels of circulating blood to transport oxygen and nutrients to the body's cells, leading to a very low oxygen concentration in the tissues (**dysoxia**). Without the oxygen and nutrients required for normal cell function, the body's organs and tissues will start to fail. Initially, the patient's physiological systems will try to compensate by triggering the sympathetic nervous system and the flight/fight response.

We tend to see the flight/fight response as a biological response that is triggered in situations of perceived stress when the body will focus on providing energy and resources to the brain, heart, and muscles to aid either running away from danger or standing and fighting. In the case of a haemorrhaging patient, the response is designed to keep the blood supply flowing to the vital organs. If the cause of blood loss is not diagnosed and treated, the patient will continue to deteriorate and move to the progressive stage of shock, or uncompensated shock, when the patient is no longer able to compensate for blood lost (the key stages are set out in Table 6.3 later in this chapter). At this stage the body is using all its reserves to try to maintain homeostasis, and if left untreated, the refractory stage of shock will be reached – the point when the body organs start to malfunction due to tissue hypoxia. You will come across shock in many clinical situations and different locations. A person may go into shock for several reasons, for example, physical trauma, dehydration, sepsis, anaphylaxis, haemorrhage, and acute cardiac failure. Such situations can occur in the person's home, outside, and in any hospital or care setting. The types of clinical shock can be classified into four categories according to the underlying clinical cause and have been described by Standl et al. (2018) as hypovolaemic, distributive, cardiogenic, and obstructive shock:

- **Hypovolaemic shock:** due to decreased circulating blood volume and includes:
  - haemorrhagic shock resulting from acute haemorrhage and/or in the presence of injury;
  - hypovolaemic shock resulting from loss of circulating volume without haemorrhage, such as in dehydration.
- **Distributive shock:** caused by altered distribution of blood in the central and peripheral circulation and includes:
  - septic shock resulting from a 'dysregulated response by the body to an infection' (Singer et al., 2016) (see Chapter 7);
  - anaphylactic and anaphylactoid shock that occurs because of either an acute systemic reaction to an allergen or by a physical or chemical hypersensitivity reaction to a specific trigger such as X-ray contrast media;
  - neurogenic shock due to widespread vasodilation associated with autonomic dysfunction (Martin et al., 2019);
- **cardiogenic shock** due to impaired cardiac function;
- **obstructive shock** caused by an obstruction to the circulating blood flow leading to impaired cardiac function.

All these situations will result in insufficient blood flow, and therefore oxygen and nutrients, to the cells. Table 6.1 lists the categories and common causes of shock in each category, with some clinical examples.

Table 6.2 provides a summary of the clinical features that are present when patients are diagnosed with a particular type of shock.

Categories of shock	Causes of shock	Clinical examples
Hypovolaemic shock associated with loss of fluid volume	Decreased blood/plasma/interstitial/cellular fluid volume due to the following: • Haemorrhage: External haemorrhage. Internal haemorrhage. • Trauma and fractures. • Hypovolaemic fluid volume loss. • Severe vomiting and diarrhoea. • Dehydration. • Major burns.	• Tom was stabbed in the leg and sustained an estimated blood loss of 750 ml. • Terry Jones was admitted with haematemesis and melaena and was diagnosed with a bleeding peptic ulcer. • Bill Holland sustained a fractured shaft of the femur in a road traffic collision. • Meera has food poisoning and has experienced vomiting and diarrhoea for 48 hours. • Betty slipped and fell and has been lying on her kitchen floor for two days with no food or water. • Jane was trapped in her car as it caught fire and she sustained 80% burns.
Distributive shock associated with a shift in distribution of fluid volume leading to relative hypovolaemia	• *Sepsis* is 'life-threatening organ dysfunction caused by a dysregulated host response to infection. Septic shock is a subset of sepsis in which underlying circulatory and cellular/metabolic abnormalities are profound enough to substantially increase mortality' (Singer et al., 2016). • *Anaphylactic shock* triggered by antibody activation and histamine-mediated vasodilation (Standl et al., 2018). • Neurogenic shock caused by: • cervical spinal cord injury leading to impaired function of the sympathetic nervous system and balance of the autonomic system; • general anaesthesia/sedation causing depression of the respiratory and circulatory system.	• Angela had been admitted to the ward in a confused state, with severe hypotension and a diagnosis of sepsis secondary to a urinary tract infection. Within an hour Angela's condition had deteriorated (R 28, SpO$_2$ 90%, HR 100, BP 80/50) and she was admitted to ITU with septicaemic shock (see Chapter 7). • Helen was admitted to A&E in a collapsed state after being stung by a bee 20 minutes earlier. • Paul sustained injuries to his cervical spine and spinal cord as the result of his car overturning. His vital signs were R 10, SpO$_2$ 90%, HR 50, BP 80/40. • Mary had been given a general anaesthetic for a surgical procedure, following which she had difficulty waking up. Her vitals signs were R 10, SpO$_2$ 92%, HR 55, BP 84/52.

(Continued)

Table 6.1 (Continued)

Categories of shock	Causes of shock	Clinical examples
Cardiogenic shock associated with pump failure	A critical reduction in the ability for the heart to pump, caused by either systolic (reduced contraction and ejection capacity) or diastolic dysfunction (impaired ventricular filling capacity). • Myocardial infarction (MI) – blocking of a coronary artery. • Myocardial contusion – bruising of the heart muscle. • Structural defects such as a ventricular septal defect – a hole in the wall of the septum between the right and left ventricles. • Cardiac arrhythmias – narrow and broad complex tachycardia.	• Harry Smith has been diagnosed with an anterior MI and when admitted to hospital he has: R 26, SpO$_2$ 95%, HR 98, BP 80/45. He is diagnosed with cardiogenic shock (see case study in Chapter 4). • Bill Holland sustained severe trauma to his sternum and myocardial contusion from the seat belt following a road traffic collision. He is breathless. Vital signs: R 26, SpO$_2$ 90%, tachycardic, HR 110, BP <90 systolic. • Fred recovered well from an ST elevation MI until two weeks after treatment, when he collapsed and was diagnosed with a ventricular septal defect secondary to an MI. • Jane was experiencing repeated episodes of broad complex tachycardia (HR 190), she was breathless with a rate of 25 bpm, SpO$_2$ 92%, and her blood pressure had fallen to 80/35.
Obstructive shock associated with obstruction of the great vessels leading from and to the heart and/or obstruction of the heart leading to reduced cardiac output	Obstruction to the circulating blood flow due to the following: • Cardiac *tamponade* – bleeding or fluid between the myocardial and pericardial layers of the heart, causing the heart to be squashed. • Pulmonary *embolus* – obstruction of oxygenated blood flowing back to the left side of the heart. • Tension *pneumothorax* – air leaking and trapped between the pleural layers of the lungs causing the lungs and heart to become squashed in the thoracic cavity.	• Bert was one hour into his post-operative care following cardiac surgery when he collapsed, becoming breathless and disorientated. His vital signs were R 26, SpO$_2$ 92%, HR 120, BP 60/30. He had a cardiac tamponade which was immediately relieved by pericardial drainage. • Jamila had been complaining at home of a red and swollen leg for two days when she collapsed with chest pain and breathlessness. A deep vein thrombosis in her leg had travelled in the circulation to the lungs causing an obstruction in blood flow (pulmonary embolism). The clot was thrombolised and she made a good recovery. • Sarah was a passenger on a flight from London to Florida when she suddenly experienced severe difficulty with breathing and she felt faint and dizzy. The change in pressure during the flight had caused a tension pneumothorax in her right lung. A medic was on board who was able to insert a temporary thoracic drain to restore optimum respiratory and cardiac function.

Table 6.1 Categories and common causes of shock

Assessment	Hypovolaemic	Cardiogenic	Obstructive	Septic	Anaphylactic	Neurogenic
					Distributive	
Airway	Is there evidence of bleeding or obstruction to the airways? Is there evidence of stridor?	Is there acute pulmonary oedema present which may impair the airway?	In severe cases the patient may go into cardiac arrest – follow basic life support guidance.	Assess airway in the context of the patient's position and in the presence of nausea and vomiting.	Redness and swelling on face and neck leading to the potential for respiratory obstruction and respiratory stridor. Requires immediate treatment with adrenaline and airway protection.	Assess for risk of airway associated with GCS and level of consciousness. If GCS is <8 protect the airway and consider the risk of a cervical injury.
Breathing	Tachypnea Reduced SpO_2, depending on cause and stage of shock Evidence of hypoxia noted on ABG analysis in the progressive stage	Tachypnea Breathlessness Reduced SpO_2 Hypoxia on ABG analysis Central and peripheral cyanosis	Tachypnea Breathlessness Reduced SpO_2 Hypoxia on ABG analysis Central and peripheral cyanosis	Tachypnea Breathlessness Reduced SpO_2 Hypoxia on ABG analysis Central and peripheral cyanosis	Tachypnea Reduced SpO_2 Hypoxia on ABG analysis Central and peripheral cyanosis as shock progresses	Slow (bradypnea) and/or shallow breathing Look for evidence of diaphragmatic breathing if the patient has a cervical injury Reduced SpO_2 Hypoxia as shock progresses
Circulation	Looks pale Dry mouth, sunken eyes related to dehydration Thirst Evidence of traumatic blood loss	Looks cold and clammy to touch Central and peripheral cyanosis Tachycardia BP <90 mm systolic pressure	Skin cool and clammy to touch Central and peripheral cyanosis Tachycardia Hypotension <90 mm systolic pressure	Skin warm to touch but this may progress to cold peripheries, central and peripheral cyanosis Tachycardia P 91–130/min Hypotension <90 systolic BP	Skin looks red and initially warm to touch, but later clammy Central cyanosis Tachycardia Hypotension <90 mm Systolic	Skin dry and warm to touch Bradycardia Hypotension <90 mm systolic Reduced urine output – consider risk of AKI

(Continued)

Table 6.2 (Continued)

Assessment	Hypovolaemic	Cardiogenic	Obstructive	Septic	Distributive	
					Anaphylactic	Neurogenic
	Tachycardia Hypotension Reduced CVP Reduced urine output – consider risk of AKI Metabolic acidosis on ABG analysis	Cardiac arrhythmias Elevated CVP Reduced urine output – consider risk of AKI	Cardiac arrhythmias Reduced CVP Reduced urine output – consider risk of AKI	Reduced CVP Metabolic acidosis Lactate >2 mmol/L Reduced urine output – oliguria Temperature <36 °C White cell count above or below the norm or other clinical signs of infection	Reduced CVP Reduced urine output – consider risk of AKI	
Disability	ACVPU: New confusion in the progressive stage and present in severe dehydration. Assess pain relative to underlying cause	ACVPU: New confusion in the progressive stage Assess pain relative to underlying cause	ACVPU: New confusion in the progressive stage Assess pain relative to underlying cause	ACVPU: New confusion in the progressive stage Assess pain relative to underlying cause	Fear/anxiety Deterioration in GCS Assess pain relative to underlying cause	Assess GCS – review sedation or anaesthetic medication if prescribed recently Assess pain relative to underlying cause
Exposure	Assess for signs of recent trauma and/or fluid loss through vomiting and diarrhoea	Assess for signs of peripheral oedema Assess for: • History of previous cardiac or circulatory events • Hypertension • Diabetes	Assess for recent history of: • Penetrating trauma leading to a tension pneumothorax or cardiac tamponade • DVT • Very recent cardiac surgery	Assess for signs of recent infection: • Respiratory • Brain • Urine • Surgical • Skin/joint/wound • Indwelling lines or catheters Assess for history of impaired immunity	Blistering/wheals/ pruritis Assess exposure to an allergen Assess exposure to X-ray contrast media Initiate treatment immediately	Assess for recent history of: • Trauma • General anaesthesia • Sedation

Table 6.2 A summary of the clinical features found on assessment of patients with different types of shock using ABCDE assessment

If any of these signs are present the patient is at risk. They should be assessed using NEWS2 criteria (RCP, 2017) and sepsis screening and you should communicate your concerns using SBAR (Chapters 2 and 7).

Activity 6.1   Reflection

With reference to Tables 6.1 and 6.2, think back to your experiences in the clinical setting and identify examples of situations where patients have been diagnosed as being in shock.

- Are any of the clinical situations you identified listed in Table 6.1?
- Did the patient deteriorate suddenly or over a period of several hours?
- What clinical signs and features were present to indicate your patient was in shock?

Hint: These reflective questions will help you to practise linking the causes and types of shock to the signs and symptoms present in the patients you have nursed.

As this answer is based on your own reflection, there is no outline answer at the end of the chapter.

Shock, regardless of the cause, has a high incidence of morbidity and mortality that increases as the length of time between the onset of clinical deterioration and treatment increases. Early recognition and anticipation of the potential for patients to develop shock is a key nursing activity that can lead to reduced morbidity and mortality of patients in your care (NICE, 2021a; RCP, 2017).

What are the stages and signs of shock?

In health, the balance between the body's physiological systems is maintained through homeostasis. This process involves the purposeful control and maintenance of the body's organs so that normal body functions can continue efficiently. These integrated systems usually operate through negative feedback systems. These are physiological control mechanisms that respond to a change in the normal range of a substance by triggering other mechanisms until the uncontrolled substance is back within normal range (Hall, 2016). The effects can be manifested through physical, emotional, and behavioural reactions to a stressor, such as haemorrhage. For example, using negative feedback, a fall in blood pressure will be identified by pressure sensors (baroreceptors) in the aorta and carotid arteries. A message will be sent to the brain via the autonomic nervous system that triggers the body to resist the fall in blood pressure by causing blood vessels in the peripheral circulation to constrict (patient becomes pale). Consequently, the volume of blood in the central circulation will increase and ensure that the heart, brain, and muscles receive oxygen. If the underlying cause of inadequate tissue perfusion is not corrected, the flight/fight response, together with the **renin-angiotensin-aldosterone system**, is able to continue to support and compensate for impaired circulation and uptake of oxygen by increasing the pulse and respiratory rate, preserving body fluids by reducing urine output, and attempting to maintain an effective supply of blood and oxygen to the tissues. This is known as the **compensatory stage of shock** (Hall, 2016). Diagnosis, support, and management of the underlying cause can reverse the progression of shock at this stage.

If the underlying cause continues to be left untreated, the compensatory mechanisms will be unable to maintain effective circulation, and the patient will collapse. Inadequate circulation leads to ischaemia (decreased blood supply to the tissues) and **tissue dysoxia**. Without an adequate supply of oxygen, the cells will no longer be able to function effectively and will start to fail. This is known as the **progressive stage of shock** (Hall, 2016). When a patient enters the progressive stage of shock, they are critically ill and need intensive support. It is during this stage that organ failure, such as acute renal failure and acute lung injury, is likely to occur. Even with intensive support of the body's systems, the damage to body organs is likely to continue, leading to multiple organ and tissue dysfunction. This is known as the **refractory stage or irreversible stage** (Hall, 2016) when shock becomes irreversible, and the patient is likely to die.

Regardless of the type and cause of shock, if the patient does not receive immediate and appropriate interventions, the ultimate outcome will be the same. However, with timely assessment and intervention, the effects of shock can be reversed before the patient progresses to the final and irreversible stage. The three stages of shock are presented in Table 6.3.

Hypovolaemic shock

Assessment and management of patients with hypovolaemic shock

As we have seen, hypovolaemic shock occurs because of the loss of a critical volume of blood, plasma, or extracellular fluid. In a healthy adult male weighing 70 kg the total blood volume is an estimated 4,900 ml (70 ml of blood/kg). This is the volume required to maintain an effective circulation (Maiden and Peake, 2019). If a patient loses up to 10% of their circulating volume, the body will respond and compensate by the movement of interstitial fluid into the circulation and no obvious clinical signs are evident. However, if the loss continues unabated, clinical signs will become evident when approximately 15% loss is reached (Martin et al., 2019). The greater the volume of loss, the more significant the clinical effects become, and cardiac output decreases exponentially (Hall, 2016). When cardiac output falls, this means that there is a reduced volume of blood being pumped into the systemic circulation every minute. To try to increase the volume and establish stability, the body will increase the heart rate. However, with a continuing loss of blood or body fluids, the body will find the task of compensating

Stages of shock	Physiological and clinical progress	Patient example
1. Non-progressive or compensatory stage	The body systems can compensate for the clinical trigger or cause. Shock is reversible with assessment and intervention. Compensation of circulation occurs by negative feedback: baroreceptors identify a reduction in blood pressure and stimulate the sympathetic nervous system (SNS) to increase: • respiratory rate • heart rate • cardiac output. Reduction in blood flow to the kidneys triggers the renin-angiotensin-aldosterone system to further stimulate SNS, release adrenaline and noradrenaline from the adrenal medulla, aldosterone triggers the retention of sodium and fluid in the body, leading to a reduction in urine output. The pituitary gland is stimulated to release vasopressin, leading to further peripheral vaso-constriction and reduction in urine output. Circulatory homeostasis is restored.	Mrs Brown has had a two-day history of severe diarrhoea and vomiting. Her GP recorded her vital signs as: R: 18/min; P: 92/min; BP: 110/65. These were within the normal range; however, if her symptoms continued to persist, she could go into hypovolaemic shock. He prescribes an intramuscular injection of anti-emetic to reduce the vomiting and suggests she contact the surgery again tomorrow if she feels no better. The following day Mrs Brown's vital signs have deteriorated. The vomiting has subsided but the diarrhoea persists. She is now anxious, cold to touch, and thirsty. Her vital signs are: R: 20/min; P: 100/min; BP: 89/58. So far, her body is just managing to compensate for her loss of fluid but there is some deterioration. Mrs Brown now requires fluid replacement, hence her feeling thirsty. If she is unable to tolerate oral fluids, she will require intravenous fluid resuscitation in order to prevent further deterioration.
2. Progressive stage	The underlying cause and impact persists. Physiologically the body has used all the compensatory mechanisms available to return to homeostasis and this has failed to compensate, and inadequate tissue perfusion continues. This leads to decreased cardiac output, decreased blood pressure, and decreased systemic blood flow to the tissues. The resultant tissue ischaemia/hypoxia leads to: • anaerobic cell metabolism • increased lactic acid production • metabolic acidosis	Mrs Brown was taken to the A&E unit where an assessment showed evidence of further deterioration. She was confused and agitated. She had not passed urine for 24 hours. Her vital signs were: R: 24/min; SpO$_2$ 90%; P: 110/min; BP: 80/50. Mrs Brown received fluid resuscitation and management of the underlying cause. Her condition improved and within four days she was discharged home.

(Continued)

Table 6.3 (Continued)

Stages of shock	Physiological and clinical progress	Patient example
	• further depression of myocardial function • inflammatory response • slow and sluggish blood flow in the microcirculation • tissue necrosis • increased capillary permeability • electrolyte imbalance leading to increased risk of disseminated intravascular coagulation, acute respiratory distress syndrome (ARDS), AKI, and liver failure. Shock is reversible in the early stages with appropriate assessment and management.	
3. Refractory or irreversible stage	Physiologically the toxic effects of acidosis, inflammatory mediators, and destructive enzymes lead to cell death, tissue death, and multiple organ dysfunction. Beyond a certain point the excessive amount of tissue damage sustained in progressive shock will lead to death. Refractory shock is irreversible.	If Mrs Brown had NOT contacted her GP and been referred to A&E in a timely manner her condition would have continued to deteriorate and, without support, she would have become severely dehydrated leading to deterioration of her circulation, GCS, and body systems. Her vital signs would have continued to deteriorate and, left unsupported, she would have developed refractory hypovolaemic shock.

Table 6.3 The stages of shock, illustrated by a clinical example

for the loss more difficult. Table 6.4 illustrates the physiological impact of hypovolaemic shock caused by haemorrhage on the patient's clinical features, based on percentage of blood loss. It is important to note that assessing patients based only on percentage of blood loss provides a limited amount of information and a complete assessment of other factors that affect the patient's oxygen delivery, such as a patient's co-morbidities and medications, should also be completed (Bersten and Handy, 2019). External blood loss leading to hypovolaemia can be measured through visual estimation on examination of the patient and environment. For example, a patient with bleeding oesophageal varices (ruptured blood vessels in the oesophagus) will have a recent history of acute and severe haematemesis. When bleeding is internal, the pattern of evidence is more complex and can only be estimated based on a physiological understanding of the patient's condition and following a clinical assessment and examination of the patient. For example, a patient with a fractured shaft of the femur can have an estimated blood and fluid loss of up to 2,000 ml, while a patient with a traumatic fracture of the tibia can lose an estimated 800 ml into the surrounding interstitial tissue around the site of the fracture. In this example, both patients have a risk of developing shock, but the patient with a fractured shaft of femur will have a much higher risk of going into shock within 30 minutes of injury than the patient with a fractured tibia. This will be manifested by evidence of patient anxiety, pale cool skin, tachycardia, tachypnoea, and reduced blood pressure and pulse pressure (difference measured between the systolic and diastolic BP).

Other causes of hypovolaemic shock are listed in Table 6.1 and include a variety of clinical conditions associated with acute loss of blood, plasma, or extracellular fluid. Patients with diarrhoea and vomiting, fever, and dehydration all experience fluid loss associated with loss of body fluids. Patients with severe burns experience loss of body fluids and plasma, and this is explained in more detail in Chapter 10. Patients who experience third space fluid shift movements suffer loss of fluid available to support the circulation. Fluid shifts into a space where it would not normally collect in such large volumes, such as with peritonitis, when fluid shifts into the peritoneal cavity, and with pancreatitis and ileus, when fluid shifts into the gastrointestinal cavity (Hall, 2016).

On assessment	No clinical evidence of shock	Compensated	Progressive	Refractory
Loss of blood or body fluid volume	0–15%, 750 ml	15–30%, 750–1,500 ml	30–40%, 1,500–2,000 ml	>40%, >2,000 ml
Measure respiratory rate	Unchanged	Tachypnea	Tachypnea	Increasing tachypnea
Observe Skin	No evidence of change	Cool skin	Pale, cool	Pale, cold to touch, central cyanosis
Measure heart rate	Unchanged	Tachycardia	Tachycardia	Increasing tachycardia
Measure pulse pressure	Unchanged	Reduced	Reduced	Reduced

(Continued)

Table 6.4   (Continued)

On assessment	No clinical evidence of shock	Compensated	Progressive	Refractory
Measure blood pressure	Unchanged	Reduced BP	Hypotension systolic arterial pressure (SAP) of <90 mmHg	Severe hypotension, SAP <70 mmHg
Measure urine output	unchanged	Reduced	Oliguria	Oliguria progressing to anuria
Disability ACVPU/GCS	Anxious	Anxious, agitated	Confused and agitated	Deteriorating ACVPU and GCS

Table 6.4   Stages of hypovolaemic shock based on percentage of blood/fluid loss for a 70 kg male, with examples of clinical signs at each stage

Source: informed by Mutschler et al., 2013 and Hooper and Armstrong, 2021.

When assessing patients with a history of excessive fluid loss it is important to assess factors such as evidence of the person feeling thirsty, dehydration, including dry mucus membranes, dry furred tongue, and sunken eyeballs. Clinical signs can determine the severity of the patient's condition and also the likely cause. Assessing and communicating all the clinical signs and information collated to the care team can improve the patient's potential for recovery and should be undertaken using a comprehensive and systematic approach recommended by NICE (2021a) and illustrated in Chapter 1. Your role as a nurse in assessing, anticipating, and interpreting the signs of a patient going into shock cannot be overestimated. In the remainder of the chapter, we have used the case study of Megan James to explore in detail the pathophysiology of shock and the nurse's role in assessing, recognising, and managing a patient as she progresses through each stage of hypovolaemic shock.

Case study: Megan's story

Sophie, a second-year student nurse, was responsible for the management of six patients on a surgical ward under the supervision of her practice facilitator. One of the patients in her care was Megan James, a 75-year-old woman who had been admitted that day with acute abdominal pain and nausea. Megan had a history of ischaemic heart disease and was routinely prescribed ACE inhibitors, statins, and aspirin 75 mg. She had been assessed by the surgical registrar, and the agreed plan was to withhold oral intake, commence intravenous fluids, manage pain relief, and monitor her progress. Megan's mouth was dry and her lips were cracked. Her blood results on admission were within the normal range and included the following: Na, 135 mmol/L; K, 4.1 mmol/L; creatinine, 75 μmol/L, and venous lactate, 1.7 mmol/L. Based on this information and Megan's two-day history of reduced fluid intake, the medical team prescribed sodium chloride 0.18% and glucose 4% at 83 ml/hour. This is consistent with NICE (2017b) guidance on fluid therapy. Sophie, on the advice of her mentor, commenced four hourly observations of her vital signs but two hours later she went to check on Megan and noticed a change in her condition.

- Megan seemed to be more restless and mildly agitated, she said 'I don't feel very well nurse'.
- R: increased from 18/min to 20/min.
- SpO_2: decreased from 97% to 96%.
- She looked pale and her hands were cold.
- Temp: 36.9 °C (no change).
- HR: increased from 90/min to 93/min.
- BP: decreased from 120/90 mmHg to 115/87 mmHg.
- Has passed urine since admission (100 ml).
- NEWS2: increased from 0 to 1 (agitation not added to the score).

Sophie shared the NEWS2 score with her practice facilitator, who reminded her that the NEWS2 was within the normal range, but if she was worried then monitor the patient more frequently. Sophie felt concerned and contacted the house officer to tell him of the change in NEWS2 (National Early Warning Score 2 – see Chapter 1). He suggested that she should keep monitoring Megan and that they would review her on the medical round later that day. Sophie decided (on her own initiative) to increase Megan's observations to hourly even though the NEWS2 indicated a low risk. Sophie was worried but she wasn't sure why.

Risk assessment, pathophysiology, and priorities of care for patients at risk of hypovolaemic shock

The way a person responds to loss of circulating volume is influenced by a number of factors. These include the cause and severity of the stressor or trauma (trigger/cause), the age of the patient, their co-morbidities, and medications. For example, the physiological effects of ageing can impact negatively on skin integrity, the musculoskeletal system, and immune system; this leads to an increased risk of the patient having multiple pathologies and increased susceptibility to the effects of shock (Bersten and Handy, 2019). In Megan's case she had been unwell for several days with abdominal pain, nausea, and indigestion and during that time she had only taken sips of water and was dehydrated. Megan had been taking 75 mg aspirin for ten years as part of her routine medication as well as anti-hypertensive drugs and statins to reduce her cholesterol. According to the BNF (2021), the side effects of aspirin include gastrointestinal haemorrhage (occasionally major), and with Megan's presenting history this should have been identified as a possible cause of her pain although there was no documented evidence of this in her medical or nursing notes.

As we have seen, a person can lose up to 15% of their circulating volume before any clinical signs become evident as fluid lost to the circulation is replaced by the movement of interstitial fluid into the central circulation. In mild fluid loss, any reduction in the volume of circulating blood is detected by pressure-sensitive baro-receptors in the arterial circulation. These receptors are in the arch of the aorta and carotid sinuses. When the receptors are triggered, impulses are relayed to the respiratory and cardiovascular centre in the medulla oblongata (brain stem), where they effect changes via the sympathetic nervous system: to increase the heart rate and force of cardiac contraction, trigger peripheral vasoconstriction, and improve blood pressure. This trigger mechanism is illustrated in Figure 6.1. In Megan's story this response was demonstrated when Sophie noticed a slight reduction in Megan's systolic blood pressure and a corresponding slight increase in her respiratory rate and pulse. Sophie risk assessed her patient using NEWS2 and identified that while physiological changes were present, they had occurred within the accepted range and, according to NEWS2, a score of 1 meant no escalation of care was required. At the time Megan had also become more restless and agitated, but Sophie had been unable to connect the subtle changes in her patient's behaviour to clinical deterioration; she was worried but didn't know why. According to the RCP (2017), evidence of agitation, confusion, and/or disorientation gives cause for concern and adds a score of 3 to the aggregated score. This would increase Megan's aggregate score from 1 to 4 and, together with a single red score (3), should have prompted

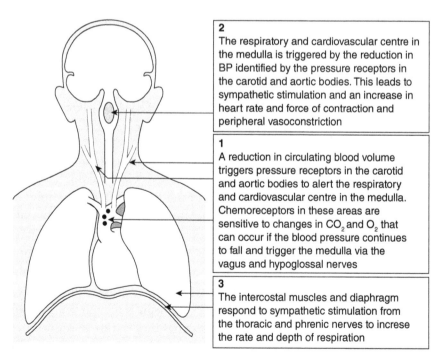

Figure 6.1 The trigger and compensatory feedback mechanisms that occur during the initial stage of shock

an immediate review from a clinician with competencies in acute illness assessment and an increase in the frequency of patient assessment.

This example highlights the importance of undertaking a detailed holistic assessment and clinical interpretation of the patient's situation, as well as having an awareness of the risks associated with the patient's illness. According to Cecconi et al. (2014) in their consensus statement on shock: physical assessment of a patient's skin (perfusion); brain (mental status); and kidneys (urine output) will provide evidence of altered tissue perfusion. They also propose that the presence of hypotension as a single indicator should not be required to define shock. If Sophie had contacted the surgeon using the SBAR approach (see Chapter 1) and given a more detailed assessment of the patient at this stage she could have identified changes in Megan's perfusion (pale skin and cold hands), mental state (anxiety, agitation, and feeling unwell), and subtle changes in her vital signs indicating the initial stage of shock. The importance of nursing skill mix has been identified as being an important factor in reducing patient morbidity and mortality and while students and carers play an important role in recognising deterioration and monitoring acutely ill people, without the support of more senior staff early signs of deterioration can go undetected until the patient becomes critically ill (Aiken et al., 2017; Quirke et al., 2011; James et al., 2010).

What can we learn from Megan's story?

Sophie had identified that Megan's condition was changing, and she had taken some correct steps to increase the monitoring of vital signs, but she had not reported that Megan had become more restless, pale, and agitated. These signs were all indicative of a patient's deteriorating condition. The very slight increase in Megan's NEWS2, without recognising agitation, meant that she was at a low risk and the surgical team did not attend. As a result, both nursing and medical staff had been unable to interpret, communicate and act on the available clinical evidence effectively. Shock is a complex condition that can manifest in many ways and, although Sophie was concerned, she didn't have the knowledge and experience to act on those concerns. To have anticipated Megan's deterioration sooner, Sophie's priorities at this stage should have been to:

- risk assess the patient for the potential to develop shock by reviewing her past and recent medical history;
- identify and understand the signs and symptoms of impending shock;
- be alert to changes in the patient's clinical condition, no matter how small;
- recognise that NEWS2 is useful when identifying a trend in vital signs but is open to interpretation and therefore should always be interpreted in the context of the patient's full clinical condition;
- prevent significant deterioration in a patient's condition by checking the patient more frequently, as illustrated by Sophie above;
- communicate any concerns using an SBAR approach (see Chapter 1);
- act in a timely manner to prevent further deterioration.

The key to successful management of patients in hypovolaemic shock is the assessment and early detection of the problem. The primary aim is to restore circulating volume while attempting to prevent further fluid loss. Fluid resuscitation of patients in hypovolaemic shock is complex and determined by a number of factors that relate to the patient and the primary cause. These include:

- the primary cause and type of fluid lost: blood, plasma, interstitial fluid;
- the age of the patient;
- evidence of co-morbidities such as heart failure, diabetes;
- fluid and electrolyte balance;
- blood glucose (Standl et al., 2018; Cecconi et al., 2014).

In Megan's case her recent history indicated that she was dehydrated and had a past medical history of hypertension and possible impaired cardiac function. She had been unable to take her prescribed anti-hypertensive medication in the last few days and this would have also had an impact on her circulatory system (BNF, 2019). Sophie was correct to feel concerned about Megan and increasing the frequency of her vital signs assessment to hourly allowed her to identify when Megan continued to deteriorate, as the story reveals.

Case study: Megan James's condition deteriorates

One hour later, as Sophie approached Megan to check her vital signs, she realised that her condition had changed significantly.

- Megan appeared pale, peripherally cyanosed, and cold to touch.
- She was agitated, confused, and appeared frightened.
- Within minutes Megan vomited 400 ml liquid that tested positive to blood (coffee ground vomit). She also asked for a bedpan and passed 300 ml of a dark liquid stool that indicated positive to blood.
- R: 25/min
- SpO_2: 91% (on air)
- Core temperature: 37.5 °C
- HR: 115/min.
- BP: 90/70 mmHg
- NEWS2: 14
- 100 ml of urine passed in the last four hours (estimated weight 60 kg)
- ABG: pH: 7.40 (n = 7.35–7.45); PaO_2: 8.9 kPa (n = 10.6–13.3); $PaCO_2$: 4.2 kPa (n = 4.7–6.7); HCO_3: 22.0 mmol/L (n = 25–30)
- Lactate 2.3 mmol/L

Sophie alerted her practice facilitator, and they called the CCOT immediately using an SBAR approach.

Risk assessment, pathophysiology, and priorities of care for the compensatory stage to prevent transition to the progressive stage of shock

The early clinical evidence of compensatory mechanisms at work includes changes in respiratory rate as a result of increased pulse, changes in skin pallor and temperature as a result of peripheral vasoconstriction, and changes in blood pressure. In Megan's case both her respiratory and heart rate have increased and blood pressure decreased. An estimation of urine output over four hours indicates that she has passed the equivalent of 25 ml/hour. Megan, with an estimated weight of 60 kg, should be passing 30 ml/hour, and her reduced urine output of <0.5 ml/kg/hr signifies oliguria (NICE, 2019b). These findings, along with a change in her behaviour and evidence of 700 ml of fluid loss, lead to a diagnosis of hypovolaemic shock with Megan's physiological systems attempting to compensate for the loss of blood volume.

The physiological response that occurs during the compensatory stage is immediate and occurs when adrenergic neurotransmitters stimulate alpha and beta 1 and 2 receptors in the smooth muscle of arterioles, cardiac muscle, and skeletal muscle to increase heart rate, cause peripheral vasoconstriction, and improve blood pressure. Stimulation of the beta 2 receptors also triggers bronchodilation and an added potential to improve lung ventilation by increasing the rate and depth of respiration, as illustrated in Figure 6.1. The sympathetic nervous system also triggers the adrenal medulla to release the catecholamines adrenaline and noradrenaline (epinephrine and norepinephrine), to continue providing the compensatory response, and this is illustrated in Figure 6.2. These are examples of negative feedback mechanisms that are used to restore homeostasis (Hall, 2016).

This stimulation of a sympathetic neural response occurs in most types of shock as part of the flight/fight response explained earlier, apart from distributive shock. For example, in neurogenic shock the sympathetic response may be impaired by spinal injury,

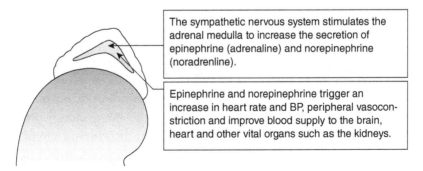

The sympathetic nervous system stimulates the adrenal medulla to increase the secretion of epinephrine (adrenaline) and norepinephrine (noradrenline).

Epinephrine and norepinephrine trigger an increase in heart rate and BP, peripheral vasoconstriction and improve blood supply to the brain, heart and other vital organs such as the kidneys.

Figure 6.2   The triggering of the adrenal medulla that occurs during the compensatory stage of shock

nerve injury, or drugs such as general anaesthetic (Martin et al., 2019). In septic shock and anaphylactic shock, the sympathetic response is challenged by a severe inflammatory response and systemic vasodilation (Martin et al., 2019). Table 6.2 provides a comparison of the different features of shock found on clinical assessment and illustrates that the cause of shock can influence the early signs and symptoms.

In Megan's case the release of catecholamines, in the form of epinephrine (adrenaline) and norepinephrine (noradrenaline), continue to affect the alpha and beta receptors and thus continue the adrenergic response. The net effect of this is to increase respiratory rate and depth, increase heart rate, and improve blood flow to the coronary arteries, skeletal muscle, heart, and brain through stimulation of the beta-adrenergic receptors. The stimulation of alpha receptors continues to increase peripheral resistance by causing peripheral vasoconstriction, leading to coolness and pallor of the skin. Figures 6.1 and 6.2 illustrate the mechanisms involved in the initial and compensatory response, and Figure 6.3 illustrates the other mechanisms involved in providing physiological compensation.

The initial fall in blood pressure also triggers a renal and a neural/adrenergic response. This response is described as the renin-angiotensin-aldosterone mechanism. Renin is an enzyme that is produced and stored in the juxtaglomerular cells of the kidneys. The juxtaglomerular cells are sensitive to changes in the responses of the sympathetic nervous system, and a reduction in blood flow to the kidneys will release renin into the circulation. Once in the circulation, renin triggers the activation of **angiotensin I** from an inactive circulating protein. Angiotensin I is then converted by an enzyme called angiotensin converting enzyme (ACE) that is found in the lungs and kidney endothelial cells to **angiotensin II**, as the blood flows through the pulmonary circulation. Once activated, angiotensin II affects short- and long-term regulation of blood pressure.

- In short-term regulation, angiotensin II:
  - causes a vasoconstrictor effect on arterioles leading to increased peripheral vascular resistance and peripheral shutdown;
  - reduces sodium excretion from the kidneys so that the body retains more sodium and water.
- In long-term regulation, angiotensin II stimulates **aldosterone** secretion from the adrenal cortex. Aldosterone increases sodium and water retention by the kidneys. This increases the volume of extracellular fluid and circulating volume.

Another hormonal response triggered by reduced circulating volume and increased plasma **osmolarity** (increased concentration of salts) is **antidiuretic hormone (ADH)** or **vasopressin**. When triggered, vasopressin is released from the posterior pituitary gland and has a powerful vasoconstrictor effect on arterioles in the systemic circulation (Hall, 2016). Vasopressin also has an antidiuretic effect and increases absorption of water from the kidneys in response to increased plasma osmolarity. These mechanisms are summarised in Figure 6.3.

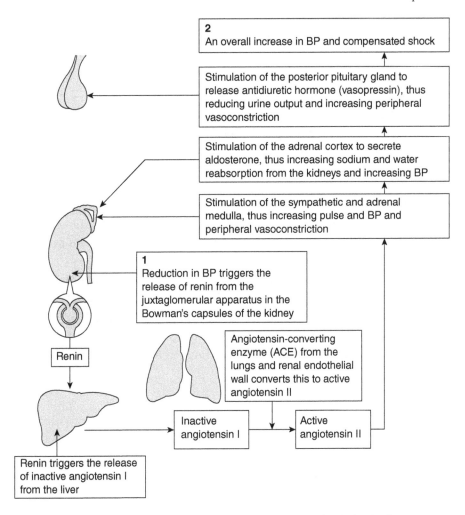

Figure 6.3 The compensatory mechanisms that occur as a physiological response to compensated shock

For Megan this meant that her peripheral temperature was cold, and there was evidence of peripheral shutdown and peripheral cyanosis (blue-tinged nails on her hands and feet). Her reduction in oxygen saturation suggests reduced perfusion and oxygenation of the peripheral circulation due to loss of circulating blood volume, and her reduced urine output is indicative of the renin-angiotensin-aldosterone mechanism and antidiuretic hormone (vasopressin). The triggering of the stress response also led to an increase in her metabolic rate manifested by an increase in her blood lactate levels as the demand for oxygen began to outstrip supply due to reduced perfusion. According to Marik (2015), as the amount of epinephrine released by the adrenal gland as part of the stress response in shock continues, so the amount of lactate produced, as a by-product of metabolism, will increase.

Case study: Risk assessing Megan at the compensatory stage of shock

The outreach team was called and following an assessment they concluded that Megan was only just compensating for her fluid loss but because of her age and cardiac history they are concerned that without more physiological support she will move to the progressive stage of shock. The following treatment regime was recommended:

- High-flow oxygen 60%, with the aim of increasing SpO_2 to 94–96%.
- Fluid resuscitation with 500 ml of 0.9% sodium chloride to be given over 15 minutes. This was to be followed by a second ABCDE assessment and further fluid boluses up to a total volume of 2,000 ml (NICE, 2017b). Based on blood lost she was also prescribed two units of blood. Fluid balance to be assessed and reviewed hourly.
- Blood samples were taken for an FBC to determine haemoglobin level (Hb) and group and cross matching; U&E to look for evidence of changes indicative of acute renal failure and an imbalance in electrolytes; LFT; **prothrombin time (PT)** and **activated partial thromboplastin (APPT)** to assess for evidence of deranged clotting.
- A urinary catheter was inserted and a further 50 ml of urine was collected, confirming oliguria.

An emergency endoscopy carried out once Megan had stabilised revealed an actively bleeding duodenal ulcer that was beginning to clot. The location of the bleeding site on the posterior wall of the duodenum made it difficult to clip and the medical team were concerned that there was a 30–40% chance of the site bleeding again based on previous clinical evidence (Simillis and Rashheed, 2019). It was agreed that Megan should be transferred to level 2 (high dependency care) for monitoring and stabilisation of her condition. She was commenced on a proton pump inhibitor via the intravenous route to reduce gastric acidity and the risk of further bleeding and continued to have nothing by mouth. Proton pump inhibitors such as omeprazole block the production of stomach acid by shutting down a system in the stomach cells known as the proton pump, which is responsible for the production of stomach acid (Ritter et al., 2020). Should Megan's condition deteriorate further with evidence of a further bleed, she would require a second endoscopy and possibly surgery.

Risk assessment, pathophysiology, and priorities of care following fluid resuscitation

Case study: Initial improvement in Megan's condition

During the first two hours of Megan's admission to the high dependency unit her condition began to stabilise. On assessment:

- She looked pale, and her hands and feet were still cool to touch.
- She described feeling very tired and she was no longer agitated or confused.
- R: 22/min
- SpO_2: 94% (40% O_2)
- HR: 105/min
- BP: 105/75 mmHg
- Core temp: 37.8 °C
- Urine output: 35 ml/hr
- She has received fluid resuscitation with saline and blood and is now in a positive balance of two litres.
- ABG: pH: 7.32 (n = 7.35–7.45); PaO_2: 9.8 kPa (n = 10.6–13.3); $PaCO_2$: 5.0 kPa (n = 4.7–6.7); HCO_3: 22.0 mmol/L (n = 25–30)
- Lactate: 2.3 mmol/L (n = 0.5–2.0)

The improvement in Megan's condition following her episode of haematemesis and melaena suggests that her peptic ulcer is no longer actively bleeding and that endoscopic haemostasis has led to her condition becoming more stable.

Activity 6.2   Decision making

1. How frequently would you assess Megan's vital signs now that she is feeling better?
2. What clinical signs would indicate that Megan's condition was getting worse?
3. What information would you give Megan at this stage about her condition?

Outline answers to this activity are given at the end of the chapter.

Risk assessment, pathophysiology, and priorities of care for a patient in the progressive stage of shock

Case study: Megan's condition deteriorates

One hour later Megan's condition deteriorated and an ABCDE assessment revealed the following:

- She is pale, peripherally cyanosed, and cold to touch.
- She is confused and drowsy.
- R: 28/min with fast shallow respirations.
- SpO_2: 88% (40% O_2)
- Pulse: 120/min, sinus tachycardia

(Continued)

(Continued)

- BP: 70/48 mmHg
- Vomited 500 ml of altered blood.
- Passed 500 ml of liquid, melaena stools.
- Urine output: 25 ml/hr
- ABG: pH: 7.23 (n = 7.35–7.45); PaO_2: 7.8 kPa (n = 10.6–13.3); $PaCO_2$: 3.8 kPa (n = 4.7–6.7); HCO_3: 15.5 mmol/L (n = 25–30)
- Urea is 11.5 mmol/L (n = 2.5–6.5).
- Creatinine is 155 µmol/L (n = 55–105).
- Lactate is 4.0 mmol/L (n = 0.5–2.0).

The clinical evidence suggests that Megan has had another bleed and is now in the progressive stage of shock. Megan is also showing signs of type I respiratory failure (see Chapter 2). The clinical signs for this include confusion and drowsiness, increased respiratory rate accompanied by oxygen saturations (SpO_2) of less than 90%, and partial pressure of arterial oxygen (PaO_2) levels of less than 8 kPa (O'Driscoll et al., 2017). Megan also has clinical evidence of a metabolic acidosis indicated by the reduced level of pH and bicarbonate in her arterial blood sample. The critical care team concludes that Megan has developed type I respiratory failure secondary to massive blood loss, hypoperfusion, and subsequent metabolic acidosis. The primary cause of her condition is progressive shock induced by a second severe gastrointestinal bleed. This has led to inadequate tissue perfusion of vital organs such as the brain, causing confusion and drowsiness, and the kidneys, leading to acute kidney injury evidenced by reduced urine output and an increasing blood level of creatinine (see Chapter 9 on acute kidney injury).

At this stage the compensatory mechanisms that the body normally recruits as short-term measures to maintain circulation have continued and are becoming detrimental to Megan's wellbeing in a number of ways. According to Hall (2016) and Martin et al. (2019), progressive shock leads to a vicious cycle of cardiac, circulatory, and nervous deterioration triggered by positive feedback loops.

1. The decrease in cardiac output caused by Megan's haemorrhage continues to reduce arterial pressure and reduce systemic blood flow carrying oxygen and nutrients. The myocardium receives blood from the coronary arteries and reduced systemic blood flow reduces oxygen and nutrients to the myocardial cells, leading to weakened cardiac muscle and a further reduction in cardiac output (CO).

2. The continued stimulation of the stress response leads to an increased metabolic demand for oxygen.

3. In the presence of a further reduction in CO the brain and central nervous system receive a diminished blood flow and the sympathetic nervous system is unable to maintain its role in the stress response, leading to vasomotor failure. For Megan a

period of prolonged hypoxia will lead to suppression of the sympathetic nervous response and the cardiac and respiratory centre in the medulla oblongata; and because of the reduced oxygen to the brain Megan's level of consciousness will continue to deteriorate.

4. The continued reduction in CO leads to slow and sluggish blood flow, blocking the micro-circulation and leading to the development of micro-clots.

5. With a marked reduction in oxygen, cells are starved of **adenosine triphosphate (ATP)** production through the aerobic (oxygen dependent) pathway and lack the energy to function effectively.

6. The cells have to rely on a less efficient process of energy production through the anaerobic pathway, which produces about 20% of the energy that is normally acquired through aerobic metabolism.

7. The anaerobic pathway produces carbonic and lactic acids as by-products of metabolism, and this leads to increased acidity in cells and a lactic acidosis. This is evidenced by a raised lactate level and a metabolic acidosis. Megan's respiratory effort has increased in response to the metabolic acidosis in an attempt to compensate for the acidity of the blood. By increasing her respiratory rate she is breathing out more carbon dioxide and water in an attempt to eliminate hydrogen ions (a measure of acidity; see Chapter 3).

8. The inflammatory response is triggered because of the ischaemia, and damage caused by anaerobic metabolism. Consequently, tissues in body organs become damaged and inflamed, leading to an increased risk of acute respiratory distress and impaired renal function.

9. Without energy the normal cell function cannot be maintained, and the cells swell due to the failure of the sodium/potassium pump to maintain the fluid balance inside the cell and increased cell permeability.

10. As shock progresses, the inflammatory mediators, **histamine** and **bradykinin**, exert their vasodilatory properties, leading to progressive hypotension and cellular hypoxia (insufficient supply of oxygen).

As the shock becomes more progressive, tachypnoea, tachycardia, and hypotension will persist, but there will also be evidence of system failure in the form of pulmonary and peripheral oedema, respiratory failure, renal failure (AKI), and cardiac failure, manifested by increased demand for oxygen, central and peripheral cyanosis, decreased urinary output, and confusion. There may also be evidence of paralytic ileus (absence of bowel sounds) and abdominal distension. The patient will have a metabolic acidosis and altered blood clotting because of the hypoxia and inflammatory response.

The extent of cellular and organ damage that occurs in this progressive stage of shock is determined by the severity of the cause and the period your patient spends in the progressive stage. If not reversed, this stage will lead to your patient developing overwhelming cellular damage and destruction, leading to the failure of organs and systems. At this stage the progress of shock becomes irreversible, their body will be unable to respond to supportive therapy and death is inevitable. In Megan's situation, due to her age and co-morbidities, her condition has become critical and at risk of progression to refractory shock.

Case study: Managing Megan's care while in progressive shock

Megan's condition is now critical, and as a result the team decides to increase her respiratory support through intubation and mechanical ventilation with biphasic respiratory support (see Chapter 3) and continue with fluid resuscitation and further transfusions. Once haemodynamically stable, Megan will have a repeat endoscopy to review and stabilise the bleeding duodenal ulcer and continue to be risk assessed for acute kidney injury (see Chapter 9).

Risk assessment, preventing refractory shock

Refractory shock could occur in Megan's case if the critical care team is unable to re-establish haemodynamic stability and prevent the progression of cellular and tissue damage that will ultimately lead to irreversible failure of the respiratory, cardiovascular, hepatic, and renal systems. It is the effect of decreased oxygenation and nutrition, the inflammatory response, and the release of toxins from ischaemic tissue that leads to refractory shock (Hall, 2016). In severe and/or prolonged shock the body is no longer able to compensate for the loss of circulating volume through the negative feedback systems illustrated in Figures 6.1, 6.2, and 6.3 and, instead, reaches a stage where an increase in the degree of shock causes a further increase in the degree of shock (a type of positive feedback) and any supportive therapy becomes incapable of saving a person's life. The priority is always to risk assess patients using the assessment strategies included in this chapter and to prevent the progression of shock before refractory shock can occur.

In Megan's story the critical care team was able to stabilise her haemodynamic state and a second attempt at endoscopic haemostasis was successful. Megan remained in hospital for a further ten days during which her medication was reviewed, and her routine anti-platelet prescription discontinued. We have identified the importance of timing, rapid and accurate risk assessment, and communication when caring for patients in shock. In Activity 6.3, you have an opportunity to practise risk assessment and decision making.

Activity 6.3 Decision making

In your bay you have two patients causing concern.

Mrs Thompson came into hospital for day surgery, but was later admitted to your surgical ward following a history of post-operative nausea and vomiting. Her nausea and vomiting have continued for 12 hours, with limited relief from anti-emetic medication. The surgical team are reluctant to commence any supportive care, such as an infusion, if the patient's nausea will settle with the medication.

Mrs Jacks has not passed urine since her return from theatre six hours ago following a **laparoscopic cholecystectomy**.

1. What would you look for when undertaking a risk assessment of Mrs Thompson?
2. What would you look for when undertaking a risk assessment of Mrs Jacks?
3. What information would you collect before informing the medical team of any concerns you have?

Outline answers for this activity are given at the end of the chapter.

Chapter summary

The aim of this chapter was to help you assess, recognise, and respond to patients who go into shock. We have focused on the assessment and management of patients in hypovolaemic shock. In all the clinical examples illustrated, the key responsibilities of the nurse are the same. They include the following:

- Carry out full ABCDE assessment and monitoring of your patients, including of their history and background. The use of NEWS2 is integral to the ABCDE assessment, but scores should always be assessed in the context of the patient's full situation and condition.
- Know your patients and notice when the situation changes, even when the change is small.
- Ensure timely diagnosis and reporting of changes in the patient's condition: time is of the essence. Any patient who shows a change in their condition that is indicative of hypovolaemic, cardiogenic, obstructive, or distributive shock should be risk assessed.
- Ensure there is continual monitoring and reporting of the patient's condition to the appropriate team.
- If unsure, act and express concern about your patient using the SBAR approach rather than hesitate and lose valuable time.

In Chapter 7 we continue to focus on assessing, recognising, and responding to patients who go into shock, and we discuss the priorities of assessment and screening patients for sepsis and septic shock.

Activities: brief outline answers

Activity 6.2: Decision making (page 171)

1. As Megan has improved and has appeared to stabilise, the temptation is to reduce her observations to two hourly. However, Megan is still at risk of further deterioration and given her co-morbidities it would be advisable to continue to monitor her hourly. If you are

concerned, increase the frequency of observation to half hourly or every 15 minutes and communicate your concern.

2. Look: Listen: Feel: Measure using ABCDE approach: the patient is pale, cool to touch, anxious; has increased respiratory rate, increased heart rate, and reduced blood pressure; the patient is complaining of nausea, vomiting, diarrhoea, haematemesis, and melaena.

3. At this stage in Megan's condition it is important to ask her what she understands about what has happened and explain what has happened and why. She will need reassurance that she is being monitored and being given treatment to promote healing and recovery. You should advise Megan to contact her nurse should she feel nauseated, unwell, faint or want to open her bowels. These are all signs that the ulcer may be actively bleeding.

Activity 6.3: Decision making (page 174)

1. Mrs Thompson has undergone minor surgery but has received nothing by mouth for an estimated 24 hours. She was probably asked to starve from midnight the night before her admission for minor surgery and has been suffering from nausea and vomiting ever since. She is in danger of developing hypovolaemic shock associated with dehydration. You need to assess the following using ABCDE and 'Look: Listen: Feel: Measure'.

   - Look, listen, and feel for signs of dehydration: dry mouth, sunken eyes, thirst, anxiety, confusion, cool skin, evidence of pain.
   - Measure: respiratory rate, SpO_2, pulse, BP, urine output and loss through vomiting, signs of negative fluid balance, time period without fluid intake, and evidence of improvement following treatment with anti-emetic medication. Is there evidence of tachypnea, tachycardia, and hypotension, NEWS?
   - Mrs Thompson is dehydrated and this is evidenced by tachypnea, tachycardia, and hypotension (respirations: 24; pulse: 98; BP: 88/58). She is reviewed based on the nurse's assessment and communication of findings and commenced on an intravenous infusion; she receives a fluid challenge of 500 ml of 0.9% saline in 15 minutes, following which Mrs Thompson's vital signs improve to: respirations: 18; pulse: 90; BP: 95/58. She continues on 125 ml/hour of intravenous saline and is encouraged to drink oral fluids as her nausea begins to subside. She feels much better the following morning and is discharged home that afternoon.

2. Mrs Jacks has not passed urine in the six hours post-operation. There could be a simple explanation in that no one has asked her or helped her to perform this activity. It could also be related to dehydration/blood or fluid loss, or post-operative pain. You need to assess the following using ABCDE and 'Look: Listen: Feel: Measure'.

   - Look, listen, and feel for signs of blood/fluid loss and/or dehydration: dry mouth, sunken eyes, thirst, anxiety, cool skin, evidence of pain.
   - Measure: respiratory rate, SpO_2, pulse, BP, urine output and loss through vomiting, signs of negative fluid balance, time period without fluid intake. Is there evidence of tachypnea, tachycardia, and hypotension?

Following an assessment of her condition Mrs Jacks reveals that she wants to pass urine but was too afraid to ask because everyone looked so busy! After some support and nursing care this patient is able to pass urine and begins to feel much more comfortable. Her vital signs are within the normal range and her pain is well managed.

3. Using SBAR you would collate the information you have collected above into:
   - the *situation*: reason for your call;
   - the clinical *background*: reason for patient's admission;
   - the changes that have occurred in the patient *assessment*: now or over time;
   - your *recommendation*: what you want the clinical team to do.

The patient causing concern was Mrs Thompson, and your prompt review has prevented this patient's condition from deteriorating and going into hypovolaemic shock.

Further reading

Higgins, C (2013) Understanding Laboratory Investigations for Nurses and Health Care Professionals. Third edition. London: Blackwell Publishing.

This textbook provides a user-friendly approach to understanding laboratory investigations.

Peate, I and Dutton, H (2012) Acute Nursing Care: Recognising and Responding to Medical Emergencies. Harlow: Pearson.

This textbook adopts a systematic approach to managing body systems during medical emergencies.

Useful websites

www.youtube.com/watch?v=Wo90bqiI5BQ and www.youtube.com/watch?v=59uO-8UVC2A

These YouTube videos demonstrate examples of endoscopic management of a person with bleeding peptic ulcers and will help to put Megan's care into context.

Chapter 7

The patient with sepsis and septic shock

Desiree Tait

Chapter aims

By the end of this chapter, you should be able to:

• define sepsis and septic shock and demonstrate an understanding of the causes;

- demonstrate an understanding of the vulnerabilities of individuals in the development of sepsis and septic shock;
- demonstrate an awareness of the complex clinical picture presented in sepsis and the importance of using a person-centred approach to risk assessment and ongoing assessment;
- recognise the importance of the clinical assessment and management of airway, breathing, circulation, disability, and exposure in the patient with sepsis and septic shock;
- demonstrate an awareness of the long-term impact of sepsis on patient morbidity and mortality and how prevention and timely risk assessment can reduce morbidity and mortality; reflect on the clinical examples used in the chapter and how they apply to your own experiences in practice.

Introduction

The aim of this chapter is to equip you with the knowledge and skills to understand the pathophysiology and triggers for sepsis, as well as recognise developing sepsis in individuals, take appropriate timely action to prevent further deterioration, and initiate prescribed treatment protocols. In 2017 the WHO adopted a resolution to 'improve the prevention, diagnosis and management of sepsis'; sepsis is now a global concern. The Surviving Sepsis Campaign (SSC) (Levy et al., 2018) is a global collaboration that was established in 2002 to raise awareness and improve the evidence-based management of sepsis. In the 18 years since their inception, they have continued to raise awareness of sepsis worldwide; developed international evidence-based guidelines and care bundles; supported service improvement; and continue to review and update evidence-based care for the management of sepsis and the subset of sepsis, septic shock (NCEPOD, 2015; Rhodes et al., 2017; NICE, 2017a; Levy et al., 2018).

In the UK between 2017 and 2018 an estimated 240,000 patients were treated for sepsis, more than double the number of cases in eight years, making sepsis more common than MIs over the same period (Daniels and Nutbeam, 2019). This pattern of increase in the incidence of sepsis is reflected worldwide and while it can be argued that this is related to the standardisation of definitions for sepsis and improved diagnostic tools worldwide, the mortality rate continues to remain high. For example, in the UK the mortality rate for sepsis is estimated to be 26%, with 22% of survivors who have received intensive care suffering post traumatic stress disorder and 17% of survivors experiencing moderate to severe cognitive decline (Daniels and Nutbeam, 2019).

What is sepsis?

The Third International Consensus Definitions for sepsis and septic shock are described in lay terms as a life-threatening condition that arises when the body's response to an infection injures its own tissues (Singer et al., 2016, p805). They go on to describe sepsis as life-threatening organ dysfunction caused by a dysregulated host response to infection. Septic shock is a subset of sepsis in which underlying circulatory and cellular metabolic abnormalities are profound enough to substantially increase mortality (p805). The Sepsis-3 full definition is presented in Table 7.1 together with clinical examples.

An infection occurs when the body has been exposed to pathogenic organisms. When this happens, the body's immune system can recognise harmful invaders and provide a defence against the attack, containing and destroying the invader. This process is called the inflammatory response, and when it occurs locally in a body region – e.g., a tooth abscess, wound infection, a urinary tract infection – it can be contained and managed. For most people, the infection will be resolved without hospitalisation and the person will make a full recovery. For some patients, however, the disease can progress from an infection to sepsis or escalate to its most severe form, septic shock.

The word sepsis originates from the Greek, *sēpein- to make rotten* (Butterfield et al., 2003, p1473), but it wasn't until 1991 that the first consensus definition of sepsis was published. This was followed by two further definitions in 2001 and the latest, Sepsis-3, in 2016 (Gyawali et al., 2019). Sepsis definitions developed in 1991 and 2001 focused on the then shared view that sepsis occurred because of the host's systemic inflammatory response to infection, referred to as Systemic Inflammatory Response Syndrome (SIRS). In 2001 it was recognised that the definition of sepsis had its limitations due to a lack of understanding of sepsis pathophysiology at that time, and the growing body of evidence to support that the pathophysiology of sepsis was more complex than demonstrated by the SIRS criteria (Singer et al., 2016). By 2016 an improved understanding of sepsis pathophysiology identified the following points:

- Sepsis is recognised as having both a pro-inflammatory response and an anti-inflammatory response and the consensus now is that the use of SIRS as part of the clinical definition of sepsis is no longer valid.
- Sepsis is recognised as involving major modifications in cardiovascular, neural, autonomic, and hormonal pathways as well as metabolic and coagulation effects in the host.
- Sepsis can lead to severe organ dysfunction.
- Age, co-morbidities and recent surgery, medications, and the source of infection impact on both the development of sepsis and the person's subsequent morbidity and mortality.

The pathophysiology of sepsis includes several processes that are triggered by the host's response to infection. These and the associated clinical signs are summarised in Figure 7.1. According to Martin et al. (2019), the initial response is triggered by immune cells called 'pattern recognition receptors' and their release leads to the production of pro-inflammatory and anti-inflammatory mediators. This systemic process of exaggerated inflammation induces collateral damage to tissues. Damage to the endothelial lining of capillaries triggers the formation of microvascular thrombi (very small clots in the capillaries), small capillaries become clogged and blood flow to those tissues becomes inhibited. Such endothelial damage also triggers the release of the inflammatory mediator nitric

Terminology	Definition	Clinical examples
Infection	The invasion of a normally sterile cavity by organisms or inflammation caused by organisms in parts of the body which are not normally sterile (Daniels and Nutbeam, 2019) A **pathogen** entering the sterile cavity of the body	Holly Jackson has been complaining of toothache and a swollen hot left cheek for several days. A visit to the dentist confirmed the presence of a tooth abscess. She was prescribed empiric antibiotics (evidence based), amoxicillin 500 mg three times a day.
Sepsis	Life threatening organ dysfunction caused by a dysregulated host response to infection. Medical diagnosis of organ dysfunction can be identified as an acute change in total Sequential Organ Failure Assessment (SOFA) score of ≥2 points because of the infection. This score is used in ICU and is the official diagnostic and prognostic tool for sepsis (Singer et al., 2016). For clinical practicality the UK Sepsis Trust (2020) and NICE (2017a) recommend that a risk of, or clinical evidence of sepsis can be identified if any of the following are present: • NEWS2 score of 5 or more or 3 in one parameter • When an identified risk factor is present (age >75, impaired immunity, recent trauma, indwelling lines/catheters) • When a carer or healthcare practitioner is unduly worried • When the deterioration could be due to infection • **Specific Red Flag Sepsis (RFS) criteria in the above contexts are:** • New confusion or altered mental state • R ≥25/min • Needs O_2 to keep SpO_2 ≥92% (88% in COPD) • Systolic BP ≤90 mmHg • HR ≥130/min • Non-blanching rash/mottled/cyanosis	Tom Parkin has COPD, is 71 years old and was discharged from ICU to a medical ward eight hours ago after receiving treatment for pneumonia. He had required IMV, invasive haemodynamic monitoring, and urinary catheterisation. ABCDE assessment data reveals: • R: 30/min, dyspnoeic (RFS, NEWS2 = 3) • SpO_2: 84% on 28% O_2 (RFS, NEWS2 = 2 + NEWS2 = 2) • Centrally cyanosed (RFS) • P: 110/min (NEWS2=1) • BP: 95/65 mmHg (NEWS2 = 2) • T: 38.8 °C (NEWS2 = 1) • Skin hot and dry • Urine output in the last six hours 100 ml, urinary catheter removed 8 hours ago • Urinary tract infection diagnosed • New confusion (RFS, NEWS2 = 3). Tom's NEWS2 score is 14 and he has 4 Red Flags for sepsis. ACT: Alert critical care outreach team, CCOT, and senior medic. Commence continuous monitoring and stay with your patient. Commence Sepsis Six interventions, see later in the chapter. Alert Tom's family of the change in his condition.

(Continued)

Table 7.1 (Continued)

Terminology	Definition	Clinical examples
	• Lactate ≥2 mmol/L • Recent chemotherapy within previous 28 days • Not passed urine in 18 hrs (<0.5 ml/kg/hr) • **Identification of one or more Red Flags assumes the presence of sepsis.**	
Septic shock	A subset of sepsis (RFS): where underlying cellular and metabolic abnormalities are severe and lead to an increased risk of mortality of more than 40% (Vincent et al., 2019; Singer et al., 2016). Medical diagnosis of septic shock is based on the following criteria: • Persisting hypotension requiring intravenous vasopressor medication (norepinephrine or vasopressin) to maintain the mean arterial pressure (MAP) of ≥65 mmHg. MAP is the average arterial pressure over the period of one cardiac cycle and is estimated as: MAP = diastolic pressure (DP) + 1/3(systolic pressure − DP). • Serum lactate level >2 mmol/L after adequate fluid volume resuscitation.	• Sarah Clark (aged 70 years) was admitted to the emergency unit with a two-day history of back and abdominal pain and vomiting. Sarah has chronic renal failure for which she receives dialysis twice a week. • On assessment: • R: 38/min (RFS, NEWS2 = 3) • SpO_2: 87% on 60% oxygen (RFS, NEWS2 = 3 + NEWS2 = 2, Total 5) • P: 136/min (NEWS2 = 3) • BP: 75/50 (NEWS2 = 3) • **MAP: 55 mmHg (despite fluid resuscitation) indicative of septic shock** • Skin warm and flushed • Lethargic and drowsy – altered mental state (NEWS2 = 3) • T: 38.5 °C (NEWS2 = 1) • Urine output 0 • **Lactate = 4.2 mm/L (despite fluid resuscitation) indicative of septic shock** Sarah is showing signs of clinical septic shock accompanied by acute respiratory failure together with existing renal failure with NEWS2 = 18 ACT: • Sarah requires referral and immediate transfer to ITU. • Continuous monitoring. • Update Sarah's family.

Table 7.1 Patient examples and clinical definitions of sepsis according to degree of progression

oxide (a powerful vasodilator) and the endothelial cells become permeable, allowing fluid to leak into the surrounding tissues. Collateral damage is also caused to the cardiac tissues, leading to myocardial depression and reduced cardiac output, and to gastrointestinal endothelial cells, leading to an increased risk of multiple organ dysfunction as gastrointestinal function becomes impaired (Spapen et al., 2017).

The pro-inflammatory burst triggered by sepsis leads to a concurrent anti-inflammatory response and an immunosuppressive state, described by Spapen et al. (2017) as 'immunoparalysis', which increases the vulnerability of the patient to ongoing or later infection. Left to continue unabated, sepsis will lead to ischaemic and toxic cell damage, dysfunction of mitochondria, and the release of free radicals, leading to further cell destruction and cell death. Mitochondria are organelles in most cells that provide each cell with energy in the form of adenosine triphosphate (ATP) to perform cellular function. Some energy can be produced by glycolysis (the breakdown of glucose) in the cytoplasm of cells while most energy is produced by the process of oxidative cellular metabolism (a complex chain of biochemical reactions) and via the citric acid cycle in the mitochondria (McCance, 2019). McCance goes on to describe oxygen as a critical component of effective energy production in the mitochondria; it facilitates the metabolism of carbohydrates, fats, and proteins to produce ATP. When cellular oxygen levels are low, cells rely on the process of glycolysis alone to produce ATP; however in these situations lactic acid is produced as a by-product and released into the circulation. An elevated level of lactic acid, therefore, becomes an indicator of cellular hypoxia and reduced perfusion. Hypoxia and reduced perfusion of tissues collectively reduce the availability of oxygen to produce ATP as part of mitochondrial activity and thus the availability of energy for normal cell function (Martin et al., 2019). Free radicals, in the form of reactive oxygen species (ROS), are unstable molecules released as part of the inflammatory response. In sepsis, ROS are released in large numbers inside cells leading to further destruction of essential organelles such as mitochondria. The net effect is further controlled cell death (apoptosis), impaired cell function, and dysfunction of body systems such as the lungs and kidneys (Spapen et al., 2017).

The pathophysiological processes associated with sepsis and septic shock can negatively impact on all body systems, leading to severe multiple organ dysfunction with an associated mortality rate of more than 40% (Shankar-Hari et al., 2016). Speed of recognition of clinical deterioration, diagnosis, and empirical clinical intervention is critical in reducing the risk of sepsis, septic shock, and associated organ dysfunction (Daniels and Nutbeam, 2019). The role of the nurse is to assess, plan, and prioritise care; to communicate effectively and to be accountable for the actions required (NMC, 2018a).

It is pertinent to note that although SIRS and the clinical criteria used in its diagnosis have been excluded from the Sepsis-3 definition of sepsis, SIRS is associated with a number of other clinical situations/conditions where an exaggerated inflammatory response is triggered, including those patients with infection and SIRS but not sepsis (Daniels and Nutbeam, 2019). Figure 7.2 offers a diagrammatic representation of the position of sepsis in relation to SIRS based on the Sepsis-3 definition (Singer et al., 2016) and Bone et al.'s (1992) definition of SIRS.

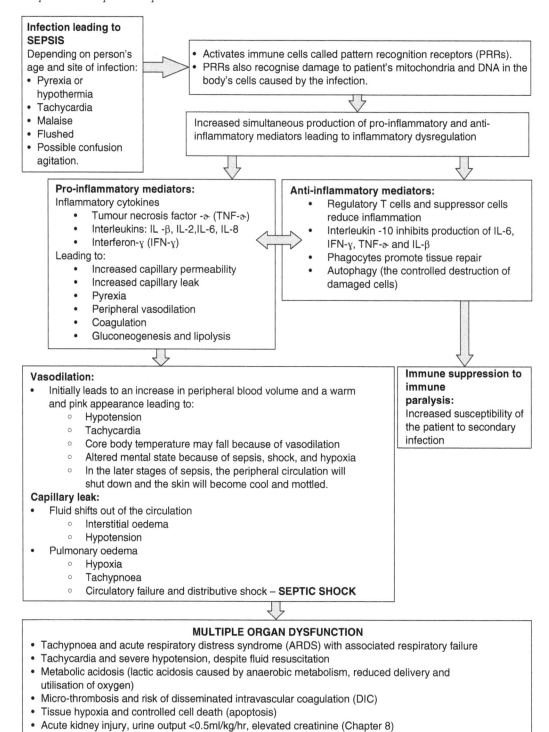

Figure 7.1 Sepsis pathophysiology linked to clinical signs of deterioration and septic shock

Source: De Daudio and Romagnoli, 2019; Tidswell and Singer, 2018.

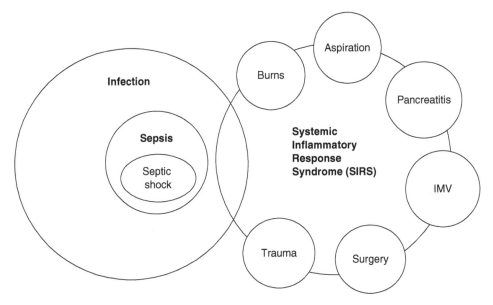

Figure 7.2 The relationship between infection, sepsis, and septic shock based on the definition of Sepsis-3 by Singer et al. (2016) and of SIRS by Bone et al. (1992)

For the remainder of this chapter the following sources and clinical guides have been used to support the assessment and management of people at risk of sepsis and those presenting with sepsis and septic shock:

- Singer et al. (2016) Consensus definitions for sepsis and septic shock;
- NICE Guideline [NG51] (2017a) Sepsis risk stratification tools;
- Daniels and Nutbeam (2019) *Sepsis Manual* (fifth edition) and the incorporated clinical tools.

An important note of caution is that when caring for patients you should always use the most up-to-date evidence to support your practice. Stating your source of knowledge to support practice ensures that if more recent evidence becomes available this can be identified and best practice can be assured.

Who is at risk of sepsis and why?

Sepsis screening, recognition, and management are the responsibility of every healthcare worker. Although it is recognised that sepsis can affect anyone, there are groups of people with a higher degree of risk (NICE, 2017a; Daniels and Nutbeam, 2019). These include:

- the very young (under 12 months) and people aged 75 years and older with evidence of frailty;

- people with weakened immune systems including:
  - people being treated for cancer, with diabetes, people who have had a splenectomy (removal of spleen), with sickle cell disease;
  - people taking systemic long-term steroids, people taking immunosuppressant drugs, for example, with rheumatoid arthritis, multiple sclerosis;
  - people who have had surgery or other invasive procedures in the previous six weeks;
  - people who have experienced a breach in skin integrity, for example, burns, blisters, skin infections, and pressure ulcers;
  - people who misuse intravenous drugs;
  - people with indwelling lines and catheters;
- women who are pregnant, have given birth or who have had a termination/ miscarriage in the last six weeks and in particular those women who:
  - have impaired immune systems (see above);
  - have diabetes/gestational diabetes;
  - have needed invasive procedures, had a prolonged rupture of membranes, or been in close contact with group A streptococcal infection;
  - have continued vaginal bleeding or an offensive vaginal discharge;
- neonates with group B streptococcal infection; premature birth (before 37 weeks' gestation).

This list identifies those people with increased risk of developing sepsis, but it is important to remember that any individual can develop sepsis. If any individual is deteriorating unexpectedly or failing to improve despite treatment, 'Think Sepsis'. Assess using ABCDE, listen to the person and their carers, hear your own personal concerns, and, if you are worried or suspicious, risk assess for sepsis.

Identifying the septic patient: what are we looking for?

The person will present with a deterioration in their clinical condition and, as recommended in Chapter 1, any patient who becomes unwell should be assessed using the ABCDE approach. This approach will help the healthcare team or carer to identify any life-threatening conditions and seek help. Once the assessment has been completed and data collected then risk assessment and management specific to the septic patient should be commenced immediately. Identifying the septic patient includes.

1. ABCDE assessment using the NEWS2 assessment tool (Resuscitation Council UK, 2015; RCP, 2017).

2. Use of sepsis screening tool to identify 'Red Flags' for sepsis (NICE, 2017a; Daniels and Nutbeam, 2019).

3. If sepsis is diagnosed commence the Sepsis Six pathway (Daniels and Nutbeam, 2019).

The SOFA (sepsis related organ failure assessment score) and qSOFA (quick SOFA) tools published as part of Singer et al.'s (2016) definition of sepsis are complex and focus on detailed measurements of clinical and haematological signs that predict the identity of organ dysfunction rather than as a risk assessment tool for identifying the probability of sepsis. 'Red Flag Sepsis' (Daniels and Nutbeam, 2019, p22) was developed by the UK Sepsis Trust in collaboration with NHS England and the Professional Royal Colleges, as a practical tool that can be used in acute settings and modified for community and midwifery settings for patients across the age spectrum. Daniels and Nutbeam (2019) argue that 'Red Flag Sepsis' is not a diagnostic tool for sepsis but evidence of one or more Red Flags in the presence of clinical deterioration and suspected infection requires immediate interventions, collectively referred to as the 'Sepsis Six' (discussed later in the chapter). The tool also identifies 'Amber Flags' that provide a second layer of risk assessment. According to NICE (2017a), evidence of a single Amber Flag should prompt action such as increased levels of monitoring, referral to a senior healthcare professional, transfer from a community setting to acute care, and haematological investigations. Therefore, sepsis screening should not end with the initiation of evidence-based treatment for sepsis but should also include the continued risk assessment for further deterioration (illustrated in Figure 7.3).

The role of the nurse is critical in relation to the identification of sepsis risk, recognition of deterioration, and escalation of care; actions that can improve patient outcomes. As a nurse you have direct responsibility for assessing and monitoring the patient's condition, even when you may have delegated the task to others. Your role when risk assessing for sepsis includes the following activities, and these activities apply wherever you meet a person who is unwell.

*   Adopt a patient-centred approach to care and know your patient where possible.
*   Listen to your patient and/or the patient's family.
*   Utilise a range of risk assessment tools (NEWS2) to monitor the patient and in the event of deterioration use the principles of ABCDE assessment.
*   Interpret the patient's clinical signs and symptoms in the context of screening for and recognition of sepsis.
*   Communicate effectively with the healthcare team and escalate using SBAR (Chapter 1).
*   Use the agreed clinical pathways and guidance to recognise and respond to clinical signs of deterioration in a timely manner.

Activity 7.1 gives you an opportunity to practise assessing patients for evidence of sepsis.

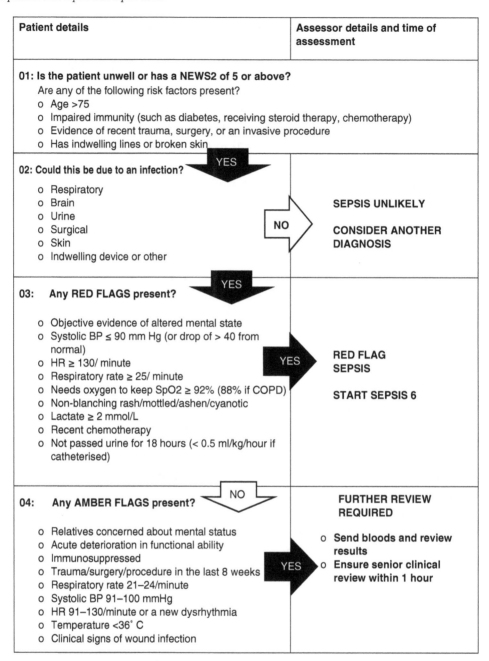

Figure 7.3 Sepsis screening tool for use in acute settings

Source: adapted from UK Sepsis Trust, 2020.

Activity 7.1   Decision making

With the aid of the sepsis screening tool in Figure 7.3, review the scenarios below and determine if any of the patients meet the criteria for sepsis.

Edward Morris

Edward Morris (69 years) has been diagnosed with inoperable carcinoma of the ascending colon. He underwent two laparoscopic bowel biopsies in a period of two weeks and finally had his diagnosis confirmed. Edward was commenced on IV chemotherapy one week later and completed the first 14-day cycle of treatment as an outpatient. Seven days later he began to experience acute abdominal pain in the right side of his abdomen and began to feel hot, shivery, and unwell. The guidance on his chemotherapy care pathway directed him to monitor his temperature and contact the 24-hour help line if it was above 38 °C. This is in line with the UK Oncology Nursing Society Treatment Toxicity Risk Assessment Tool (2017) and NICE guidance (2012). Edward's temperature was 38.6 °C and his pulse, taken by his daughter, was 95/min. He contacted the ward staff for advice.

1.   Did Edward meet any of the screening criteria?
2.   What advice would you give Edward?

Molly Taylor

Molly Taylor (73 years) has been admitted to an acute medical ward with a history of falls. On this occasion she had been found by the milkman, who heard her calling for help through the bathroom window. She had got up to go to the toilet at 02.00 hours and had lost consciousness. When she regained consciousness, she was disorientated and frightened to move. Molly had no evidence of bone fractures apart from bleeding from her nose and signs of bruising. There appeared to be no clear reason for her loss of consciousness. Nine hours after admission to hospital, she became short of breath and disorientated. Her daughter was visiting at the time and said that Molly did not normally suffer from confusion and that the only relevant thing that had happened in the last few weeks was that Molly had been suffering from a heavy cold.

Using the principles of 'Look: Listen: Feel: Measure' Molly presented with:

- confusion
- R: 28/min
- SpO_2: 88%
- P: 95/min
- BP: 100/60
- T: 37.9 °C

1. Did Molly meet any of the screening criteria for Red Flags?
2. How would you respond to Molly's condition?

Outline answers for this activity are given at the end of the chapter.

Why are changes in vital signs important?

In this section we will explore in more detail the significance of clinical signs and focus particularly on respiration, heart rate, blood flow and systolic blood pressure (SBP), evidence of new confusion, temperature, and signs of infection, by exploring the story of Cathy Price. Figure 7.1 provides a summary of the relationship between physiological factors and clinical signs, and Table 7.2 provides a summary of the clinical signs of infection for body systems most likely to be associated with the development of sepsis.

Case study: Cathy Price

Situation

Catherine (Cathy) Price, aged 41 years, has been admitted to hospital via the emergency department (ED) at 20.00 hours on Friday evening. She has been complaining of a three-week history of general malaise, lethargy, nausea, vomiting, and some abdominal discomfort, with three episodes of vomiting and diarrhoea in the last 12 hours. Cathy had been finding it increasingly difficult to breathe and cough over the last couple of hours; she was pyrexial and breathless. Her husband had become extremely worried about his wife and had made the decision to take her straight to ED.

Background

Three weeks prior to this event, Cathy had visited her GP complaining of lower abdominal discomfort, loin pain, and feeling generally unwell. Her GP had prescribed the antibiotic trimethoprim for a urinary tract infection and requested a urine specimen. The specimen proved to be negative. Despite this she remained unwell and returned to her GP a week later with a high temperature, shortness of breath, and a chesty cough. She was diagnosed with a chest infection and was prescribed a different antibiotic: amoxicillin. Since then, Cathy had been at home, feeling tired and nauseous, which she had put down to possible side effects of the antibiotics, and as the week went on she felt increasing discomfort in her central abdomen. The vomiting and diarrhoea had commenced on the day of admission together with increasing dyspnoea. Cathy had no significant past medical history apart from two normal pregnancies (two daughters aged 10 and 13 years). Cathy worked part time as a teaching assistant, was not allergic to anything, did not smoke, and only drank alcohol on social occasions.

Assessment

A:

- Airway was patent with bilateral chest movements, able to talk and respond to questions

B:

- R: 32/min, regular respiratory pattern;

- on auscultation she had shallow breaths with widespread crackles when asked to take a deep breath and the chest X-ray showed pulmonary infiltrates;
- SpO_2: 91%, oxygen was administered at 15 L/min via a non-rebreathing mask to elevate O_2 levels to 94–98%.

C:
- HR: 136/min, regular;
- BP: 108/46 mmHg;
- cool peripheries, peripheral pulses were present;
- her skin was pale and clammy;
- central capillary refill time (CRT) was four seconds;
- an ECG revealed sinus tachycardia;
- Cathy hadn't passed urine for at least 12 hours, urinary catheter inserted and 150 ml of residual urine was obtained, an hourly urometer was attached following catheterisation;
- catheter specimen of urine was sent for culture;
- blood was also obtained for culture;
- arterial blood gases (ABGs):

    o pH: 7.24;
    o $PaCO_2$: 6.39 kPa;
    o PaO_2: 8.59 kPa;
    o HCO_3: 17 mmol/L;
    o oxygen saturations: 91%;
    o lactate: 4.7 mmol/L;
    o WBC: 18.4×10^9/L;
    o haemoglobin (Hb): 8.7 g/dL;
    o platelets: 70×10^9/L;
    o potassium (K): 4.2 mmol/L;
    o calcium: 4 mmol/L;
    o urea: 14.1 mmol/L;
    o creatinine: 190 mmol/L.

D:
- ACVPU was 'A' – alert, able to answer all questions appropriately;
- Blood sugar 6.4 mmol/L.

E:
- on examination Cathy was tender over her mid-abdominal area with some distension felt;
- core temp 38.9 °C.

NEWS2 Score 13

Following an ABCDE assessment, Cathy was screened for sepsis and there was evidence of clinical deterioration with a NEWS2 score of 13, recent history of respiratory infection, and four Red Flags for sepsis. These were:

- respiratory rate: ≥25/min;
- needs oxygen to keep SpO$_2$ ≥92%;
- heart rate: ≥130/min;
- lactate: ≥2 mmol/L.

Signs of infection

The changes in clinical signs, together with evidence of infection, provide vital information when screening for sepsis or clinical deterioration. The most common sites for infection that are associated with the development of sepsis are:

- respiratory – pneumonia;
- cardiac – endocarditis;
- skin – cellulitis;
- abdomen – intra-abdominal sepsis;
- renal – urinary tract infection;
- invasive vascular access devices;
- septic arthritis;
- osteomyelitis;
- meningococcal sepsis.

The clinical signs of infection related to these sites are identified by Daniels and Nutbeam (2019) and are listed in Table 7.2, together with risk assessment and early interventions to reduce the risk of sepsis.

Body system	Signs of infection: 'Look: Listen: Feel: Measure'	Risk assessment and early interventions
Respiratory: pneumonia	<ul><li>R: >20/min.</li><li>Dyspnoea.</li><li>Temperature >38°C.</li><li>Yellow/green sputum when expectorating.</li><li>Noisy air entry during auscultation and/or no air entry to some lung quadrants.</li><li>Evidence of consolidation on chest X-ray.</li></ul>	<ul><li>Is the pneumonia community-acquired or hospital-acquired (assess for evidence of recent admissions to hospital in the last 48 hours and/or residence in a care home).</li><li>Assess the severity of illness using NEWS2, CURB65 score (BTS, 2015) and screen for AMBER or RED FLAG SEPSIS.</li><li>Act on findings using an ABCDE approach and Sepsis Six guidance.</li><li>Obtain blood and sputum cultures.</li><li>Aim for commencement of empirical antibiotics within 4 hours following blood cultures (BTS, 2015).</li><li>Use SBAR to communicate concerns.</li></ul>

Body system	Signs of infection: 'Look: Listen: Feel: Measure'	Risk assessment and early interventions
Skin: cellulitis	• Cellulitis: inflamed, red, hot, and swollen area of skin that is spreading from a focal point. • Petechial rash (rash of blood spots). • Temperature >38 °C. • Wounds: pain, tenderness, inflammation, pus. • Increased risk in diabetes.	• Risk assess for severity of illness using NEWS2 and AMBER or RED FLAG SEPSIS. • Act on findings using an ABCDE approach. • Support the commencement of empirical antibiotics following blood cultures. • Risk assess for necrotising fasciitis indicated by rapidly spreading cellulitis and severe pain (a rare but severe infection with high associated mortality (Daniels and Nutbeam, 2019)). This is a surgical emergency and rapid assessment by the senior surgical team is required. • Take wound swab as able. • Use SBAR to communicate concerns.
Abdomen	• Abdominal pain or tenderness. • Abdominal distention. • Guarding (tensing of muscles to prevent pressure from palpation). • Temperature >38 °C. • Nausea/vomiting. • Diarrhoea/constipation.	• Risk assess for severity of illness using NEWS2 and AMBER or RED FLAG SEPSIS. • Act on findings using an ABCDE approach and Sepsis Six guidance. • Assess for recent background and history. • Use SBAR to communicate concerns to the surgical team. • Faecal specimen.
Urinary tract	• Cystitis/pain on passing urine (dysuria). • Loin pain. • Frequency and/or urgency when passing urine. • Cloudy urine with a characteristic smell. • Haematuria.	• Risk assess for severity of illness using NEWS2 and AMBER or RED FLAG SEPSIS. • Act on findings using an ABCDE approach. • Obtain a mid-stream or catheter specimen of urine, blood cultures. • Support the commencement of empirical antibiotics straight away. • Assess for recent bio-psychosocial history. • Use SBAR to communicate concerns to the surgical team. • Manage catheter care and risk assess for further signs of infection (RCN, 2019). • Monitor fluid balance.

(Continued)

Table 7.2 (Continued)

Body system	Signs of infection: 'Look: Listen: Feel: Measure'	Risk assessment and early interventions
Meningococcal sepsis	• Headache, photophobia, drowsiness and altered mental state/confusion. • Rigors. • Muscle rigidity. • Cold hands and feet often with severe pain. • Myalgia (muscle pain). • Purpuric non-blanching rash (like small bruises) in late stages. • Circulatory shock and reduced urine output.	• Risk assess for severity of illness using NEWS2 and AMBER or RED FLAG SEPSIS. • Act on findings using an ABCDE approach. • Monitor GCS. • Assess for recent bio-psychosocial history. • Use SBAR to communicate concerns to the surgical team. • Support the initiation of intravenous antibiotics following blood cultures, without delay.

Line sepsis (vascular access device)	• In the advanced stage of thrombophlebitis (Jackson, 1998):
	  ○ Pain along the path of the cannula.
	  ○ Redness, exudate and swelling around the site.
	  ○ Palpable venous cord.
	  ○ Pyrexia.
		• Risk assess and reduce the risk of phlebitis through effective management and prevention of infection.
		• Adopt universal infection control measures.
		• Use the Visual Infusion Phlebitis Scale (Jackson, 1998).
		• Risk assess for severity of illness using NEWS2 and AMBER or RED FLAG SEPSIS.
		• Act on findings using an ABCDE approach and Sepsis Six if indicated.
		• Use SBAR to communicate concerns to the surgical team.
		• Line culture/possible removal and line tip for culture.

Septic arthritis (inflammation of a joint caused by infection)	• Severe joint pain. • Heat, redness and swelling around the affected joint. • Recent history of trauma or surgery may be present. • Evidence of infection following joint aspiration and imaging.	• Risk assess for severity of illness using NEWS2 and AMBER or RED FLAG SEPSIS. • Act on findings using an ABCDE approach and initiate Sepsis Six as appropriate. • Assess for recent bio-psychosocial history. • Use SBAR to communicate concerns to the surgical team.
Osteomyelitis (infection of the bone)	• Pain felt over the affected site. • Swelling and tenderness. • Often identified as secondary to a primary infection or injury; for example, discitis.	• Risk assess for severity of illness using NEWS2 and AMBER or RED FLAG SEPSIS. • Act on findings using an ABCDE approach and Sepsis Six interventions as appropriate. • Assess for recent bio-psychosocial history.

Body system	Signs of infection: 'Look: Listen: Feel: Measure'	Risk assessment and early interventions
	• (infection and abscess formation around a spinal disc), infected diabetic foot ulcer.	• Use SBAR to communicate concerns to the surgical team.
Endocarditis (infection of the cardiac endocardium)	• Rare condition associated with a history of rheumatic fever in childhood or heart valve disease. • Dyspnoea. • Weight loss. • Intermittent fever associated chills and sweats. • Heart murmur may be present. • Some patients may present with pulmonary emboli from vegetations broken off from the right side of the heart and carried to the lungs.	• Risk assess for severity of illness using NEWS2 and AMBER or RED FLAG SEPSIS. • Act on findings using an ABCDE approach and Sepsis Six interventions as appropriate. • Assess for recent bio-psychosocial history. • Use of SBAR to communicate concerns to the surgical team.

Table 7.2 Clinical signs of infection in body systems, risk assessment, and early management

Source: informed by Daniels and Nutbeam, 2019.

When assessed for a history of infection and signs of a new infection, Cathy had a three-week history of infection and had received two courses of antibiotics. She was now presenting with abdominal pain, distention, and diarrhoea consistent with an abdominal infection (see Table 7.2). She now meets the criteria for sepsis. In the following section we interpret Cathy's clinical signs and blood results so that we can begin to understand what is happening to her and what is likely to happen next, starting with respiration.

Respiration

One of the earliest clinical signs of sepsis is an increase in the patient's respiratory rate. According to Daniels and Nutbeam (2019), this increase may be triggered by several factors related to the patient's condition and include:

*   evidence of respiratory infection or existing disease including pyrexia, elevated WBC;
*   pulmonary oedema triggered by increased capillary permeability and leaking of fluid into the alveoli as part of the inflammatory response to infection;
*   fight/flight response triggering the respiratory centre to increase the rate of respiration to respond to reduced O_2 in the arterial blood (Chapter 6);
*   respiratory compensation for Cathy's metabolic acidosis (Chapter 3).

When Cathy was assessed, her respiratory rate was 32/minute, her breathing was shallow and on auscultation widespread crackles were heard. She had been treated for a chest infection a week before admission and this may have exacerbated her respiratory problems. The ABG results revealed evidence of a combined respiratory and metabolic acidosis and potential for type II respiratory failure (Chapter 2). The presence of pyrexia indicates the presence of bacterial pathogens (infective organisms) and this triggers the stress response and a corresponding increase in respiratory rate. Evidence of respiratory crackles on auscultation further raised concern and, with evidence of pulmonary infiltrates visible on the chest X-ray, Cathy was showing signs of pulmonary oedema due to increased capillary permeability and movement of fluid into the pulmonary interstitial and alveolar spaces (Murray, 2011). Thus, with a respiratory rate of more than 25/min, and evidence of bilateral pulmonary infiltrates, Cathy already meets the criteria for sepsis and requires Sepsis Six interventions (Figure 7.3).

Heart rate, blood flow, and blood pressure

When an inflammatory response is triggered, key changes stimulated by the release of pro-inflammatory mediators include vasodilation, capillary leak, hypovolaemia, and hypoxaemia (Figure 7.1). Vasodilation increases the blood flow to the affected area to transport the chemicals needed to fight the infection. In sepsis, widespread vasodilation can initially lead to patients having warm peripheries followed by evidence of peripheral shutdown as blood pressure falls. In addition to vasodilation, capillaries have increased permeability to allow pro- and anti-inflammatory mediators and leucocytes to the site of the infection. Clinically patients can present with interstitial oedema, diarrhoea, and vomiting. In sepsis the delicate balance that needs to be maintained between pro- and anti-inflammatory mediators becomes disordered leading to circulatory and organ dysfunction. This triggers the stress or flight/fight response (Chapter 6) and the heart rate, cardiac output, and blood pressure will initially increase to compensate for the fall in central circulating volume as a result of the inflammatory response. However, this will be difficult to maintain in the presence of continued inflammatory dysfunction. Cathy has been able to maintain a BP of 108/46 mmHg and does not yet meet the criteria for septic shock (Table 7.1). Her heart rate of 136/minute, however, is high and once again meets one of the criteria for sepsis (Figure 7.3). When there is loss of central circulating volume the body will continue to try to maintain its homeostatic balance by drawing on fluid reserves in the liver, spleen, and mesenteric circulation. A central capillary refill time (CRT) (measured by placing a thumb over the sternum and pressing for five seconds; when the thumb is removed the patient's skin should return to normal in under three seconds) of more than three seconds indicates reduced perfusion. Cathy's CRT was four seconds and, if the inflammatory mediators continue unabated, Cathy will be unable to maintain a systolic blood pressure over 90 mmHg and could progress to septic shock.

A further complication with sepsis is the damage caused to the endothelial lining of the capillaries (micro-circulation), discussed earlier in the chapter. Blood flow that would normally be diverted to the tissues that need it most as part of the fight/flight response fails, and the micro-circulation can become blocked with micro-clots. As more micro-clots form the number of available clotting factors is reduced, leading to bleeding and disseminated intravascular coagulopathy. Therefore, vigilance in continuously monitoring Cathy's vital signs is required, and commencement of Sepsis Six (Daniels and Nutbeam, 2019).

Altered mental state

When a patient presents with an altered mental state, it can include a range of signs, such as:

- sudden new confusion as in delirium, a sudden reduction in the GCS (Chapter 11);
- lethargy, sleepiness, with disorganised movements;
- disorientation, restlessness;
- being bewildered, having difficulty with obeying commands;
- stuporous (having reduced alertness), comatose.

In relation to sepsis this altered state may be due to one or more of the following:

- hypoxia;
- hypovolaemia and electrolyte imbalance.

The significance of acute confusion as an indicator for clinical deterioration, and particularly for sepsis, has been identified by the RCP (2017) as part of their evaluation of NEWS and by Seymour et al. (2016) as part of their review of criteria for sepsis. Thus, according to Williams (2019), acute confusion could be misinterpreted when using the standard APVU scale during a NEWS assessment. This led to the NEWS2 chart changing the AVPU scale to ACVPU, where C denotes new confusion and a score of three on the NEWS2 scale (RCP, 2017). When Cathy was admitted, she was tired but alert and was able to answer questions appropriately. At that stage she was showing no signs of an altered mental state even though her oxygen saturation levels had reduced to 91%.

Temperature

A fever or pyrexia occurs in response to the release of pyrogens from the infective organism and inflammatory mediators or chemicals that trigger inflammation. These include cytokines (prostaglandin E2) and histamine, which are triggered by an event that causes damage to body tissues and cells, including infection (Hall, 2016). This process can be initiated within minutes or hours of damage by pathogens. Not all patients with sepsis or SIRS will present with pyrexia; exceptions include patients who have impaired temperature regulation, such as patients with cervical spinal injury, people who are taking anti-inflammatory medication, and patients where there is evidence of systemic inflammatory response but no evidence of infection. There are benefits from having a fever and these include the creation of a chemical environment that helps to destroy the invading organisms and facilitation of the immune response. This response is part of a negative feedback loop that includes, first, peripheral vasoconstriction and elevation of temperature, and second, periods of peripheral vasodilation and sweating (McCance and Huether, 2019).

According to Daniels and Nutbeam (2019), there is evidence that pyrexia could be a protective response to sepsis and that patients presenting with higher temperatures can have better clinical outcomes. They go on to propose that a temperature below 36 °C can be associated with poor patient outcome. For Cathy, evidence of a fever (38.9 °C) and a raised WBC count of 18×10^9/L was further evidence of inflammation and infection. In summary, Cathy is presenting with evidence of infection, deterioration of three body systems including respiratory, abdominal, and renal, and four Red Flags for sepsis.

What are the priorities of care for a patient diagnosed with sepsis?

So far in this chapter we have focused on risk assessment, recognition, and diagnosis of a patient with sepsis. We will now continue with Cathy's story and examine nursing and medical interventions required to support her care. During the ABCDE assessment it is important to assess the patient's situation, which includes questioning whether there are any limitations of treatment that exist for your patient and whether these limitations are still valid. It is important not to make assumptions about a patient's care and, if possible, always to involve the patient and family in the decision-making process (see Chapter 1). In Cathy's case she was a previously young and fit mother with no limitations on her treatment and she and her husband were actively informed and involved in her management.

When a patient is diagnosed with sepsis, the speed of response is critical to prevent further deterioration. Rhodes et al. (2017) and Daniels and Nutbeam (2019) recommend that resuscitation and further diagnostic interventions should be initiated immediately and follow the Sepsis Six protocol for initial resuscitation and management in the first hour from diagnosis. The UK Sepsis Trust (Daniels and Nutbeam, 2019) and NICE (2017a) prescribe a set of six tasks (Sepsis Six) that should be completed within the first hour following recognition of sepsis. These interventions support the international sepsis bundle produced as part of the Surviving Sepsis Campaign (Levy et al., 2018) but have been adapted to reflect the clinical setting and age range of the patient (UK Sepsis Trust, 2020). This group of multidisciplinary interventions is called the Sepsis Six and adopting this plan in a timely manner can reduce patient mortality by preventing the patient's progression towards septic shock. The aim of Sepsis Six is to ensure timely interventions managed by specialist teams, to measure and correct problems with oxygen delivery and perfusion of tissues to reduce the likelihood of inadequate tissue perfusion and shock, and finally to monitor and support body systems for optimum outcome. According to Daniels and Nutbeam (2019, p55), *delivering the sepsis 6 within one hour is the most effective life saving treatment in medicine.*

The Sepsis Six include the following:

1. *Ensure senior clinician attends*

Sepsis is a complex condition and the Red Flags for sepsis are not always specific to sepsis. It is essential that a senior clinician or the CCOT assess the patient and confirm diagnosis as a priority. Sepsis Six interventions should be utilised collaboratively with the NEWS2 guidance on escalation of response (RCP, 2017).

2. *Give oxygen if required*

Oxygen should only be commenced if SpO_2 is less than 92% and titrated to maintain SpO_2 of 94–98%. If the patient has a history of chronic respiratory disease a target range of 88–92% should be maintained. Monitoring Hb as well as SpO_2 will identify whether the patient is anaemic (see below). The use of ABG analysis, as well as oxygen saturation and Hb, will give a more detailed picture of the underlying condition, as discussed in Chapters 2 and 3, but waiting for a full set of results should not delay the commencement of high-flow oxygen. Practical tips from Daniels and Nutbeam (2019) include:

- If the patient is critically ill, commence initial oxygen therapy with a reservoir mask at 15/L/min (O'Driscoll et al., 2017). Once the patient is stable, reduce the oxygen to maintain an SpO_2 range of 94–98%. Patients with COPD or other risk factors (neuromuscular problems, thoracic spinal deformities, obesity) should have the same initial target saturations as any critically ill patient and be monitored closely. Hypoxia will kill a patient before hypercapnoea!
- Use humidified oxygen if the oxygen is required for more than four hours to maintain hydration and prevent drying of secretions.

3. *Obtain IV access and take bloods*

- Blood cultures: The sampling of blood cultures and other possible sites of infection should be completed before antibiotic therapy has commenced unless this is contraindicated.
- Glucose: To manage the risk of secondary infection associated with high glucose levels and for the risk of hypoglycaemia.
- Lactate: A raised arterial lactate is associated with circulatory failure, insufficient oxygen delivery to the micro-circulation (anaerobic metabolism), mitochondrial dysfunction, or excessive oxygen demand that exceeds oxygen delivery. Lactate can reduce following fluid resuscitation because of improved circulation.
- FBC: Generally, a raised total white cell count indicates inflammation rather than specific infection. An elevated neutrophil count can indicate infection.
- Platelets: An elevated platelet count in the early stages of sepsis is indicative of inflammation. Later thrombocytopenia (a low platelet count) as sepsis progresses is indicative of the severity of the situation as coagulation dysregulation leads to clots in the micro-circulation and multiple organ dysfunction (Figure 7.1).
- Haemoglobin: A patient with a low Hb will have a lower oxygen-carrying capacity overall even when fully saturated with oxygen. Each haemoglobin molecule can carry four oxygen molecules. Fewer haemoglobin molecules mean less oxygen available to the tissues.

- U&E including creatinine: To monitor evidence of elevated creatinine as a sign of acute kidney injury (Chapter 7). **Hyperkalaemia** (elevated potassium) and hypokalaemia (low potassium) are associated with a risk of cardiac arrhythmias. C-reactive protein, an acute phase protein, is elevated in conditions that cause acute and/or chronic inflammation.
- Clotting screen: Disseminated intravascular coagulation (Figure 7.1) is associated with a severe depletion of clotting factors together with evidence of bleeding from mucus membranes. It may also indicate the presence of liver ischaemia. Both situations are associated with multi-organ dysfunction and a poor patient prognosis.

4. *Give intravenous antibiotics:*

The use of prescribed broad spectrum **empirical antibiotic therapy** can be initiated before the infecting organism is identified, following blood cultures, and reviewed when more information is available.

5. *Give IV fluids:*

- Administer a fluid bolus of 500 ml and repeat if clinically indicated. Use lactate levels to guide further therapy (NICE, 2017). Fluid resuscitation 30 ml/kg.

A functioning circulation is critical to ensure body tissues receive oxygen and nutrients. The aims of fluid resuscitation therapy are to correct hypovolaemia, maintain pulse, BP, and urine output within agreed parameters, and to do so without triggering the symptoms of fluid overload. Crystalloids are the first choice for fluid resuscitation and include: Hartmann's solution (however, avoid if the patient has hyperkalaemia), and 0.9% sodium chloride if there is evidence of hyperkalaemia.

6. *Monitor:*

- Use NEWS2 and monitor every 15 minutes or continuously.
- Monitor urine output hourly (catheterise the patient if necessary) to achieve a target of 0.5 ml/kg/hr.
- Repeat lactate hourly if clinical condition changes.

A patient with sepsis can improve dramatically with the initiation of Sepsis Six, but they can also deteriorate with equal speed. Continuous monitoring and evaluation of clinical findings is critical in the effective management of sepsis.

Case study: Cathy Price – medical recommendations and management in ED within one hour of admission

Let us return to Cathy's story and review her medical recommendations following a diagnosis of sepsis.

- Commence oxygen therapy to maintain SpO$_2$ between 94 and 98%.

- Monitor continuously using ABCDE approach.
- Obtain venous access: sample for blood cultures, a full blood screen including U&E, LFT, FBC, coagulation studies, and lactate.
- Take an arterial sample of blood to monitor acid-base balance and respiratory function.
- Commence intravenous fluid bolus of 500 ml of Hartmann's solution and review based on second lactate result.
- Review respiratory function and initiate non-invasive or mechanical ventilation to support failing respiratory function and manage pulmonary oedema.
- Insert a urinary catheter to monitor hourly urine output to achieve 0.5 ml/kg/hr.
- Commence empirical antibiotics.
- Arrange a CT scan.
- Move to ICU for management of sepsis.

When we return to Cathy's case and review the recommendations and management, we can see that all the Sepsis Six interventions were initiated in the first hour of her admission and, at that stage, hypotension had been avoided although her lactate level and respiratory function remain a concern.

Activity 7.2   Decision making

Henry Mason is 76 years old. He used to smoke 20 cigarettes a day but gave up 20 years ago when he was diagnosed with type 2 diabetes. He has very poor eyesight due to bilateral cataracts and is waiting for surgery. He has had hypertension and been on ACE inhibitors for ten years. Henry has already been in hospital for a week. He was originally admitted with pneumonia, and following a respiratory arrest on the medical ward, he spent five days in ICU. During his stay in ICU, he required MV (Chapter 3) to support his respiratory function as well as intravenous antibiotic therapy, physiotherapy, haemodynamic and nutritional support. To monitor and support his condition he had an arterial line, a central line, a urinary catheter, and intubation with an endotracheal tube. By the time Henry was discharged from ICU, he was breathing with the support of 40% oxygen, and his urinary catheter, central line, and arterial line had been removed. He was making good progress, but 48 hours after his discharge to the ward, Jan, the nurse looking after him, noted that he was reluctant to eat and drink, he was lethargic, and his chest sounded noisy. Henry's respiratory rate had increased to 21/min from 18/min with a fall in SpO_2 from 97% to 94%, but otherwise his vital signs remained unchanged (P: 89/min; BP: 130/85 mmHg, T:37.5 °C). Jan communicated her concerns to the medical team at 18.00 hours using NEWS2 and SBAR and recorded them in the notes.

1.   What were Henry's risk factors for developing sepsis?

(Continued)

(Continued)

2.	With reference to the sepsis screening tool in Figure 7.3, can you identify whether Henry met any of the criteria for sepsis?

3.	Using the screening tool and the recognition and response bundles identified in Chapter 1 (Table 1.2), plan what you would do to support optimum management of Henry from 18.00 hours to 19.00 hours.

Outline answers for this activity are given at the end of the chapter.

How should patients with septic shock be managed?

As we have seen, when a patient is diagnosed with sepsis, it is important to escalate to the CCOT and transfer the patient to ICU as soon as possible because these patients will need intensive support of their respiratory, cardiovascular, and circulatory systems to support their body organs, prevent multiple organ dysfunction, and improve their chances of survival. In the following sections we will explore how Cathy was managed in relation to the Surviving Sepsis Campaign's international guidance on managing sepsis (Rhodes et al., 2017). This guidance recommends that the resuscitation and management bundles for patients with sepsis should be completed within one hour of diagnosis to improve survival and this was achieved for Cathy. A summary of the International Guidelines for the Management of Sepsis and Septic Shock are illustrated in Table 7.3.

When we return to Cathy's story after her transfer to ITU we can see that her condition has been critical and her care complex.

Stages of management	Interventions
Initial resuscitation and infection issues	
Initial resuscitation:	• Should begin immediately.
	• Commence fluid resuscitation with 30 ml/kg of IV crystalloid solution and review based on clinical condition.
	• Continue monitoring of ABCDE using invasive haemodynamic monitoring as appropriate.
	• Target MAP of 65 mmHg in patients with septic shock and apply vasopressors if the patient remains hypotensive after fluid resuscitation.
	• Guide resuscitation to achieve a normalised level of lactate as an indicator of improved perfusion.
Diagnosis	• Take blood cultures before antibiotic therapy commences where this means there will be no significant delay in commencing antibiotics.

Stages of management	Interventions
Antimicrobial therapy	• Administer empiric broad spectrum antibiotics as soon as possible or within one hour of recognition of sepsis and septic shock. • Empirical antibiotics are reviewed on the basis of microscopy and monitored on a daily basis.
Source control	• Locate/diagnose source of infection and treat. • Remove any lines (culture) that may be associated with cause and send the tip for culture.
Haemodynamic support and adjunctive therapy	
Fluid therapy	• Crystalloids are the initial fluid of choice. • Initial fluid challenge in sepsis-induced hypotension to achieve a minimum of 30 ml/kg.
Vasoactive medications	• Infuse norepinephrine (vasopressor) via a central line to maintain a MAP of 65 mmHg if fluid resuscitation is refractory. • Vasopressin 0.03 units/minute can be added with norepinephrine when an additional agent is needed to maintain MAP. • Dobutamine (inotrope) infusion (up to 20 mcg/kg/min) may be infused to improve cardiac contractility and output. • MAP measured with invasive arterial monitoring via a pressure transducer for continuous monitoring.
Other supportive therapy	
Corticosteroids	• Recommended only if fluid resuscitation and vasopressor therapy do not restore haemodynamic stability. • IV hydrocortisone 200 mg/day.
Blood product administration	• Red blood cell transfusion should occur when Hb <7.0 g/dL to target Hb of 7.0–9.0 g/dL.
Mechanical ventilation (MV)	• Target a tidal volume of 6 ml/kg predicted body weight. • Inspiratory plateau pressure should be ≤30 cm H_2O. • Add positive end expiratory pressure (PEEP) to avoid alveolar collapse at the end of expiration and reduce oxygen demand. • Consider recruitment manoeuvres to re-expand lung tissue in patients with severe unchanged hypoxaemia (prone positioning). • Prone positioning is recommended over supine positioning for patients with acute respiratory distress syndrome (ARDS). • Have a weaning protocol in place.
Sedation, analgesia, and neuromuscular blockade	• Minimise continuous or intermittent sedation for patients receiving MV. • Avoid neuromuscular blockade, particularly after the first 48 hours.
Glucose control	• Commence continuous intravenous insulin when two consecutive blood sugars are >10 mmol/L. • Monitor blood glucose hourly using arterial sample if available.

(Continued)

Table 7.3   (Continued)

Stages of management	Interventions
Renal replacement therapy	• Commence when clear evidence of acute kidney injury.
DVT prophylaxis	• Commence daily.
Stress ulcer prophylaxis	• Commence daily for patients with risk factors that will contribute to a GI bleed.
Nutrition	• Initiate early enteral nutrition.
Setting goals of care	• Discuss goals of care with the patient and their family.

Table 7.3   A summary of the Surviving Sepsis Campaign International Guidelines for the Management of Sepsis and Septic Shock bundle

Source: based on Rhodes et al., 2017.

Case Study: Cathy Price is transferred to ICU for management of septic shock

When Cathy was transferred to ICU, she was commenced on BIPAP (Chapter 3) to improve her PaO_2 and promote oxygen delivery to the tissues. The SSC guidance for initial resuscitation and supportive therapy for sepsis was followed (Rhodes et al., 2017; Daniels and Nutbeam, 2019). Over the following 24 hours, Cathy developed acute respiratory distress syndrome (ARDS) and her condition deteriorated further (Chapter 3). ARDS is associated with inflammation of the lung parenchyma that leads to impaired gas exchange with associated systemic release of inflammatory mediators causing inflammation, reduced lung compliance, poor gas exchange, and hypoxia (Bersten and Bihari, 2019). Cathy received support, including IMV and renal replacement therapy, in ICU for three weeks before she was transferred to high dependency care and eventually to the ward. A year later, Cathy is a sepsis survivor but is still suffering from the impact of sepsis in the form of nightmares and panic attacks, poor concentration, memory loss, and extreme fatigue consistent with post-sepsis syndrome (Sepsis Alliance, 2015; Daniels and Nutbeam, 2019).

Managing the patient in ICU

The role of the nurse in ICU when supporting patients with sepsis and their families focuses on three key areas.

1. Assessing, recognising, interpreting information, and timely escalation of changes in your patient's condition.

2. Providing interventions to support goal-directed therapy.

3. Providing information and reassurance to the patient and family.

Airway and breathing

For some patients, pneumonia may be the primary cause of sepsis, but this is not the case for all patients. Patients who develop sepsis develop respiratory failure associated with a dysregulated inflammatory response, developing increased respiratory rate (tachypnea), pulmonary oedema, and hypoxia (ARDS). Cathy developed ARDS and the guidance for mechanical ventilation for sepsis-induced ARDS was followed (Table 7.3). The aim of management is to support the patient's respiratory function and reduce the risk of ventilator-associated injury (Chapter 3, Table 3.6) by providing respiratory support to achieve PaO_2 at >8 kPa and adhering to the ventilator bundle explained in Chapter 3 and the Sepsis Bundle (Table 7.3).

Cardiac and circulatory system

Patients with sepsis, and particularly septic shock, have hypotension associated with vasodilation and increased capillary permeability (Figure 7.1). The aims of cardiovascular support are to ensure the patient has accurate, safe, and continuous monitoring of their heart rate, blood pressure/mean arterial pressure (MAP) (arterial line), **central venous pressure** (CVP), temperature, and urinary catheter to manage their fluid requirements. Fluid requirements for patients with sepsis are high during the period of fluid resuscitation but this may change depending on the evidence of fluid volume deficit or overload. Within 24 hours of her admission, Cathy was commenced on renal replacement therapy to manage her severe metabolic acidosis, stabilise her fluid balance, and support renal function during acute kidney injury (Chapter 9).

The goals of this early directed therapy to support Cathy's cardiac and circulatory system include maintenance of the following:

- CVP >8 mmHg (>12 mmHg if ventilated);
- systolic blood pressure >90 mmHg (MAP >65 mmHg);
- fluid replacement should continue until the patient's systolic blood pressure is above 90 mmHg.

If the patient's blood pressure does not respond to fluid resuscitation, they have progressed to septic shock. Management in this situation involves the commencement of a group of drugs known as vasopressors, which work by increasing peripheral vasoconstriction and improving blood pressure. Many of these occur naturally in the body. They include adrenaline (epinephrine), vasopressin, and noradrenaline (norepinephrine). These drugs are given intravenously via a central line as they cause peripheral vasoconstriction and extravasation will cause necrosis. They are delivered as a continuous infusion because the half-life of these medications is short (90 seconds). There are significant patient safety issues when changing a syringe or altering dose and strength, with profound hypotension or hypertension and arrhythmias identified as side effects (Mallet et al., 2013). Noradrenaline (norepinephrine) is the first drug of choice and is infused until the patient can maintain a blood pressure above systolic 90 mmHg (MAP 65 mmHg) (Rhodes et al., 2017).

Disability and exposure

It is important to assess and review the patient's mental state and level of consciousness hourly as this can be a sign of improvement or deterioration. Sedation levels should also be assessed daily (Chapters 3 and 11). To reduce the risk of further infection and control existing infections, it is essential to continue with core interventions related to infection prevention and control.

These include:

- hand washing;
- appropriate use of uniforms and personal protective equipment;
- safe disposal of sharps;
- aseptic procedure and adherence to bundles of care such as the central line bundles (IHI, 2015);
- assessment for evidence of developing infection at infusion sites and catheters;
- isolation of patients with healthcare-related infection;
- vaccination of healthcare staff.

Finally, when caring for a patient with sepsis or septic shock, it is important to support the patient's mobility, positioning, and hygiene in order to reduce the risk of pressure ulcers, impaired circulation, and muscle tone. The use of the skin bundle in ICU provides a systematic approach to assessment and management of the patient's skin, nutrition, and mobility and can reduce the incidence of pressure ulcers in critically ill patients (Whitlock et al., 2011).

Chapter summary

The aim of this chapter was to help you to assess, recognise, and respond in a timely manner to patients who develop sepsis and septic shock. It is also important to note that Covid-19 is a viral infection that can lead to multiple organ dysfunction. Based on the information available at the time this chapter was written, this means that Covid-19 can cause sepsis (UK Sepsis Trust, 2020) and early assessment and interventions are essential. The responsibilities of the nurse when caring for patients at risk of sepsis can be summarised as follows:

- Undertake a rigorous assessment and monitor the patients in your care.
- Know your patients and recognise that any change in their condition is significant.

- Provide evidence-based care and support decision making using national and international guidance in the context of local policy.
- Use SBAR to structure your communication when escalating patients causing concern.
- Anticipate and be prepared to support a patient's deteriorating condition.

Activities: brief outline answers

Activity 7.1: Decision making (page 189)

Edward Morris

1. Edward did meet some of the screening criteria on both the UK Oncology Nursing Society (UK ONS, 2016) and the sepsis screening tool.
   - The UK ONS (2016) recommend that patients who are receiving chemotherapy with a pyrexia and signs of malaise and infection should dial 999 for urgent ED assessment for neutropenic sepsis. Edward met this criterion.
   - Using the sepsis screening tool Edward has a risk of impaired immunity, and recent chemotherapy indicates a Red Flag for sepsis.
2. Advice to give Edward:
   - Neutropenic sepsis is a medical emergency, so Edward should be advised to call 999 and ask for the ambulance service. Patients in Edward's situation need an urgent FBC to confirm neutropenic sepsis, screen for sepsis, and implementation of the Sepsis Six if positive.
   - While he is waiting for the paramedics, advise his daughter to collect an overnight bag and a summary of the chemotherapy drugs and any other medications he has taken.

Molly Taylor

1. Molly presented with a NEWS2 score of 11 with evidence of a respiratory infection. She had three Red Flags for sepsis including:
   - New confusion.
   - R: 28/min.
   - SpO_2: 88%.
2. A NEWS2 score of 7 or more is a key trigger threshold for emergency action. Molly is critically ill and requires an emergency assessment from a senior clinician and the CCOT.
- Using the SBAR framework, you should contact the senior clinician and outreach team and summarise Molly's current situation, background, and most recent vital signs.
- You should respond by anticipating the needs of the patient and outreach team when they arrive. While one person stays with the patient, someone can collect any equipment necessary.

Activity 7.2: Decision making (page 201)

1. An examination of Henry's care plan showed that he was at high risk of developing sepsis for the following reasons.
   - He has co-morbidities including diabetes, and is recovering from pneumonia.
   - He had required invasive lines and catheters to support his respiratory and cardiovascular function in ICU.
   - He is on antibiotic therapy for pneumonia.
   - His NEWS2 score is 6.
2. The increase in Henry's respiratory rate meant that he met a Red Flag for sepsis and evidence of a deterioration in his respiratory function could indicate a new infection.

3. Based on Henry's recent medical history and his high risk of developing sepsis, the priorities for care would include:

- contact senior medical staff to ask for an urgent review of Henry's condition, using an SBAR approach;
- sit Henry up in the bed and promote a position to support effective respiration, ensure the oxygen mask was fitted securely and encourage him to take deep breaths;
- monitor his observations every 30 minutes and if his condition deteriorates any further then escalate the urgency of the situation;
- continue to screen for sepsis, sputum sample, assess IV access if any, refer to physiotherapist for productive chest.

Further reading

EB Medicine. (2018) Calculated decisions: clinical decision support for *Emergency Medicine Practice* subscribers. Accessed at: www.ebmedicine.net/media_library/files/Calculated%20 Decisions%20E1018%20Sepsis.pdf

This paper offers a brief explanation of the SOFA score, qSOFA and the Glasgow Coma Scale. The digital version provides access to the relevant calculators.

Daniels, R and Nutbeam, T (2019) *The Sepsis Manual.* Fifth edition. Birmingham: UK Sepsis Trust.

This book offers up-to-date explanations on the risk assessment and pathophysiology of sepsis and would be of interest to those who have placements in critical care areas. It can be downloaded as a PDF from: https://sepsistrust.org/professional-resources/education-resources/

Useful websites

https://sepsistrust.org/

The UK Sepsis Trust website has information for professionals on sepsis learning resources and information for the public on how to cope with and survive sepsis. Information about COVID-19 and its relationship to sepsis continues to be updated.

www.nice.org.uk/guidance/ng51/resources/algorithms-and-risk-stratification-tables-compiled-version-2551488301

This link provides a comprehensive list of risk stratification tools for sepsis along the age continuum and a link to the full NICE guideline for further details. The tools have been developed with the cooperation of the UK Sepsis Trust.

https://jamanetwork.com/journals/jama/fullarticle/2492881

This link provides the full article on the Third International Consensus Definitions for sepsis and septic shock – Sepsis-3. Always remember that evidence-based practice requires constant review and updating so make sure you use the most recent advice.

www.ncepod.org.uk/2015report2/downloads/JustSaySepsis_FullReport.pdf

This report sets out the recommendations for good practice and is based on a national confidential enquiry into the assessment and management of patients admitted to hospital with sepsis.

Chapter 8 The patient with delirium

Desiree Tait

Chapter aims

By the end of this chapter, you should be able to:

- describe the term delirium;
- identify the common causes of delirium;
- demonstrate an awareness of how to risk assess for, and prevent, delirium;

(Continued)

(Continued)

- demonstrate an awareness of how to manage patients with delirium and provide them with a safe environment;
- reflect on, and rehearse, the risk assessment and management of patients with delirium.

Introduction

Delirium is an acute confusional state that can develop in both acute and long-term care settings. Acute new confusion can be triggered by clinical deterioration and is recognised as part of the NEWS2 (see Chapters 1 and 11). In this chapter we will focus on exploring the various clinical definitions, types, and causes of delirium, how to risk assess for and prevent delirium, and discuss how to provide safe and effective care using a collaborative approach. We will examine two patient scenarios, Jack Porter, an 85-year-old gentleman residing on a ward for older adults with medical problems, and Paul Chapman, a 28-year-old gentleman being cared for in ICU. We will begin by reading Janet's description of events when she first met Jack Porter.

Case study: Jack Porter

My name is Janet and I have been a registered nurse (adult) for one year. I was working a bank shift one night and I found I had been allocated to work on an acute medical ward for the elderly. I had never worked on this ward before and did not know the patients, but after a few hours I began to feel that I was comfortable with the layout and had assessed the patients I had been allocated. That was until midnight when I heard a scream coming from the female section of the ward followed by several shouts for help. When I arrived, a gentleman from the male section was attempting to get into bed with one of the female patients. The gentleman was pushing Joan (the female patient) out of bed to make room. I pulled her buzzer to call for assistance and tried to calm the situation down. The gentleman's name was Jack Porter (85 years), and at the time I knew nothing about him. I tried to reason with him and explained that he should go back to his bed where he would be more comfortable. He looked at me and nodded, and then walked over to another patient and tried to get into bed with her. I tried to talk to him again and gently held his elbow to guide him away. When I did this, he resisted in an aggressive manner, pushing me and pinning me against the wall. The other staff again tried to reason with him, but he began shouting and pushing them away. The on-call medical team attended, and together we were able to calm Jack and persuade him to go back to bed. The medical team prescribed haloperidol and said they would perform a detailed assessment in the morning.

The female patients were terrified by this time and particularly frightened of the fact that it took three nurses and two medical staff to resolve the situation. No person came to physical harm that night, but the psychological distress felt by the female patients led to a disturbed and sleepless night for them. Jack was also clearly distressed and appeared to believe that we were trying to harm him.

Janet's story is not uncommon and describes an example of a patient with delirium. The incidence of delirium in acute and critical care settings is high and can increase the risk of morbidity and mortality (European Delirium Association and American Delirium Society, 2014).

According to NICE (2019a), in the UK the prevalence of delirium is 20–30% of patients admitted to medical wards and 10–50% in surgical wards. Similarly, an epidemiological review of the incidence of delirium on medical wards identified that 11–15% of older patients who are admitted will have delirium on admission (prevalent delirium) and a further 29–31% of older patients admitted to medical wards will develop delirium (incident delirium) during their time on the ward (Vasilevskis et al., 2012). In ICU the incidence of delirium in ventilated patients is 22–83% (Vasilevskis et al., 2012).

According to NICE (2019a) and Morandi et al. (2012), patients who develop delirium have:

- a higher-than-average incidence of complications such as falls and pressure sores;
- an increased risk of self-removal of an endotracheal tube supporting ventilation and removal of invasive devices used in critical care settings;
- a correspondingly increased length of stay in hospital;
- an increased risk of long-term cognitive impairment associated with critical illness;
- an increased incidence of dementia either as related to existing delirium or dementia that can occur as a later consequence of delirium;
- an increased risk of mortality associated with delirium co-morbidities such as falls, pressure sores, and tissue injury.

The importance of recognising, responding to, and, where possible, preventing delirium cannot be overestimated.

What is delirium and how should it be described?

Delirium is a term used to describe an altered state of consciousness that is accompanied by a change in cognition or perception. The onset is acute, developing over one to two days and the course of the condition fluctuates according to time and other factors (NICE, 2019a). NICE (2019a) describes delirium as having two subtypes, hyperactive and hypoactive, and these are described in Table 8.1. A third subtype of delirium is a mix of hyper- and hypoactive symptoms (Mulkey et al., 2018). The core features of delirium found in patients include:

- a reduced awareness and understanding of their immediate environment;
- an impaired ability to focus their attention, sustain and change their attention to something else;
- altered cognition, including memory impairment, disorientation, paranoia, language or perceptual disturbances including hallucinations.

These disturbances develop over several days and tend to fluctuate over a 24-hour period. Sundowning syndrome describes a state of acute mental confusion equivalent to delirium that takes place towards the end of the day. It is precipitated by diminished illumination as natural light diminishes (Silva et al., 2017).

The International Classification of Disease (ICD-10) (2016) states that delirium not induced by alcohol and other psychoactive substances is

An etiologically nonspecific organic cerebral syndrome characterized by concurrent disturbances of consciousness and attention, perception, thinking, memory, psychomotor behaviour, emotion, and the sleep-wake schedule. The duration is variable and the degree of severity ranges from mild to very severe.

The American Psychiatric Association (2013) updated their classification of delirium to focus more on disturbance in attention and awareness, although the European Delirium Association and American Delirium Society (2014) argue that the understanding of delirium must extend beyond cognitive testing of attention and that medical assessments must consider both attention and arousal. Thus, the DSM-5 Classification of Delirium (European Delirium Association and American Delirium Society, 2014, p2) is defined as:

A. *Disturbance in attention (i.e., reduced ability to direct, focus, sustain, and shift attention) and awareness (reduced orientation to the environment).*

B. *The disturbance develops over a short period of time (usually hours to a few days), represents an acute change from baseline attention and awareness, and tends to fluctuate in severity during a day.*

C. *An additional disturbance in cognition (e.g., memory deficit, disorientation, language, visuospatial ability, or perception).*

D. *The disturbances in Criteria A and C are not better explained by a pre-existing, established or evolving neurocognitive disorder and do not occur in the context of a severely reduced level of arousal such as coma.*

E. *There is evidence from the history, physical examination or laboratory findings that the disturbance is a direct physiological consequence of another medical condition, substance intoxication or withdrawal (i.e., due to a drug of abuse or to a medication), or exposure to a toxin, or is due to multiple etiologies.*

This definition does, however, offer a clinically specific focus to support a more consistent diagnosis than the more generic ICD-10 classification.

For some patients, delirium will last a few days; for others it can continue for months, depending on the predisposing and precipitating factors listed in Table 8.2. The two subtypes of delirium described by NICE (2019a) are set out in Table 8.1 and are consistent with understanding delirium from a psychomotor behavioural perspective (Morandi et al., 2012).

Delirium subtype	Clinical signs and symptoms	Patient examples
Hyperactive *People who have heightened arousal and can be restless, agitated or aggressive.* NICE (2019a, p7)	Agitation and restlessness • Fidgeting. • Pulling at clothes, catheters, or tubes. • Moving from side to side. • Shouting and calling out. Confusion • Does not know who or where they are. • May have difficulty following commands. Paranoia • Sees some members of staff as a threat. • Expresses fear and distress as the environment appears hostile. • May try to escape.	Charlie Thomas (70 years) was admitted to a cardiac ward after feeling light-headed and dizzy. He was later diagnosed with an anterior (STEMI) myocardial infarction. When he was admitted, his heart rate was 35/min and the ECG showed he had a bradycardia and complete heart block. A temporary pacing wire was inserted, and his heart rate and blood pressure improved. Later that night the nurse noticed that his ECG trace had gone flat. She rushed to his bedside to find Charlie out of bed and looking for the exit. He had disconnected himself from the ECG leads but the pacing wire and equipment were still connected, and he was holding the temporary pacing box. He pushed past the nurse and made his way along the corridor to the exit and the bus stop. When the nurse caught up with him, he could not understand why he had to go with her because he needed to go home – they were expecting him. The nurse sat at the bus stop with Charlie for ten minutes before he agreed to come back to the ward and wait there.
Hypoactive *People who become withdrawn, quiet and sleepy.* (NICE, 2019a, p7)	Confusion • Does not know who or where they are. • May have difficulty following commands. Withdrawn • Lying quietly with evidence of reduced mobility and movement. • Looking away and avoiding opportunities for human contact. • Slow responses to questions or conversation. • Change in appetite.	Margaret Adams (83 years) was admitted yesterday evening with a fractured neck of femur and was waiting for surgery to stabilise the fracture. On admission she was alert and keen to know who everyone was and much happier now that she had been rescued from her fall. Twelve hours later, Margaret did not want to talk and when asked about her home arrangements she began to give information that was contradictory to what was in the nursing notes. When Margaret was asked to roll on her side she did not move or attempt to help with the procedure, and she appeared not to understand simple commands. The nurse noted that this was very different from what she was like on admission and undertook an ABCDE assessment of her condition.

Table 8.1 Subtypes of delirium with clinical examples

What causes delirium?

Delirium appears to occur when a single factor, or a combination of factors, leads to a reversible organic mental syndrome. This means that in more than 90% of patients the underlying cause is physiological and related to the impact of disease and/or the impact of hospitalisation (Aldemir et al., 2001). The pathophysiology of delirium is complex and a number of theories have been proposed which involve the triggering of neurotransmitter imbalances in the brain. Related and arguably complementary theories focus on the impact of physiological stress, the inflammatory response, and oxygen deprivation on the balance of neurotransmitters in the brain (Mulkey et al., 2018).

According to Mulkey et al. (2018), the main neurotransmitters and chemicals associated with the onset of delirium include:

- *Dopamine:* helps to control the brain's reward and pleasure centres, regulates movement and emotional response. Dopamine levels increase in the presence of hypoxaemia.
- *Acetylcholine:* plays a role in enhancing sensory perceptions when we wake up and in sustaining attention as well as regulating digestion and muscle movement. Acetylcholine levels decrease with older age, in the presence of hypoxaemia, when associated with a previous diagnosis of cognitive impairment, and with the use of sedatives and opioids.
- *Serotonin:* plays a role in sleep, memory and learning, mood, behaviour, and depression. Serotonin levels decrease in the presence of alcohol withdrawal, older age, Parkinson's disease, and when there is an abrupt discontinuation of antidepressants.
- *Gamma-aminobutyric acid (GABA):* is a primary inhibitory neurotransmitter that prevents over-stimulation, stress responses, and relaxes muscle tone. Fluctuations in GABA levels are associated with alcohol use, sedatives, infection, and electrolyte imbalance.
- *Endotoxins:* endotoxins released as bacteria break down following a bacterial infection, can alter cell function in the brain and increase cortisol levels.

Some factors that trigger delirium are *predisposing factors*, in that some patients have increased risk of developing delirium before they have been admitted to hospital. This may be due to existing dementia, old age, pre-existing illness, or functional impairment including vision or hearing loss, malnutrition, drug and/or alcohol abuse, and depression (Vasilevskis et al., 2012). Delirium can also be caused by potentially modifiable *precipitating factors* associated with the severity of the patient's illness, the use of certain drugs, electrolyte and/or chemical imbalance, severe infection including Covid-19 and sepsis (British Geriatric Society, 2020; Vasilevskis et al., 2012). A full list of the predisposing and precipitating factors can be found in Table 8.2, which includes some clinical examples. In the next section we will put these factors into context by returning to Jack Porter's story.

Predisposing factors	Clinical examples
• Increasing old age >65 years. • Existing cognitive impairment/dementia. • Evidence of increasing severity of illness. • Existing physical impairment. • Pre-existing alcohol/substance misuse.	• Any person, male or female, who is 65 years or older has an increased risk of developing delirium. • Patients with existing dementia or depression have an increased risk of developing delirium. • A patient with bronchitis who develops an acute chest infection has an increased risk of developing delirium. • Patients with visual and/or hearing impairments, or with limited mobility, can experience sensory deprivation in hospital, and this predisposes them to developing delirium. • A person who may have misused drugs in the past, but has not taken them for several years, is still at risk of developing delirium as addiction can effect permanent changes on brain cells.
Precipitating (modifiable) factors	**Clinical examples**
Severe illness, or a person at risk of deteriorating • Respiratory disease and associated hypoxia (Chapters 2 and 3). • Cardiovascular disease. • Hypotension. • Severe infection and/or sepsis. • Head injury. • Acute admission for hip fractures. Physiological imbalance • Imbalance of electrolytes particularly sodium and potassium. • Increased levels of creatinine, urea. • Anaemia. • Metabolic acidosis. • Dehydration. • Vitamin deficiency. • Blood glucose. • Pharmacology • Polypharmacy. • Drug withdrawal. • Drug side effects that cause an altered balance of the neurotransmitters, acetylcholine, and dopamine. • Pain.	Hanna Mera (67 years) developed hyperactive delirium after her oxygen saturations fell to 87% as the result of an acute exacerbation of her chronic respiratory disease. Harold Jones (70 years) developed delirium following a delayed diagnosis of MI and hypotension. Sarah Moon (65 years) developed delirium after developing sepsis from a wound infection. Fred Holloway (78 years) fell and fractured his hip. He had to wait 48 hours after admission before he had surgery to stabilise the fracture. He developed delirium post-operatively and he was found to have an imbalance in sodium and potassium, dehydration, and an increase in his creatinine levels. Maryam Abdul (57 years) was admitted to hospital with cellulitis and sepsis. She was suffering from hypoxia and metabolic acidosis. She was disorientated and distressed. Ryan Sheppard (20 years) was involved in a road traffic collision. He sustained multiple fractures. He was intubated and ventilated for 24 hours in the post-operative period, after which attempts were made to reduce his respiratory support. As he awoke, he appeared to be hyper alert and tried to get out of bed. He was unable to respond to requests to stay in bed and became very agitated.

(Continued)

Table 8.2 (Continued)

Predisposing factors	Clinical examples
Use of physical and invasive therapy Physical restraint caused by clinical equipment. • Indwelling catheters. • Immobilisation. • Lack of sleep. • Alien environment such as ICU.	Ryan was a regular user of illegal substances and that, together with his critical illness, had triggered delirium. Barry Jones (54 years) had been a patient in ITU for 14 days, during which time he had been both physically restrained by catheters and tubes as well as chemically restrained by sedation to support respiratory function. He slept all day and was awake all night. At night he became very agitated and would regularly disconnect his ventilator tubing and attempt to get out of bed.

Table 8.2 Predisposing (vulnerability) and precipitating (modifiable) factors for the development of delirium with clinical examples

Source: based on NICE, 2019a and Vasilevskis et al., 2012.

Why did Jack Porter develop delirium?

Jack Porter presented with hyperactive delirium. On assessment the following predisposing and precipitating factors were found:

Predisposing factors

- Age: Jack is 83 years old.
- Loneliness and isolation: He has been married to his wife for 62 years, and during that time they have never been separated for more than a few days and he is lonely and isolated from his family.
- Existing physical impairment: Jack has type 2 diabetes and hypertension for which he takes beta blockers (slows the heart rate and reduces cardiac output).
- Pre-existing cognitive impairment: Jack has been diagnosed with dementia, and his main carer is his wife.
- Clinical deterioration: Jack has been admitted to hospital with a recent history of blackouts and falls.

Precipitating factors

- Time in hospital: Jack has been in hospital for five days.
- Medication review and changes: His dose of beta blocker has been reviewed and reduced.
- Infection: He has been diagnosed with a urinary tract infection and prescribed antibiotics.
- Electrolyte imbalance: His blood results from earlier today showed raised sodium (Na) and potassium (K) levels, and an elevated creatinine level consistent with a risk of acute kidney injury (see Chapter 9).
- Deteriorating vital signs: When Jack settled, his respirations were 20/min, SpO_2 94%, his pulse was 58/min, and his blood pressure was 110/65 mmHg (lower than normal for Jack); his temperature was 37.5 °C and his blood sugar was 7.4 mmol/L.

- Dehydration and possible acute kidney injury: Jack has only passed 500 ml of urine in the last 18 hours (see Chapter 9).

He was reviewed by the on-call medical team and commenced on oxygen therapy to maintain oxygen saturations of 94–98% (BTS, 2017), an intravenous infusion of 0.9% saline to improve hydration, and was catheterised to monitor his urine output. His medication for hypertension was discontinued with a view to assess Jack's renal function in the morning. The number of predisposing and precipitating factors identified in Jack's case would have increased his overall risk of developing delirium and a full list of predisposing and precipitating factors can be found in Table 8.2.

Activity 8.1   Developing clinical decision-making skills

When you are next on placement in a hospital setting:

- review the patients that you have been allocated for risk factors associated with developing delirium;
- if you identify a patient who is at risk, collaborate with the healthcare team and discuss possible options for prevention as shown in Table 8.3;
- continue to observe your patients to monitor any change in their condition that may increase the risk of them developing delirium.

As this activity is based on your own observation, there is no outline answer at the end of the chapter.

How is delirium risk assessed and prevented?

When a patient is admitted to the ward, or unit, part of their assessment on admission should include an assessment of the predisposing and precipitating risk factors for developing delirium.

As with all other elements of assessment, patients should be assessed using the 'Look: Listen: Feel: Measure' and ABCDE criteria and this should be followed by a full holistic assessment, to include information from the patient's friends and relatives to develop a picture of the patient as a person before they were admitted to hospital. Plan and organise the patient's care so that they see familiar faces among the carers, as this will provide continuity of care and continuity of assessment and monitoring. Assess for the core features of delirium (Table 8.1), and if any of these are present, your findings need to be validated by a more comprehensive clinical assessment based on the Diagnostic and Statistical Manual of Mental Disorders criteria (NICE, 2019a) and, in critical care settings, a tool such as the Confusion Assessment Method for ICU (CAM-ICU) (Ely, 2014; Ely et al., 2001; NICE, 2019a). In older people with delirium, Dixon (2018) recommends the use of the 4AT to assess for delirium and cognitive impairment. The 4AT tool (Bellelli et al., 2014) focuses on four parameters:

- Alertness
- Abbreviated Mental Test (AMT4) (age, date of birth, place, current year)
- Attention (listing the months of the year backwards)
- Acute change or fluctuating course in cognition.

Links to these tools can be found at the end of this chapter.

According to Mistraletti et al. (2012), the correct way to approach delirium is to suspect its presence whenever a change in health status occurs, and according to NICE (2019a), patients should be assessed for delirium at least once a day. If a diagnosis of delirium is confirmed, the next step is to adopt a multidisciplinary approach to prevent further deterioration and treat any underlying precipitating factors. This process may be summarised as follows:

- Assess the patient and family using a holistic approach to care.
- Risk assess for predisposing factors for developing delirium.
- Promote continuity of care.
- Assess for features of delirium daily and/or if the patient's condition deteriorates.
- If present, validate with the use of an assessment tool (CAM-ICU in critical care and 4AT with older adults – links to these tools can be found at the end of the chapter).
- Risk assess daily for evidence of any changes in risk factors.
- Develop a multidisciplinary plan to risk assess and adopt preventative interventions.

Table 8.3 provides an example of a multidisciplinary plan for assessing and preventing delirium, using Jack Porter as an example. Jack Porter remained in hospital for three weeks, and he remained in a state of delirium for a week before a gradual improvement was seen. After his discharge Jack was able to go home to his wife with support from community and social services. For patients in acute care, and particularly those patients who have undergone surgery, identifying the risk of delirium and preventing long-term problems for patients has become a priority (NICE, 2019a). Your role as a nurse is to be vigilant in the holistic assessment of the patient and family to identify the potential for delirium and, if possible, prevent it.

In summary the key messages when assessing and managing people who are at risk of delirium and/or who present with delirium include:

- Risk assess the person for predisposing and precipitating factors associated with delirium and manage any underlying factors present.
- Ensure there is effective communication between the healthcare team, the patient, and their family and work collaboratively to reduce the risk factors and prevent progression to delirium.

Factors on assessment	Preventative interventions	Management interventions for Jack Porter

Cognitive impairment disorientation	• Reorientate the person by explaining:
	  o where they are
	  o who they are
	  o who you are: 'My name is …'
	  o what your role is.
	• Provide:
	  o a clock
	  o a calendar
	  o appropriate signage.
	• Provide cognitive stimulation:
	  o reminiscence.
	• Encourage regular family visits.
		• When Jack awoke the next morning, we reminded him where he was and why.
		• We introduced ourselves and our roles.
		• We found his watch in the locker and put it on his wrist, checking it was the right time.
		• We explained what day it was and encouraged him to talk about his wife and family.
		• We contacted Jack's family to explain that he had become confused in the night and encouraged them to visit.

Hypoxia	• Assess for hypoxia and treat as necessary with oxygen, other medication, positioning, and physiotherapy.	• Jack's oxygen saturations were 94% and we encouraged him to sit up and take regular deep breaths to help his breathing and circulation, while continuing to encourage him to keep his oxygen mask on.
Dehydration Constipation	• Assess fluid balance and bowel activity daily. • Encourage the person to take oral fluids; however, if necessary, supplement with subcutaneous or intravenous fluids.	• Because of Jack's reduced urine output and elevated blood levels of sodium, potassium, and creatinine, he was given an infusion of fluids to improve his fluid and electrolyte balance (NICE, 2017b). He was risk assessed for acute kidney injury (Chapter 9). • Jack had a history of cardiovascular disease, so his respirations, pulse, and fluid balance were monitored closely in case of fluid overload. • Jack's blood results were checked the next day to review the situation.
Imbalance in electrolytes and creatinine Metabolic acidosis	• Monitor blood levels of electrolytes, liver, and renal function. • Assess for signs of metabolic acidosis (Chapter 3).	

(Continued)

Table 8.3 (Continued)

Factors on assessment	Preventative interventions	Management interventions for Jack Porter
Infection	• Undertake daily infection and sepsis screening and escalate care as necessary (Chapter 7). • Implement infection control procedures. • Avoid invasive catheterisation unless necessary.	• The results from Jack's catheter specimen of urine directed a change in antibiotic therapy. • The presence of the urinary catheter was reviewed daily. • The catheter was removed three days later. • All infection control procedures were followed.
Multiple medications	• Review the person's medications and assess the risks of side effects and continued requirement for the drugs.	• Jack resumed a reduced dose of antihypertensive medication as he recovered, and metformin continued for his diabetes.
Medications that alter the balance of neurotransmitters • Anticholinergics: atropine, ipratropium bromide. • Analgesics: opioids such as morphine. • Corticosteroids: hydrocortisone. • Antihistamines: chlorphenamine. • Cardiovascular agents: digoxin. • Hypnotic drugs: benzodiazepines such as **midazolam**.	• Many of the drugs on this list will be vital for the patient's safety and well-being. • It is important that the drugs are only given when necessary and reviewed daily.	• These were reviewed daily by checking blood glucose levels and vital signs.
Pain	• Assess for pain using a holistic approach and manage effectively.	• We continued to assess Jack for evidence of pain and discomfort (Schofield, 2018).
Poor nutrition	• Undertake a nutritional assessment and assess factors that may be affecting adequate nutrition such as ill-fitting teeth.	• Jack's appetite had reduced since being diagnosed with a urinary tract infection. However, over the next few days he gradually improved.

Factors on assessment	Preventative interventions	Management interventions for Jack Porter
Limited mobility	• Encourage patients who have had surgery to mobilise as soon as possible after surgery. • Encourage people to walk, with support if necessary, as often as possible during the day. • Encourage all patients to carry out active range of movement exercises every day.	• Jack was encouraged to walk around his bed and do a range of motion exercises during the day.
Sensory impairment	• Ensure hearing impairments are assessed and managed with a hearing aid. • Ensure people have the appropriate glasses for reading and long-distance vision. • Provide regular stimulation for those patients who are physically isolated.	• We encouraged the family to bring in Jack's reading glasses as well as his regular spectacles so that he could read the paper.
Sleep disturbances	• Avoid undertaking medical and nursing procedures during sleep periods. • Reduce noise to a minimum.	• We kept Jack in the same section of the ward that he was used to and provided an environment to promote restful sleep.

Table 8.3   Clinical assessment factors and interventions to prevent delirium

Source: NICE, 2019a.

NICE (2019a) guidance recommends that if a person with delirium becomes distressed and/or a risk to themselves or others, always attempt communication interventions to de-escalate the situation. If the person's distress or risk to themselves or others continues, the antipsychotic drug haloperidol can be prescribed in the short term until the underlying factors have been resolved (NICE, 2019a).

Delirium in ICU

The incidence of delirium among patients in ICU is up to 30% higher than found in acute medical and surgical wards (Vasilevskis et al., 2012; Alce et al., 2014). In the UK, Page (2008) identified that a diagnosis of delirium can occur in up to 69% of patients receiving IMV. Delirium can also be an independent predictor of morbidity, in the form of post ICU cognitive impairment, and mortality in ventilated patients (Ely et al., 2003). In the next section we will explore the relationship between the ICU environment and the development of delirium by exploring Paul Chapman's story.

Case study: Paul Chapman

Paul Chapman (28 years) was walking home from a night out when he was hit from behind by a hit-and-run driver. He was found by a passer-by who called the emergency services. Paul was taken to A&E where he was stabilised and transferred to the operating theatre. Paul's injuries included:

- facial fractures;
- fractured ribs (3 and 4) on the left side and contusion on the right side of his chest;
- fractured pelvis;
- fractured right shaft of femur, tibia, and fibula.

In theatre Paul received the following:

- external fixation of a fractured pelvis;
- internal fixation and pinning of his right shaft of femur, tibia, and fibula.

Paul was transferred to ICU from theatre in an unconscious state, intubated and ventilated.

When Paul was admitted to the ED, in addition to his fractures he was suffering from hypoxia, hypovolaemic shock, and a metabolic acidosis. When assessed against predisposing and precipitating modifiable factors (Table 8.2), Paul was already considered to be at risk of developing delirium on the basis of hypoxia, hypotension, and traumatic fractures. He was resuscitated with oxygen, respiratory support, and fluid replacement, including a blood transfusion. Paul had been conscious at the scene, but his level of consciousness had deteriorated by the time he was admitted to hospital, and this again is a predisposing factor for delirium (European Delirium Association and American Delirium Society, 2014).

In ICU Paul received a tracheostomy tube to prevent destabilisation of his facial fractures and was supported by IMV. Intravenous medication for the purposes of pain relief and sedation included: fentanyl, which is a potent synthetic opioid used for analgesia and anaesthesia (Marik, 2015), and midazolam for the purpose of sedation. According to Marik (2015) and Vasilevskis et al. (2012) the use of benzodiazepines such as midazolam have been shown to increase the risk and severity of delirium in patients at risk and they recommend that early mobilisation and reduction of sedation can reduce this risk. An alternative sedative is dexmedetomidine or propofol (Marik, 2015). For people with critical illness requiring sedation, there is evidence from a systematic review and meta-analysis to suggest that the drug dexmedetomidine can reduce the incidence of delirium and agitation in this patient group (Ng et al., 2019). Paul had several invasive and restricting devices inserted to monitor his haemodynamic state including central and peripheral intravenous infusion lines, arterial line, urinary catheter, a chest drain to drain a pneumothorax on his left side, and ECG monitoring. All these interventions and devices can be described as physically restrictive and invasive forms of therapy and are precipitating factors for delirium (Table 8.2). In summary, the risk of precipitating factors for the development of delirium for Paul were high and it was imperative that he was risk assessed and managed to limit the onset of delirium on a shift-by-shift basis (NICE, 2019a; Ely, 2014).

When Paul was assessed for predisposing factors for the development of delirium, the nurse's initial assessment revealed that the only predisposing factor was that of his severity of illness. This was reviewed, however, when Paul's mother confided in the nurse at the bedside that Paul had experimented with drugs as a teenager but had told his mother that he had given them up eight years ago when he met his wife. This highlights the requirement to continually review your assessments – often not all the relevant information is available from the outset. This finding became significant when 48 hours later Paul was stable enough for the team to reduce his sedation and respiratory support.

Case study: Paul Chapman's sedation is reduced

As Paul started to wake up, he became very agitated, and despite the use of reorientation and reassurance from Jennie, his nurse, Paul tried to pull at his peripheral and arterial line and ECG leads. Jennie continued to reassure him, explaining where he was and what had happened. She asked him if he had any pain, and Paul responded by beckoning to her to come closer. As Jennie leant forward Paul grabbed her round the waist and would not let go. Jennie instinctively leant back and, as she did, Paul came forward in the bed and was in danger of falling out. Jennie shouted for help, and with gentle reassurance from several members of staff Paul eventually let go and appeared to relax. A few minutes later, however, Paul was again trying to pull at anything that appeared to be attaching him to the bed. Jennie decided to invite Paul's wife to the bedside in the hope that this would reassure him. She explained to his relatives why he was more awake and that he was quite agitated at times, but if he were able to settle, they would be able to continue to reduce the sedation and respiratory support as the next step in his recovery. When Paul saw his wife, he held out his arms and she leant forward to hold his hands. Paul, seeing her come closer, made a grab for her, and pulled her onto the bed. We advised her to stay still and tried to persuade Paul to let her go. Paul resisted, and a team decision was made to recommence sedation and review the plan for weaning Paul from respiratory support. Paul's wife was tearful and upset by what had happened, and Jennie tried to reassure her that this situation can occur in critically ill patients and that, as Paul began to improve, he would become less confused about what had happened.

Treating delirium

For some patients, risk assessment and preventative interventions are not enough to prevent severe cases of hyperactive delirium. In the case study, Paul Chapman was suffering from severe symptoms of hyperactive delirium triggered by multiple pre-disposing and precipitating factors. In cases such as Paul's, a plan of management would begin by dealing with the immediate problem of his distress. Paul was placing himself and others in danger by his actions, and the only option available was to recommence sedation to stabilise his condition and protect the safety of others. This can be described as a form of chemical restraint, which in Paul's case was justified to protect his safety in the short term (Bray et al., 2004).

When patients develop delirium, a treatment plan should always begin with an assessment of the underlying causes and the provision of open and reassuring communication to both the patient and family (Borthwick et al., 2006; NICE, 2019a). The causes of Paul's delirium were related to a history of drug misuse and factors related to his condition, such as fear and anxiety, physical and chemical restraint from his multiple therapeutic interventions such as the tracheostomy tube, ECG, infusions and urinary catheter, and the risk of physiological imbalance associated with his critical illness. The most effective method for managing Paul's delirium was to promote recovery and rehabilitation and the subsequent removal of trigger factors.

According to Borthwick et al. (2006), patients with a history of drug abuse and who undergo sedation with benzodiazepines such as midazolam for seven days or more are very likely to experience delirium when the drug is withdrawn. For Paul, a plan for recovery included a gradual reduction of sedation over several days and a daily review of his risk factors for developing delirium. Five days later, Paul was awake and no longer requiring respiratory support. He was transferred to the orthopaedic ward, where his rehabilitation continued. Paul continued to experience episodes of confusion for several months following his accident and, according to Arend and Christensen (2009), Paul may experience prolonged neuropsychological side effects that can extend beyond his physical recovery.

Key steps in managing delirium include:

- assess patient safety immediately;
- risk assess underlying causes and avoid where possible medication that increases the severity of delirium;
- communicate with, reorientate, and reassure the patient;
- involve family and friends;
- encourage early mobility;
- ensure stability and continuity of care using a team approach;
- if the patient is distressed, try verbal and non-verbal reassurance to calm the patient.

A systematic toolkit to operationalise interventions to promote prevention of delirium and safety of patients in ICU is accessible through the American Association of Critical Care Nurses (2015) and is based on work by Vasilevskis et al. (2012) and Balas et al. (2012) on their development and evaluation of the ABCDEF bundle for delirium prevention and safety. The bundle of care addresses six key areas and includes the following.

- A: Assess, prevent, and manage pain.
- B: Both spontaneous awakening trials and spontaneous breathing trials (this involves daily cessation of sedation to assess the patient's suitability for weaning from respiratory support and sedation using, for example, the Richmond Agitation and Sedation Scale) (Taran et al., 2019).
- C: Choice of analgesia and sedation should be patient orientated and goal directed.
- D: Delirium – assess, prevent, and manage using validated assessment tools such as CAM-ICU.
- E: Early mobility and exercise.
- F: Family engagement and empowerment.

Alternatively, Ely et al. (2016) propose a multidisciplinary empirical protocol for the assessment, prevention, and management of delirium in intensive care settings incorporating the use of sedation scales (Chapter 3) followed by assessment for delirium using CAM-ICU, minimising the use of sedation and avoiding benzodiazepines unless specifically needed to treat specific conditions. Both approaches can be used synergistically to prevent psychological trauma and suffering in ICU.

Activity 8.2 Evidence-based practice and research

This activity encourages you to think about how you might update and improve practice. Go to the website **www.icudelirium.org/medicalprofessionals.html** or alternatively search for 'CAM-ICU' and the 'ABCDEF' bundle for delirium and explore the toolkits and guides that are available. When you are on your next placement ask the clinical staff how they assess for delirium. The importance of asking questions like this is that it opens avenues of inquiry that the clinical staff may not have considered and has the potential to improve practice. The website: www.idelirium.org/ also provides resources to support evidence-based practice.

As this answer is based on your own reflection, there is no outline answer at the end of the chapter.

Chapter summary

Within this chapter we have considered the common causes of delirium in patients placed in acute and critical care settings. We have explored ways in which patients can be risk assessed for developing delirium and how it may be prevented and treated. The key messages from this chapter to apply to your practice are the following:

(Continued)

(Continued)

- Patients who develop delirium have increased risk of morbidity and mortality.
- Daily risk assessment of patients for developing delirium can prevent its onset and should be considered a priority of care.
- Think delirium in patients who show signs of deterioration as part of managing their care.
- Promoting good communication and continuity of care is an important factor in preventing delirium.
- If delirium cannot be prevented, then strategies and interventions used must be person centred and enhance the safety of the patient and others.

Further reading

Bray, K, Hill, K, Robson, W et al. (2004) British Association of Critical Care Nurses' position statement on the use of restraint in adult critical care units. *Nursing in Critical Care*, 9(5): 199–212.

This paper provides advice by the BACCN on the use of physical and chemical restraint for patients who become agitated and combative.

Useful websites

icudelirium.org

This website offers general information about the assessment, prevention, and management of delirium.

www.icudelirium.org/medicalprofessionals.html

This website has educational resources on how to assess patients using the Confusion Assessment Method, CAM-ICU, and the ABCDEF bundle for delirium prevention and safety. The site also provides links to videos that demonstrate the assessment in practice.

www.nice.org.uk/cg103

This website provides you with all NICE guidance documentation of assessing and treating delirium, including a guideline for patients and carers. The guidance was last updated in 2019.

the4at.com

This website introduces the 4AT rapid clinical test for delirium, the validation of the tool, and guidance on clinical implementation.

Chapter 9

The patient with acute kidney injury

Desiree Tait

(Continued)

NMC Annex B Nursing procedures

This chapter will address the following procedures:

Part 2: Procedures for the planning, provision, and management of person-centred nursing care

5. Use evidence-based, best practice approaches for meeting needs for care and support with nutrition and hydration, accurately assessing the person's capacity for independence and self-care and initiating appropriate interventions.
5.1 Observe, assess, and optimise nutrition and hydration status and determine the need for intervention and support.
5.4 Record fluid intake and output and identify, respond to, and manage dehydration or fluid retention.

Chapter aims

By the end of this chapter, you should be able to:

*   describe the functions of the kidney and recognise the signs and symptoms of abnormal renal function that can lead to renal failure;
*   describe and differentiate between acute kidney injury and chronic kidney disease;
*   identify and describe risk factors that lead to acute kidney injury;
*   demonstrate an awareness of how to risk assess people for acute kidney injury in primary and secondary care settings;
*   recognise and interpret the clinical signs and symptoms of a person suffering from acute kidney injury and identify appropriate nursing interventions;
*   describe the signs and symptoms and nursing management of a person with renal failure in a critical care setting;
*   reflect on the clinical examples referred to in this chapter and relate to your own clinical practice.

Introduction

Within this chapter we will explore how to assess and interpret situations where people may be at risk of acute kidney injury (AKI), how to prevent patients from developing AKI and, finally, how to manage patients who develop AKI. The chapter will begin with a summary of the functions of the kidney and what happens when those functions fail.

Impaired renal function is described as either acute, known as AKI or chronic as in chronic kidney disease (CKD). AKI occurs as an acute onset renal impairment occurring within a few hours or days, depending on the severity of the underlying trigger. AKI is potentially both preventable and reversible when risk assessed for, and the underlying cause (such as hypotension) managed effectively. Timely intervention is essential to prevent or reduce the risk of progression to end-stage kidney disease. CKD describes the progressive decline of renal function, developing over months or years. CKD is often associated with co-morbidities including hypertension, diabetes, pre-existing renal disease, and cardiovascular disease. Someone living with CKD is also at a high risk of developing AKI secondary to an acute exacerbation of new or existing co-morbidities. Some people can develop AKI without any associated co-morbidities while others may present with a more complex picture of health needs. The importance of a person-centred holistic approach to assessing and managing care cannot be underestimated and this is explored through the analysis of Tim Hunter's story later in the chapter.

What are the functions of the kidney and what happens when they fail?

The main function of the kidney is the formation of urine, which is produced at a rate of approximately 1.5 L/day, although this will depend on a person's level of hydration. This process occurs within the functional units of the kidney, the nephrons, and involves the processes of filtration, reabsorption, and secretion.

The formation of urine begins in the glomerulus. The afferent arteriole subdivides into many smaller capillaries as it enters the Bowman's capsule and arterial pressure within the capillary bed forces water and low molecular weight substances from the blood into the Bowman's capsule. The **glomerular filtration rate** (GFR) is a measure of the volume of fluid that is filtered by all the functioning nephrons in the kidneys. In a healthy person this is 180 L/day or equal to approximately 90 ml per minute of blood flow. However, to maintain homeostasis, 80% of this volume is reabsorbed as it flows through the proximal and distal tubules and collecting duct (McCance and Huether, 2019).

The concentration of urine occurs in the loop of Henle and involves the diffusion and reabsorption of sodium and reabsorption of water. The secretion of ions, including hydrogen and potassium, from tubular capillaries, occurs in the proximal and distal tubules. A summary of this process is illustrated in Figure 9.1.

Other functions of the kidney include the following (McCance and Huether, 2019).

- The production of hormones, such as:
  - renin: produced by the juxtaglomerular cells in the Bowman's capsule close to the afferent capillary, triggers the renin-angiotensin-aldosterone system if there is a reduction in blood flow to the kidney;

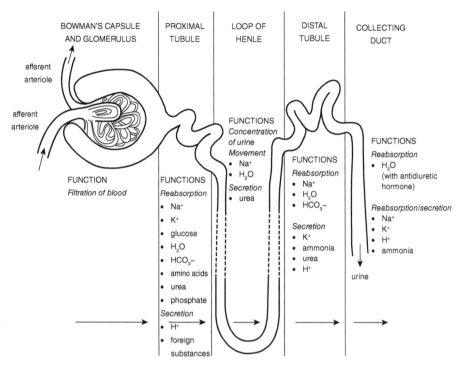

Figure 9.1   Major functions of the nephron

- o   erythropoietin: produced by interstitial cells in the kidney, controls red cell production;
- o   calcitriol: produced in the proximal tubules of the nephron, promotes the absorption of dietary calcium.
- •   Excretion of the by-products of metabolism, including:
  - o   creatinine (produced as a by-product of energy production from muscle contraction);
  - o   urea (produced as a by-product of protein metabolism);
  - o   sodium (Na);
  - o   potassium (K);
  - o   bicarbonate (HCO_3).
- •   Maintenance of acid-base balance (see Chapter 2).

The signs and symptoms of impaired kidney function depend on several factors, including the progression of the damage (50% of nephrons can be destroyed before signs and symptoms begin to occur), and whether the person is suffering from AKI or CKD (McCance and Huether, 2019). This is explored in more detail later in the chapter. Regardless of the speed of onset, as renal function becomes impaired pathophysiological changes occur. Table 9.1 provides a general summary of physiological signs of renal malfunction.

Normal renal function	Signs and symptoms of renal malfunction
Formation of urine	<ul><li>Reduction in urine production and output.</li><li>Fluid overload.</li><li>Hypertension.</li><li>Heart failure.</li><li>Increased risk of pulmonary and interstitial oedema.</li><li>Reduction in estimated GFR.</li></ul>
Production of renin	<ul><li>Inability to control the renin-angiotensin-aldosterone system, leading to loss of control over:<ul><li>blood pressure</li><li>fluid balance</li><li>sodium balance.</li></ul></li></ul>
Excretion of the by-products of metabolism	<ul><li>Inability to excrete ammonia in the form of urea, leading to uraemia and encephalopathy (eventually coma).</li><li>Inability to excrete creatinine, leading to increased creatinine levels.</li><li>Inability to excrete potassium, leading to hyperkalaemia.</li><li>Anorexia, nausea, and vomiting.</li><li>Muscle weakness.</li><li>Sexual dysfunction.</li></ul>
Maintenance of acid-base balance (see Chapter 2)	<ul><li>Metabolic acidosis (see Chapter 2).</li></ul>
The production of erythropoietin	<ul><li>Anaemia, tiredness, and lethargy.</li><li>Prolonged bleeding time.</li></ul>
The production of calcitriol	<ul><li>Increased risk of calcium loss and osteoporosis.</li><li>Bone pain.</li></ul>

Table 9.1 Kidney functions and the signs and symptoms of renal malfunction

What is AKI?

AKI, previously known as acute renal failure, can be described as a syndrome involving an acute, rapid deterioration in renal function resulting in the patient being unable to maintain fluid, electrolyte, and acid-base balance (Fliser et al., 2012). Patients can present with mild reversible AKI or at any point on a continuum that leads toward a severe syndrome that can progress to end-stage kidney disease. According to the available evidence, even mild AKI can be accompanied by permanent decline in kidney function and an increased risk of CKD (Ostermann et al., 2020).

The best treatment for AKI is therefore prevention; this is reflected in the clinical guidance offered by NICE Guideline 148 (2019b) and supported by the European Renal Best Practice (ERBP) group (Fliser et al., 2012) and the Kidney Disease: Improving Global Outcomes (KDIGO) Group (Ostermann et al., 2020).

The medical definition of AKI is based on the following three key physiological factors:

- urine output (<0.5 ml/kg/hr, oliguria);
- serum creatinine (SCr) level increase;
- the severity of urine output decline and increase in SCr level from the patient's baseline level at the onset of their current condition.

The ERBP workgroup recommend that each patient should be assessed according to the severity of the AKI rather than an absolute definition of whether AKI exists or not. Table 9.1 provides a summary of the ERBP recommendations and KDIGO severity score (Fliser et al., 2012). The criteria and severity score are due for review by 2022; however there is growing evidence that the KDIGO recommendations published in 2012 have been effective in preventing and managing AKI with a relative improvement in clinical outcomes (Ostermann et al., 2020).

Degree of severity of AKI from 1–3, with 3 as the most severe	Criteria
Stage 1	**One of the following**
	Serum creatinine (SCr) increased to 1.5–1.9 times the baseline or SCr increase >26.5 µmol/L.
	Urine output <0.5 ml/kg/hr during a 6-hour block.
Stage 2	**One of the following**
	SCr increase 2.0–2.9 times baseline.
	Urine output <0.5 ml/kg/hr during two 6-hour blocks.
Stage 3	**One of the following**
	SCr increase >3 times baseline or SCr increase >353 µmol/L.
	Urine output <0.3 ml/kg/hr during more than 24 hours.
	Anuria (no urine output) for more than 12 hours.
	Initiation of renal replacement therapy to substitute kidney function.

Table 9.2   Criteria for determining the severity of AKI in a patient at risk based on ERBP and KDIGO guidance

Source: Fliser et al., 2012; KDIGO AKI Work Group, 2012

Why does AKI occur?

AKI occurs because of factors leading to:

- extracellular volume depletion and decreased renal blood flow (pre-renal);
- toxic inflammatory injury to kidney cells (intra-renal);
- obstruction to the flow of urine in the urinary system, usually bilateral (post-renal).

The most frequent cause of the syndrome is transient hypoperfusion leading to decreased renal blood flow and is referred to as pre-renal AKI. For example, if a patient goes into physiological shock, the body's natural regulatory mechanisms will activate the autonomic nervous system and the renin-angiotensin-aldosterone mechanism (described in Chapter 6). Consequently, renal blood flow and GFR are reduced to preserve circulating volume and maintain tissue perfusion. At this stage, AKI is preventable and/or reversible by treating the cause of the shock. However, if the underlying cause of shock is not diagnosed and corrected in a timely manner, renal blood flow will continue to be reduced and the kidney will become ischaemic, leading to cell damage and the inflammatory response. This more severe form of the syndrome is referred to as intra-renal AKI. Other causes of intra-renal AKI include toxic damage caused by nephrotoxic drugs such as non-steroidal anti-inflammatories, and iodinated contrast agents. Post-renal AKI is rare and usually occurs when there is bilateral obstruction to both kidneys or when there is obstruction to the flow from a single functioning kidney. Regardless of cause, all types of AKI lead to oliguria, a reduction in urine output to less than 0.5 ml/kg/hr (see Figure 9.2).

According to McCance and Huether (2019), AKI progresses through three phases:

- **The initiation phase**: caused by reduced perfusion or toxicity and during which AKI is evolving. This phase lasts for 24–36 hours and accurate risk assessment and monitoring can prevent further progression at this stage. If this phase is left to progress, ischaemia and cell injury will lead to a renal inflammatory response.
- **The maintenance phase**: the oliguric phase is the period where there is established renal injury and dysfunction which will continue after the initial cause is resolved and can continue for weeks or months. Clinical signs of renal malfunction include: oliguria, elevated levels of serum creatinine, potassium, and blood urea nitrogen, metabolic acidosis, high sodium, and water overload (see Table 9.1).
- **The recovery phase**: renal injury goes through a process of repair and normal renal function is established. Initially while GFR returns to normal, the renal tubules are initially unable to concentrate the urine. This leads to polyurea, a decline in creatinine and urea levels, **hyponatraemia** (low sodium), and hypokalaemia (low potassium) and a risk of dehydration.

The phases of AKI and nursing management are explored further as part of Tim Hunter's story.

Who is most at risk?

AKI is common in hospitalised patients experiencing acute illness and there is a risk of mortality ranging from 20–60% (Wiersema et al., 2020). However, in patients where AKI is complicated by multiple failure of their body organs the mortality rate is likely to be more than 50% (Lewington and Kanagasundaram, 2011). The risks associated with AKI are high and the severity of the problem for people at risk has been highlighted by a report published by NCEPOD (2009) where they identified serious deficiencies in the care of patients who developed AKI, reporting that only 50% of the patients reviewed received good care. Deficiencies reported include poor attention to detail and inadequate risk assessment of factors for AKI. The recommendations from this report have informed NICE guidance (2019b).

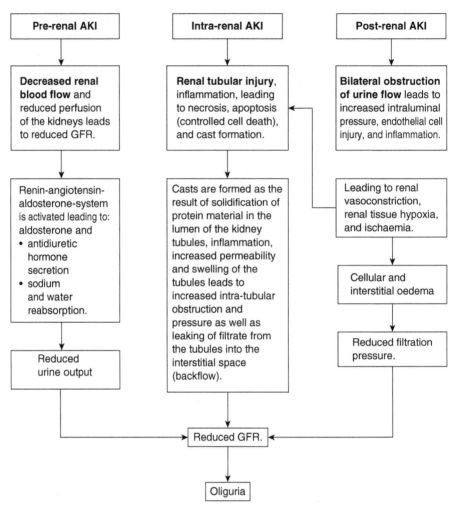

Figure 9.2 A summary of the physiological mechanisms involved in the development of AKI and oliguria

Source: informed by McCance and Huether, 2019.

Some patients have a higher degree of risk for developing AKI and, according to NICE (2019b), these include people:

- with acute illness;
- with evidence of deteriorating vital signs, particularly hypotension;
- with urine output of less than 0.5 ml/kg/hr (oliguria);
- with sepsis;
- receiving iodinated contrast agents in the previous week;
- having surgery and at risk of hypovolemia and/or infection;
- with co-morbidities including heart failure, diabetes, and liver disease;
- who have a history of previous episodes of AKI;

- with CKD;
- aged ≥65 years;
- who are regularly prescribed nephrotoxic drugs such as NSAIDs, aminoglycosides such as gentamycin, ACE inhibitors, angiotensin II receptor antagonists (ARBs), and diuretics;
- with a history of, or a condition that may lead to, urinary obstruction.

NICE (2019b) guidance prioritises assessing risk of AKI based on the following:

- identifying AKI in people with acute illness;
- identifying AKI in people with no obvious acute illness;
- assessing risk factors in those people receiving iodine-based contrast media;
- assessing risk factors in adults having surgery.

Once risk assessed, ongoing prevention should focus on assessment and monitoring of individuals using NEWS2 criteria and the detection of AKI using clinically recognised definitions of AKI such as KDIGO (2012). Table 9.3 illustrates clinical examples of patients at risk of developing AKI.

What are the nursing responsibilities when assessing patients at risk?

The role of the nurse in risk assessing the patient for the potential, existence, and severity of AKI is to:

- Know your patients, including their past and recent medical history, physiological observations at admission, recent investigations, prescribed medication, and when they last had renal function tests.
- Identify if your patient is at risk of AKI (see Table 9.3).
- Risk assess and monitor your patients for evidence of deteriorating respiratory function.
- Risk assess and monitor your patients for evidence of deteriorating circulation using the ABCDE approach and NEWS2, paying particular attention to:
  - deterioration in fluid balance;
  - deterioration in urine output with evidence of oliguria (urine output less than 0.5 ml/kg/hr);
  - deterioration in BP;
  - evidence of sepsis (see Chapter 6).
- Perform urine dipstick testing for blood, protein, leucocytes, nitrites, and glucose and monitor for haematuria and proteinuria as well as infection.
- Monitor for signs of an increase in blood creatinine levels according to, for example, the KDIGO criteria (2012), reduction in estimated GFR (as evidence of CKD), urea, and electrolyte levels.
- Communicate your concerns to the relevant medical practitioner using an SBAR approach (see Chapter 1).

People at risk	Why	Clinical example
With acute illness	People with an acute episode of illness are more likely to present with fluid volume depletion due to haemorrhage, diarrhoea and vomiting, burns, acute cardiac failure, and failure of other body systems. They are also more likely to need emergency surgery and have a higher associated risk of infection than people receiving elective surgery.	Jenny Brown (19 years old) is admitted following a four-day history of acute diarrhoea and vomiting. She refused help from her university friends, initially because she was too embarrassed. On admission Jenny was pale, weak, and lethargic: R: 24; P: 97; BP: 89/55. She had not passed urine that day and did not want to.
With evidence of deteriorating vital signs, particularly hypotension	If the early signs of clinical deterioration are missed the patient is likely to experience transient reduced perfusion of the kidneys because of hypotension. 55% of people who develop AKI have a transient period of hypotension (Patschan and Müller, 2015).	Terry Jones (35 years old) – a coach driver – had collapsed in a local hotel with haematemesis and melaena. Vital signs on admission were R: 23/min; P: 100/min; BP: 85/58. He received fluid resuscitation as he was assessed as having a low risk of a further bleed. Four hours later he became restless: R: 28/min; P: 120/min; BP: 70/40. He received further fluid resuscitation and blood transfusions before his BP stabilised at 110/65. Following a review of Terry Jones's fluid balance since admission the nurse estimated that his urine output had been less than 0.5 ml/kg/hr for the last three hours, increasing his risk of AKI.
With urine output of (less than) <0.5 ml/kg/hr (oliguria)	Possible reasons include: • hypovolaemia and urine output should be assessed with evidence of deteriorating vital signs; • obstruction to the flow of urine (see below).	
With sepsis	Sepsis can cause AKI because of: • hypotension • the triggering of a dysregulated response to infection associated with injury to cells and organs (discussed in Chapter 7).	William Butler (73 years old) had a past medical history of ischaemic heart disease, diabetes, and hypertension. Several days ago, he cut and bruised his upper arm on a kitchen door and was admitted with cellulitis. Twenty-four hours later he was risk assessed and diagnosed with sepsis (Chapter 7). His BP fell to 70/30 and he had passed <0.5 ml/hr for three hours.
Receiving iodinated contrast agents in the previous week	Potential toxicity of these agents increases if patients have any other risk factors listed in the table. Therefore, careful assessment of the risk benefit of undertaking the investigation, e.g., percutaneous intervention (PCI) and effective management of other risk factors should be undertaken before the procedure is undertaken (Fliser et al., 2012). NICE (2019b) recommends:	Harry Smith (58 years old) has a medical history of diabetes, hypertension, and hyperlipidaemia. He is prescribed ACE inhibitors, statins, and aspirin. This afternoon he was found by his wife in a state of collapse at home. On admission he was diagnosed with ST elevation myocardial infarction (STEMI) and cardiogenic shock. On assessment: R: 24/min; SpO₂: 85%; P: 120/min; BP: 83/55.

People at risk	Why	Clinical example
	Encourage oral hydration before and after the procedure, or intravenous fluid replacement if other risk factors are present. • Discuss the temporary discontinuation of drugs with renal toxicity with the medical team.	His estimated GFR was 29%, indicating he had stage 4 CKD. He was risk assessed by the cardiac and renal specialist to determine the risks/benefit of PCI and it was decided that without percutaneous intervention and insertion of vascular stents he had a high risk of mortality and they proceeded with the PCI. His co-morbidities, including CKD, PCI, and cardiogenic shock, all increased his risk of developing AKI.
With chronic kidney disease (CKD)	AKI can occur in patients with existing CKD making the risk of morbidity and mortality higher in this group (Carville et al., 2014).	
Having surgery and at risk of hypovolaemia and/or infection	These patients have a higher risk of hypotension, and/or surgical complications and infection (Aitken et al., 2013; Borthwick and Ferguson, 2010; NICE, 2019).	Martha Brown (75 years old) lived alone and suffered with congestive heart failure, hypertension, thyroid disorder, and rheumatoid arthritis. Her medication included: amiodarone, furosemide, levothyroxine, and NSAIDs. She was admitted following a fall at home and sustained a fractured neck of femur. During the surgery she sustained moderate to severe blood loss and an episode of hypovolaemia. She was admitted to ITU for post-operative care because the following factors put her at risk of further clinical deterioration and AKI. • her age; • co-morbidities; • medication of NSAIDs and diuretics; • episode of hypovolaemia.
With co-morbidities including heart failure, hypertension, diabetes, and liver disease	Progressive disease increases the risk of chronic inflammatory damage to the nephrons and stimulation of the renin-angiotensin-aldosterone system (McCance and Huether, 2019).	
Age ≥65 years	Increased risk of CKD and co-morbidities as indicated above.	

(Continued)

Table 9.3 (Continued)

People at risk	Why	Clinical example
Who are regularly prescribed nephrotoxic drugs such as: • non-steroidal anti-inflammatory drugs (NSAIDs); • aminoglycosides such as gentamicin; • angiotensin converting enzyme (ACE) inhibitors; • angiotensin II receptor antagonists (ARBs); • diuretics.	Nephrotoxic drugs increase the risk of inflammatory and vascular damage to the functioning nephrons, particularly in patients with existing co-morbidities and with increasing age.	
Who have a history of previous episodes of AKI	This indicates the kidney will have some existing damage from previous episodes, thus making the patient more susceptible to further injury.	Barry Taylor (65 years old) has been admitted for a second time in five years to the ITU with acute pancreatitis. On the first occasion he developed AKI secondary to systemic inflammatory response syndrome. On this occasion he was admitted following a period of depression and an increased intake of alcohol. He was diagnosed with acute necrotising pancreatitis, sepsis, and AKI.
With a history of, or a condition that may lead to, urinary obstruction	This is a rare cause of AKI unless the patient has only one functioning kidney left or if obstruction affects both kidneys at the same time. For example, a kidney stone can lead to inflammatory damage in the nephrons. A tumour may cause an obstruction to the one ureter or the urethra.	Matthew Richardson (42 years old) presented himself in the emergency unit with a 12-hour history of blood-stained urine and severe lower abdominal and loin pain. He was diagnosed with renal colic and advised to increase his fluid intake and was prescribed strong analgesics to manage the pain. He then said: 'Oh by the way I only have one kidney'. He was then admitted, and risk assessed for AKI.

Table 9.3   Clinical examples of people at risk of developing AKI

Activity 9.1 Reflection

With reference to Table 9.3, think back to your experiences in the clinical setting: can you identify a patient that you have nursed who was at risk of AKI?

If so, now consider the following questions.

- Did your patient fit into one or more of the high-risk groups?
- Did you consider them to be at risk of AKI?
- Was your patient identified as being at risk by the clinical team?
- If so, how was the patient managed?
- What was the outcome for the patient?

These reflective questions will help you to link the chapter content to patients you have nursed.

As this answer is based on your own reflection, there is no outline answer at the end of the chapter.

How can we prevent progression to established AKI?

The first priorities of the nurse when preventing patients from progressing to established AKI are the same as the nursing responsibilities for assessing patients at risk of AKI (page 233). The medical responsibilities for preventing a patient's progression to established AKI include:

- fluid resuscitation and maintenance of intravascular volume in order to restore blood pressure and cardiac output;
- temporarily discontinuing and removing nephrotoxic substances from the circulation;
- identifying and treating any related trigger factors such as hypoxia, infection, anaemia (NICE, 2019b; Bellomo, 2019).

Swift action within the first 24–26 hours of the patient being identified as at risk is critical to preventing AKI. Prescott et al. (2012) identify ten top tips that describe points along the patient's pathway where we can make a difference.

1. Empower people to take charge of their healthcare in primary care if they become acutely ill by advising them to increase their fluid intake.

2. The use of regular updates for healthcare staff on risk assessing for AKI and the use of computer support decision-making systems if available.

3. The effective use and interpretation of NEWS2.

4. All patients should have a consultant review their care within 12 hours of admission (NCEPOD, 2009).

5. The use of an electronic alert system to identify when abnormal serum creatinine levels increase.

6. Follow NICE (2019b) guidance for the management of AKI.

7. The use of the NICE (2019b) AKI care pathway and timely referral of patients from primary and secondary care for a renal review.

8. Effective communication and handover of care between practice areas and disciplines.

9. Effective clinical coding and audit of the incidence of AKI.

10. The medical follow-up of patients who have been diagnosed with AKI to manage their risk of developing CKD.

How is AKI different from CKD?

According to Ostermann et al. (2020), AKI and CKD are related and arguably represent a continuum of disease leading to end-stage kidney failure. For patients experiencing AKI, the syndrome can progress very rapidly, occurring within a few hours or days, depending on the severity of the underlying trigger. Patients will experience signs and symptoms based on the acuteness of their clinical condition and recent medical history as well as deterioration in urine output. Serum creatinine levels will increase correspondingly as the urine output deteriorates (see Table 9.2). The extent of changes in creatinine level and urine output determines the severity of, and stage of, AKI (Fliser et al., 2012). When a patient develops AKI, they progress through three clinical phases: the initiation phase, the maintenance phase, and the recovery phase. Later in the chapter we will introduce you to Tim Hunter and discuss how the syndrome impacted on him and his family as he progressed through the stages of AKI.

For patients experiencing CKD, the disease is progressive, developing over months or years. According to the National Kidney Foundation (2006) and KDIGO (2012) there is progressive loss of renal function associated with systemic diseases such as:

• hypertension;
• diabetes mellitus;
• systemic lupus erythematosus;
• existing kidney disease or injury;
• cardiovascular disease.

In the early stages of the disease, patients will experience no specific symptoms apart from those of the related disease, such as diabetes. The progression of CKD is instead measured by the patient's estimated glomerular filtration rate (eGFR) and urine albumin to creatinine ratio (Carville et al., 2014). As the disease progresses from mild to moderate CKD, the patient will begin to show more signs and symptoms of renal malfunction (Table 9.1), these becoming more severe as CKD progresses to stage 5 (end-stage kidney disease). CKD is not reversible but early screening and management of underlying co-morbidities, nutrition, vitamin D, fluid and electrolyte balance, and erythropoietin, as necessary, can delay its progression. Table 9.4 provides a summary of the key differences in diagnosis and disease progression.

Criteria	AKI	CKD
Onset of the condition	Acute onset over hours/days	Progressive onset over months/years
Prognosis	Potentially reversible	Progressive/not reversible
Classification of severity measurement	>SCr <urine output (see Table 9.2)	<GFR >urine albumin : creatinine ratio

Risk assessment	• Identify people at risk (see Table 9.3).
	• Monitor and prevent the development of AKI where possible.
	• Recognise early signs and provide physiological support.
		• Identify people at risk with:
		 o hypertension
		 o diabetes mellitus
		 o systemic lupus erythematosus
		 o existing kidney disease or injury
		 o cardiovascular disease.
		• Monitor GFR and urine albumin : creatinine ratio.
		• Stages of CKD based on GFR (ml/min) include:
		 o Stage 1: ≥90
		  Normal kidney function
		 o Stage 2: 60–89
		  Mildly reduced kidney function
		 o Stage 3: 30–59
		  Moderately reduced kidney function
		 o Stage 4: 15–29
		  Severely reduced kidney function
		 o Stage 5: <15
		  End-stage kidney failure
		(Renal Association, 2013)
		• Refer patients in stage 4 for specialist assessment (Carville et al., 2014).

Table 9.4   A summary of key differences in the diagnosis and risk assessment of AKI and CKD

The nursing management of a person with AKI

In the case study below, we explore Tim's story as he progresses through the initiation, maintenance, and recovery phases of AKI.

Case study: Tim Hunter in the initiation phase of AKI

Tim is a 78-year-old gentleman who lives with his wife Daphne (aged 76) in a small bungalow in the suburbs of the local town. They used to have a good social life, but this has dwindled in the last few years and Daphne has recently taken over the driving because of Tim's poor eyesight.

Situation

- Tim has been feeling generally unwell for a few weeks and Daphne has been concerned that he has not been eating properly and seemed tired and lethargic. Tim has been reluctant to go to his GP but was eventually persuaded to go after he became increasingly lethargic with a history of passing small infrequent amounts of red-stained urine and complaining of abdominal discomfort. The GP assessed Tim and was concerned that he had developed an ascending urinary tract infection because of a neurogenic bladder. Tim's blood glucose level in the surgery was 18 mmol/L. Considering his co-morbidities, the GP arranged his admission to the medical admissions unit.

Background

Tim has a past medical history of:

- type 2 diabetes for 20 years (prescribed metformin and glipizide);
- atrial fibrillation (prescribed digoxin and aspirin);
- hypertension for which he is prescribed an ACE inhibitor (ramipril);
- awaiting surgery for bilateral cataracts;
- he used to smoke but gave up 10 years ago.

Assessment

On admission to hospital the following assessment data were collected.

- **Airway and Breathing:**
  - R: 22/min, regular rate (NEWS2 = 2)
  - SpO_2: 97%
- **Circulation:**
  - HR: 87/min
  - pulse appeared irregular

- o ECG confirmed atrial fibrillation
- o BP: 115/65 mmHg
- Urine output: passed 100 ml of urine on admission, tested positive to blood and protein
- Complaining of nausea
- **Disability and exposure:**
  - o blood glucose 18.2 mmol/L
  - o lethargic but alert
  - o skin and mucous membranes dry and skin cracked
  - o T: 38.2 °C
  - o NEWS2 = 2

Recommendations and ongoing care

- Commence antibiotic therapy for a suspected urinary tract infection.
- Encourage Tim to drink and commence intravenous fluids to correct dehydration.
- Insert a urethral catheter and send a catheter specimen of urine (CSU) for culture and sensitivity.
- Monitor fluid balance.
- Assess serum creatinine and U&E and eGFR.
- Follow NEWS2 guidance for frequency of assessment and monitoring and increase frequency of observations if you are concerned.

Tim's blood results confirmed a high blood glucose of 18.7 mmol/L and an elevated potassium (K) of 6.4 mmol/L. His sodium level was within the normal range (137 mmol/L). Tim's creatinine level was 128 µmol/L, slightly elevated but not indicative of AKI at this stage (see Table 9.2). However, according to NICE (2019b), Tim continued to be at high risk of developing AKI due to the following reasons:

- acute illness;
- co-morbidities of hypertension and diabetes;
- nephrotoxic drug prescription (ACE inhibitor) (see Table 9.3);
- stage 3 CKD.

Tim's immediate problem was hyperkalaemia, and he was prescribed an insulin/ dextrose regime (GAIN, 2014). The insulin works by moving potassium from the circulation back into the cells, thus lowering serum potassium levels. The 50% dextrose is given to prevent hypoglycaemia. Once this treatment is complete, the patient's potassium should drop by 0.6–1 mmol/L within 15 minutes (GAIN, 2014). Later that day Tim's serum potassium had reduced to 4.7 mmol/L and his blood glucose level was reduced to 8.9 mmol/L. According to GAIN (2014), hyperkalaemia is commonly associated with AKI and/or CKD and with patients prescribed ACE inhibitors. Tim's eGFR was less than 60 ml/min, indicating moderately reduced kidney function. Based on this finding Tim continued to be at high risk of developing AKI and could be in the initiation phase of the syndrome.

The following morning Tim was beginning to feel much better; his vital signs were within the normal range, and he was in an equal fluid balance. His urethral catheter was removed, and he was encouraged to continue to drink a glass of water every hour. He was referred to the dietitian for advice on how to reduce his dietary intake of potassium and the diabetic specialist nurse to monitor his management of the diabetes. He was advised to stay for a further 24 hours to monitor his renal function (because of his risk of developing AKI) but Tim insisted he felt better, he had had enough and decided to discharge himself without further consultation and treatment. Daphne became very distressed by the idea of self-discharge and argued that this just was not like Tim! However, in the end a taxi was called, and Tim and Daphne left the hospital. What Tim and Daphne did not receive before discharge was the planned information and advice on how to prevent further deterioration in his kidney function and a medical review of his medication. Following discharge Tim continued to take his ACE inhibitors, anti-diabetic medication, and NSAIDS that he had been prescribed several months before for arthritic pain. Once at home he became reluctant to drink despite being encouraged to do so in the hospital, arguing that he was better now, and it was too much effort to keep going to the bathroom so often.

During the last few weeks, according to Jin et al. (2008), certain aspects of Tim's behaviour could be described as non-compliant or non-concordant with his long-term therapy. For example, his hesitance to seek healthcare advice from his GP, his hesitance to follow advice from the medical team, and his insistence on early self-discharge. Psychological factors that could have influenced this include Tim's feelings of distress around the emotional burden of his disease and possible depression (Walker et al., 2015). In this instance it has led to a further deterioration in his condition and his progression to the maintenance phase of AKI.

Activity 9.2 Communication

Identify three communication strategies you could use to defuse a situation such as when Tim Hunter insisted he was going home.

A sample answer is found at the end of this chapter.

The maintenance phase of AKI

The maintenance, or oliguric, phase of AKI is synonymous with established renal injury and dysfunction. This period may last weeks or months and its severity is measured by the degree of elevated serum creatinine and evidence of reduced urine output (see Table 9.2). The impact on the patient is severe and the risk of mortality increases correspondingly with rising creatinine levels and reduction in renal function (Fliser et al., 2012). Let us return to Tim's story after he experienced a deterioration in his condition.

Case study: Tim Hunter in the maintenance phase of AKI

Situation

Tim discharged himself from hospital 48 hours ago, after being admitted with a urinary tract infection and hyperkalaemia. He took his own discharge against medical advice and has been readmitted with abdominal pain, headache, and nausea. He has not passed urine since late yesterday evening (14 hours ago). His wife said that since returning home he had taken to his bed and been reluctant to eat and drink.

Background

Past medical history remains unchanged.

- Has been continuing to take NSAIDS for pain.
- Recently diagnosed with neurogenic bladder and urinary tract infection.

Assessment

- **Airway and Breathing:**
  - R: 25/min, regular rate (NEWS2 = 3), (Red Flag sepsis)
  - SpO_2: 95% (NEWS2 = 1)
- **Circulation:**
  - HR: 92/min (NEWS2 = 1)
  - pulse appeared irregular, confirmed as atrial fibrillation on ECG
  - BP: 98/63 mmHg (NEWS2 = 2)
- Urine output: not passed urine for 14 hours, urethral catheter inserted, drained 80 ml of cloudy urine (80 ml over 14 hours) (Red Flag sepsis)
- CSU sent for culture and sensitivity
- Complaining of nausea
- **Disability and exposure:**
  - blood glucose 17.4 mmol/L
  - lethargic but alert
  - skin and mucous membranes dry and cracked
  - T: 38.5°C (NEWS2 =1)
- NEWS2 = 8
- Red Flags for sepsis = 3
- **Blood biochemistry and haematology:**
  - Na: 132 mmol/L
  - K: 5.3 mmol/L
  - creatinine: 630 µmol/L
  - white cell count: 25×10^9/L

(Continued)

(Continued)

- o lactate: 2.9 mmol/L (Red Flag sepsis)
- o eGFR <60 ml/min

Recommendations

- Continue to risk assess for AKI and sepsis.
- Commence Sepsis Six.
- Alert a senior clinician to attend.
- Take blood for culture and commence intravenous antibiotic therapy.
- Review oxygen saturations and requirement for oxygen therapy.
- Commence fluid resuscitation.
- Monitor urine output hourly, vital signs using ABCDE, and review after 1 hour.
- Contact the CCOT for transfer to ITU.

When Tim was risk assessed for sepsis and AKI, he was found to meet the criteria for both.

These included:

- R >20/min;
- urine output <0.5 ml/kg/hr;
- lactate >2 mmol/L.

Tim's diagnosis of stage 3 AKI was confirmed by (see Table 9.2):

- serum creatinine (SCr) increase >353 µmol/L (630 µmol/L);
- anuria (no urine output) for more than 12 hours (immediately prior to admission).

Tim was transferred to intensive care for monitoring and treatment of his condition.

What is the clinical impact of established AKI?

When a patient moves into the maintenance phase of AKI they present with evidence of intra-renal damage, and while the precise pathophysiological mechanisms can only be theorised, there does appear to be some consensus over the following three events (Patschan and Müller, 2015; Hammer and McPhee, 2014). A summary of the processes leading to the maintenance phase or established AKI can be found in Figure 9.2.

1. Initially renal ischaemia leads to renal tubular dysfunction and damage. This triggers apoptosis (programmed cell death) and, in severe cases, necrosis (un-programmed cell death) and an increase in oxidative damage from the release of free radicals. A direct consequence of this damage is that the endothelial linings of the tubules are unable to maintain their functions of secretion and reabsorption,

and this triggers the functioning tubules to further reduce GFR through a tubule–glomerular feedback mechanism. There is also evidence of backflow of fluid into the interstitial space of the kidney, increasing the risk of more generalised damage.

2. Second, the ischaemic damage causes an interstitial inflammatory response and the release of pro-inflammatory chemicals, such as cytokines, and activation of the immune response, which leads to both pro- and anti-inflammatory effects. The triggering of the pro-inflammatory response can aggravate interstitial tissue damage in AKI but the anti-inflammatory effects are essential for facilitating tissue repair (Patschan and Müller, 2015).

3. Finally ischaemic damage can also lead to renal interstitial micro vasculopathy. This occurs when swelling of the endothelial cells in the peritubular capillaries leads to prolonged ischaemia because of microvascular occlusion, even when the primary cause of the renal ischaemia has been resolved (Patschan et al., 2012).

Overall, the combined impact of these mechanisms leads to acute loss of renal function and the signs and symptoms illustrated in Table 9.1. When we return to Tim's story, the clinical impact of his renal damage becomes evident as his story unfolds.

Case study: Tim arrives in ITU

Situation

Tim Hunter has been diagnosed with sepsis and AKI. He commenced the Sepsis Six Care Pathway (UK Sepsis Trust 2020) 30 minutes ago and was in the process of being transferred to ITU when his condition deteriorated.

Assessment

- **Airway and Breathing:**
  - R: 28/min, rapid shallow breathing
  - central cyanosis
  - producing pink frothy sputum
  - inspiratory crackles heard
  - SpO_2: 80% on high-flow oxygen (100%)
  - chest X-ray: pulmonary oedema
- **Circulation:**
  - HR: 98/min
  - BP: 70/50 mmHg (MAP 56.7 mmHg)
- Urethral catheter 10 ml in 30 minutes
- **Disability and exposure:**
  - blood glucose 18.4 mmol/L

(Continued)

(Continued)

- o   anxious, disorientated, acute confusion
- o   GCS: 12
- o   T: 38.5 °C
- **Blood biochemistry and haematology:**
  - o   Na: 138 mmol/L
  - o   K: 5.4 mmol/L
  - o   creatinine: 630 µmol/L
  - o   urea: 36.8 mmol/L
  - o   WCC: 28 × 10^9/L
  - o   lactate: 2.9 mmol/L
- **Arterial blood gases:**
  - o   pH: 7.166
  - o   PaO$_2$: 7.9 kPa
  - o   PaCO$_2$: 5.8 kPa
  - o   HCO$_3$: 17.2 mmol/L

Recommendations

- Commence positive pressure respiratory support to relieve pulmonary oedema and support respiratory function.
- Assess Tim's clinical condition against the criteria for continuous renal replacement therapy (CRRT).
- Monitor for drug toxicities.
- Maintain nutrition.

By the time Tim arrived in ITU his condition had become critical. The combination of impaired renal function, oliguria, and fluid resuscitation had led to fluid overload, culminating in an increase in pulmonary capillary hydrostatic pressure and pulmonary oedema. Hammer and McPhee (2014) describe the signs and symptoms of pulmonary oedema as: rapid shallow respirations, hypoxaemia, and the presence of pink frothy sputum; a pulmonary chest X-ray usually reveals evidence of interstitial and alveolar oedema and inspiratory crackles may be heard on auscultation. These signs and symptoms were consistent with the clinical findings identified on Tim's assessment. He was also demonstrating evidence of increased respiratory and cardiac workload with an increased respiratory and heart rate, but accompanied by reduced perfusion and a failing BP. Tim's cardiovascular and respiratory systems were struggling to cope with his body's increased demand for oxygen and nutrients, and his capillary oxygen saturation fell to 80% despite high-flow oxygen; he was becoming anxious and disorientated. An arterial blood sample confirmed that Tim was suffering from type I respiratory failure with a PaO$_2$ of 7.9 kPa and PaCO$_2$ of 5.8 kPa (see Chapter 2). The arterial sample also revealed that Tim had a severe metabolic acidosis with a pH of 7.166 and HCO$_3$ of 17.2 mmol/L, consistent with a diagnosis of both sepsis and AKI.

It was imperative that as a priority Tim received interventions to support his respiratory and cardiovascular system. He now met the criteria for endotracheal intubation and IMV for several reasons, including:

- type I respiratory failure and pulmonary oedema;
- confusion;
- exhaustion.

(For more information about IMV, see Table 3.3, on page 88.)

Tim was intubated and commenced on bilevel positive airways pressure ventilation with an inspiratory pressure of 20 cm H_2O, an expiratory pressure of 5 cm H_2O and an assisted rate of 18 bpm with 80% oxygen. The use of bilevel positive airways pressure, or continuous positive airways pressure support, via a non-invasive route is usually recommended for a patient experiencing pulmonary oedema as it provides a constant flow of positive pulmonary airways pressure in the alveoli to a level higher than the capillary hydrostatic pressure, thus pushing the leaking fluid back into the capillaries (Hammer and McPhee, 2014; Marik, 2015). However, in Tim's case he was unable to cope with NIV due to acute confusion with a GCS of 12, and IMV was prescribed. Tim also met the criteria for continuing with resuscitation and maintenance therapy for sepsis (Rhodes et al., 2017). This includes mechanical ventilatory support and assessment for renal replacement therapy when there is clear evidence of AKI (see Table 7.3).

If one of the criteria below is present, consider the use of continuous renal replacement therapy (CRRT)	If two or more criteria are present CRRT is essential	Tom's assessment for readiness to commence CRRT
Oliguria (<200 ml in 12 hours)		Yes
Anuria (0–50 ml in 12 hours)		
Creatinine >400 µmol/L		Yes
Urea >35 mmol/L		Yes
Potassium >6.5 mmol/L		
Pulmonary oedema		Yes
Uncompensated metabolic acidosis pH <7.1		
Sodium <110 or >160 mmol/L		
Temperature >40 °C		
Uraemic complications (encephalopathy, myopathy, neuropathy, pericarditis)		
Overdose with a toxin that can be removed by dialysis (e.g., lithium)		

Table 9.5 Modern criteria for the initiation of renal replacement therapy in ITU (based on Bellomo, 2019) and a column indicating the results of Tom's assessment for readiness to commence CRRT

Assessing Tim for readiness to commence CRRT

AKI in critically ill patients like Tim frequently develops in situations where there is another critical underlying pathology such as shock, sepsis, major surgery, and/or trauma, and where there is an increased risk of multiple organ dysfunction. In Tim's case the underlying pathology was sepsis, and the AKI has occurred simultaneously with evidence of an ascending renal infection and circulatory failure. The criteria for initiation of CRRT are listed in Table 9.5 (Bellomo, 2019). An assessment of these criteria in relation to Tim indicated that he met four of the criteria listed and CRRT was deemed essential to provide a balanced and controlled removal of fluid and waste products from Tim's circulation.

CRRT in the form of continuous haemodiafiltration can remove plasma water in a controlled process to achieve a desired fluid balance, correct electrolyte abnormalities, remove waste products, and correct metabolic acidosis (Richardson and Whatmore, 2014). The two main processes through which this is achieved are:

- **Haemofiltration**: the movement of water across a semipermeable membrane from an area of high pressure (the patient's blood) to an area of low pressure (the filter) at a measured rate of flow. Replacement fluids are titrated in order to maintain the desired fluid balance.
- **Haemodialysis**: the selected diffusion of waste molecules (solutes) from an area of high concentration to an area of low concentration across a semipermeable membrane. For example, dialysis fluid usually contains haemodynamically normal levels of sodium and potassium, to ensure the levels in the patient's blood remain within the normal range, but may have higher than normal levels of bicarbonate to increase bicarbonate levels in the patient's blood and so resolve a metabolic acidosis. Dialysis fluid will contain no creatinine or urea, thus increasing the flow of both solutes out of the body and into the dialysis fluid.

The nursing management of a patient who requires CRRT is complex and highly specialised and includes the following principles (Richardson and Whatmore, 2014).

- To assess for indications for CRRT (see Table 9.5).
- To assess, monitor, and ensure effective venous access:
    - check patency and flow of the central venous catheter;
    - ensure the catheter is secured with a suture and dressing;
    - monitor the outgoing and return pressures of the blood flow.
- To avoid unnecessary interruptions to CRRT:
    - make sure the pump speed to direct the flow from the patient to the circuit is adequate as prescribed;
    - monitor the use of anticoagulants to maintain blood flow and check for blood clots;
    - ensure the alarm limits have been set.

- To reduce the risk of complications associated with CRRT:
  - reduce the risk of air embolism by flushing the circuit before its use;
  - monitor for fluid and electrolyte imbalance;
  - monitor for haemodynamic stability/instability;
  - reduce the risk of hypothermia;
  - reduce the risk of infection.

Tim continued CRRT together with full respiratory and cardiovascular support and intravenous antibiotic therapy for five days in ITU. The team were able to reduce his respiratory support and sedation after 24 hours and he became more involved in his recovery. According to Wahlin (2017), the development of a mutual and supportive relationship with a critically ill person, together with feelings of self-power and autonomy supports feelings of reduced strain and increased comfort when experiencing critical illness. Daphne had thought Tim was going to die and seeing him winking at her and holding her hand made her cry and gave her hope. Tim's renal function was slower to return and it was another 10 days before his renal function improved enough to further reduce his respiratory and renal support. He was progressing toward the recovery phase of AKI.

The recovery phase of AKI

The recovery phase of AKI is the period when renal injury is repaired, and normal renal function becomes re-established. As renal function begins to improve there is a progressive increase in urine volume and GFR, and there is a gradual decline in blood urea and creatinine levels. In this early recovery phase, however, the renal tubules are unable to concentrate the filtrate, and this leads to increased losses of sodium, potassium, and fluid in the urine (McCance and Huether, 2019). The patient becomes at risk of:

- fluid volume depletion due to polyuria (passing large volumes of urine);
- hypokalaemia.

The nursing responsibilities when caring for patients during the recovery phase include the following.

- Assessment of vital signs for dehydration (Thomas et al., 2008):
  - thirst;
  - dry skin and mucous membranes;
  - > pulse;
  - < BP;
  - confusion;
  - negative fluid balance.
- Assessment of vital signs for hypokalaemia (McCance and Huether, 2019):
  - slow or irregular pulse;
  - muscle weakness.

- Risk assess for signs of infection and deterioration in renal function by checking:
  - serum urea;
  - creatinine;
  - electrolyte balance;
  - white cell count;
  - temperature.
- Inform the medical team if there are any signs of deterioration.
- Patient and family education:
  - the process of renal recovery can take from three to 12 months and continues after the patient has been discharged;
  - encourage the patient and their family to understand and work in partnership with the medical team to support recovery and reduce the risk of a decline in renal function and CKD.

Activity 9.3   Decision making

Assess the patients below and based on what you have learned from this chapter, discuss your recommendations for care.

(a) Mr McDonald

- **Situation:** Mr McDonald (aged 65 years) presented in the ED with a history of three days of shortness of breath and wheezing.
- **Background:** known hypertensive, prescribed atenolol.
- **Assessment:**

  R: 26/min, SpO$_2$: 92%

  Respiratory wheeze

  Chest X-ray: pulmonary oedema

  HR: 98/min, BP: 140/95

  Urine output: 100 ml on admission

  T: 37.5 °C

  Patient very agitated and confused

  Creatinine: 1504 µmol/L

  Urea: 14.2 mmol/L

  K: 9.2 mmol/L

  Na: 132 mmol/L

  Weight estimated at 70 kg

(b) Mrs Kumar

- **Situation:** Mrs Kumar (aged 75 years) has been admitted to the high dependency unit post-operatively following a surgical repair for a fractured hip sustained after a fall. During the surgical procedure Mrs Kumar required a transfusion and fluid resuscitation following severe blood loss. She was breathing spontaneously on 60% oxygen.
- **Background:** history of chronic heart failure, hypertension, rheumatoid arthritis, and hypothyroid dysfunction. Medication includes: amiodarone, levothyroxine, furosemide, and NSAID.
- **Assessment:**

R: 40/min, SpO$_2$: 89%

HR: 120/min, BP: 190/110

Urine output: 25 ml/hr

Chest X-ray: pulmonary oedema

T: 37.5 °C

Patient very agitated and confused

Creatinine: 216 µmol/L

Urea: 16.9 mmol/L

K: 4.9 mmol/L

Na: 151 mmol/L

Weight estimated at 60 kg

Sample answers can be found at the end of the chapter.

Finally, returning to Tim's story, he continued to make a good recovery and 11 days after being admitted to ITU he was transferred to the high dependency unit for 48 hours before he was fit enough to return to the ward. He was discharged from hospital a week later. Tim and his wife were informed that because of his critical illness and AKI, diabetes, and hypertension he was at an increased risk of deteriorating kidney function and would need careful monitoring of his kidney function by the GP as part of his annual diabetes check. Tim admitted that he now realised that he should have sought help sooner and he would be more aware of what to do should he feel unwell again.

Chapter summary

In this chapter you have been introduced to patients who are at risk of developing AKI and what happens if AKI becomes established: acute and severe deterioration in the patient's

(Continued)

(Continued)

condition with an increased risk of developing CKD should they survive. The important messages to gain from this chapter are:

- Risk assessing patients for AKI, particularly when they are in the initial stage of the syndrome, can prevent established AKI and improve patient morbidity and mortality.
- Assessing and knowing your patient's situation and background is necessary to prioritise assessment of patients who have a high risk of developing AKI.
- Working in partnership with patients, particularly those with chronic conditions, encourages patients to feel empowered and more in control of their care.

Activities: brief outline answers

Activity 9.2: Communication (page 244)

Communications strategies you can use when diffusing a situation include the following:

- Be open and questioning: ask Tim what the problem is and whether you can help.
- Use an assertive but democratic approach to the conversation.
- Stay professional.
- Encourage Tim to sit down in a quiet and more private area so that his concerns can be discussed.
- Listen and value what Tim has to say.
- Offer possible solutions.
- Discuss each solution with Tim.
- Encourage Tim to make his decision in a calm environment.

Activity 9.3: Decision making (page 252)

(a) Recommendations – Mr McDonald

- There is evidence of acute respiratory failure associated with pulmonary oedema: recommend commence bilevel positive pressure ventilation.
- AKI severity is stage 3.
- Meets the criteria for CRRT: creatinine: 1504 µmol/L, presence of pulmonary oedema, K: 9.2 mmol/L. Commence CRRT.
- Assess history for evidence of the use of nephrotoxic drugs or X-ray contrast media.

(b) Recommendations – Mrs Kumar

- Evidence of acute respiratory failure due to fluid overload and existing heart failure: commence invasive respiratory support.
- Urine output is currently below the required 0.5 ml/kg/hr. Monitor urine output following commencement of mechanical invasive ventilation (MIV) and diuretic therapy over the next five hours and review.
- Monitor creatinine levels in an hour for increasing severity of AKI.

Further reading

Woodrow, P (2019) *Intensive Care Nursing*. Fourth edition. London: Routledge.

This book offers further insight into the care of patients with AKI in a critical care setting (Chapter 38) and further information on haemodialysis (Chapter 39).

Useful websites

https://renal.org/health-professionals/guidelines/guidelines-commentaries

The Renal Association website offers links to clinical guidance for managing patients with both AKI and CKD.

www.youtube.com/watch?v=MH1DCCqLGps

This recording describes the pathophysiology of AKI and can be used to support the content of this chapter.

www.youtube.com/watch?v=88ajR62XEcg

Please watch this recording if you are interested in exploring the process of CRRT in more detail.

Chapter 10 The patient with physiological trauma

Catherine Williams

7.5   understand and recognise the need to respond to the challenges of providing safe, effective, and person-centred nursing care for people who have co-morbidities and complex care needs.

7.7   understand how to monitor and evaluate the quality of people's experience of complex care.

7.8   understand the principles and processes involved in supporting people and families with a range of care needs to maintain optimal independence and avoid unnecessary interventions and disruptions to their lives.

7.10   understand the principles and processes involved in planning and facilitating the safe discharge and transition of people between caseloads, settings, and services.

Annexe A: Communication and relationship management skills.

Annexe B: Nursing procedures Part 2: Procedures for the planning, provision, and management of person-centred nursing care.

At the point of registration, the registered nurse will be able to safely demonstrate the following procedures:

Use evidence-based, best practice approaches to undertake the following procedures:

2.1   take, record and interpret vital signs manually and via technological devices

2.2   undertake venepuncture and cannulation and blood sampling, interpreting normal and common abnormal blood profiles and venous blood gases

2.3   set up and manage routine electrocardiogram (ECG) investigations and interpret normal and commonly encountered abnormal traces

2.4   manage and monitor blood component transfusions

2.5   manage and interpret cardiac monitors, infusion pumps, blood glucose monitors and other monitoring devices

2.10   measure and interpret blood glucose levels

2.12   undertake, respond to and interpret neurological observations and assessments

2.13   identify and respond to signs of deterioration and sepsis

4.8   assess, respond and effectively manage pyrexia and hypothermia

8.2   manage the administration of oxygen using a range of routes and best practice approaches

8.6   manage airway and respiratory processes and equipment

9.9   safely assess and manage invasive medical devices and lines

Chapter aims

By the end of this chapter, you should be able to:

- interpret the mechanisms of injury to form individualised patient care;
- demonstrate the systematic approach to physiological trauma care;

(Continued)

(Continued)

- describe the primary and secondary surveys;
- list the indications for intravenous fluid replacement therapy;
- reflect on clinical examples illustrated in the chapter and apply this to your own clinical situation.

This chapter provides an overview of the general causes and treatments of physiological trauma and examines the care of a patient with physiological trauma and the metabolic response to trauma. The chapter proceeds with an overview of the knowledge and skills required to assess, differentiate, and manage the care of a patient who sustains any form of physiological trauma. The underlying physiology and implications of the patient's care will be discussed in the context of diagnostic tests, treatments, and collaborative management of care and highlighted through the chapter. The assessment and management of patients with shock is touched upon in this chapter; for a detailed assessment of cardiogenic and distributive shock (including sepsis and septic shock), please refer to Chapters 4, 6, and 7.

Trauma care starts at the point of injury and continues through to the end of rehabilitation to ensure the best possible outcome; in any trauma an organisational approach is essential.

We will now introduce you to the physical and psychological impact of trauma and about how to help patients and their families in their own processes of healing, recovery, and restoration, beginning with Doris Daniels's story.

Case study

Mrs Doris Daniels, aged 74, is admitted to A&E after tripping over a raised paving slab while running for a bus. Lily, a student nurse, is working with her mentor, who is triaging patients in A&E. It is the first day of Lily's placement. On admission Mrs Daniels is carefully holding her left wrist and can give her own account of the accident, although she speaks slowly and deliberately as though she is trying to speak with loose dentures. She has an abrasive graze to her swollen nose and chin and a runny nose. Mrs Daniels appears embarrassed by her facial injuries and focuses on her wrist injury.

Lily did not carry out an accurate primary assessment, GCS, and history but focused upon the secondary survey assessment of Mrs Daniels. Lily assumes that Mrs Daniels' wrist probably has a **Colles fracture** because of the classic dinner fork deformity presentation. An X-ray will be needed to confirm this with subsequent reduction of the fracture.

However, Lily's mentor is a very experienced A&E nurse, and she prioritises Mrs Daniels more urgently. After completing accurate primary and secondary surveys she believes that Mrs Daniels may have sustained maxillofacial injuries based on the abnormal facial mobility, and may have a leak of cerebrospinal fluid (CSF) from her nose. CSF is clear and has a high sugar (clinistix) and low protein content (electrophoresis) compared to nasal or lacrimal fluid. An individual with a CSF leak may have clear watery fluid draining from their nose or ears when they move their head, especially when bending forward. CSF may also drain down the back of the throat and is described as a salty metallic taste. A CSF leak is a serious issue that can cause complications such as headaches, meningitis, and seizures.

Neurological observations are commenced on Mrs Daniels and she is admitted to the resuscitation bay for urgent medical attention. The GCS allows healthcare professionals to consistently evaluate the level of consciousness of a patient. It is commonly used in the context of head trauma, but it is also useful in a wide variety of other non-trauma-related settings. Regular assessment of a patient's GCS can identify early signs of deterioration.

There are important messages to learn from Lily's story and we must always implement these into our nursing practice; they are:

- Always be alert to changes in your patient's clinical condition, no matter how small.
- Use the ABCDE approach to assess and treat the patient. Do a complete initial assessment and reassess regularly.
- Errors are often made in the early management of the trauma in the critically ill patient; depressed consciousness often leads to airway obstruction.
- A systematic approach is required to identify and treat the immediately life-threatening and potentially life-threatening conditions.
- Timing is of the essence: your patient will continue to deteriorate if prompt action is not taken.
- Communicate effectively – use the SBAR (Chapter 1) or Reason, Story, Vital signs, Plan (RSVP) approach.

What do we mean by physiological trauma?

We will now review the stress response sustained from physical and psychological trauma.

A physiological stress response is initiated the moment the body recognises the presence of a stressor. The response is designed to be rapid and to reduce the impact of the stress on the body and maintain homeostasis in the short term.

When the body senses that a particular stressor is present, signals about that stimulus are sent to the brain. The master gland, called the hypothalamus, is then alerted to arouse the autonomic nervous system (ANS). The ANS is the system that controls most of the major organs of the body: the heart, lungs, stomach, glands, and blood vessels.

Other than the nervous system, the body's stress response also includes the help of the adrenal glands. Situated on top of each kidney, the adrenal glands are also included in the physiologic stress response because the adrenal medulla (the central part of the glands) has nerves that connect the gland to the sympathetic nervous system (SNS). The SNS stimulates the adrenal medulla to start releasing adrenaline and noradrenaline into the blood circulation. This action results in the 'fight or flight' response, which is manifested by the increase in heart rate, dilation of bronchial airways, and an increase of the metabolic rate (Sincero, 2012).

After the amygdala sends a distress signal, the hypothalamus activates the SNS by sending signals through the autonomic nerves to the adrenal glands. These glands respond by pumping the hormone epinephrine (also known as adrenaline) into the bloodstream. As epinephrine circulates through the body, it brings on several physiological changes. The heart beats faster than normal, pushing blood to the muscles, heart, and other vital organs. Pulse rate and blood pressure go up. The person undergoing these changes also starts to breathe more rapidly. Small airways in the lungs open wide. This way, the lungs can take in as much oxygen as possible with each breath. Extra oxygen is sent to the brain, increasing alertness. Sight, hearing, and other senses become sharper. Meanwhile, epinephrine triggers the release of blood sugar (glucose) and fats from temporary storage sites in the body. These nutrients flood into the bloodstream, supplying energy to all parts of the body.

Below we will look at trauma in more detail.

What is trauma?

Eckes-Roper (cited in Saunderson Cohen, 2002) defines trauma as a blunt or penetrating force to the body resulting in actual injury.

Irrespective of the cause of trauma, the medical team must make a systematic assessment to ensure that the most important injuries are prioritised. Courses such as the **Advanced Trauma Life Support (ATLS)**/European Trauma Course (ETC) provide a means of assessing patients that is widely accepted worldwide as a framework of rapid assessment for trauma. Broadly speaking, this comprises a **primary survey** and a **secondary survey** of the patient to ensure that less obvious serious injuries are not missed while healthcare staff deal with more visually apparent patient problems.

During the primary survey, life-threatening injuries are identified and simultaneously resuscitation is begun. A simple mnemonic, ABCDE, is used for the order in which problems should be addressed.

When the primary survey is completed, resuscitation efforts are well established, and the vital signs are normalising, the secondary survey can begin. The secondary survey is a head-to-toe evaluation of the trauma patient, including a complete history and physical examination, including the reassessment of all vital signs. Each region of the body must be fully examined. X-rays indicated by examination are obtained. If at any time during the secondary survey the patient deteriorates, another primary survey is carried out as a potential life threat may be present (NICE, 2016).

Case study

Danny, a seven-year-old boy, was a front-seat passenger in his uncle's car. He was not in a car seat and he was not wearing a seatbelt. As they drove along the road at around 30 mph, Danny stood up and turned around to wave to the people in the car behind. At that point, his uncle braked heavily and swerved to avoid a car that had pulled out from a junction without looking. While the impact was not particularly serious, Danny was catapulted into the dashboard and had an obvious ankle deformity requiring a visit to hospital for X-rays. An ambulance was called and arrived promptly. On arrival at the hospital, Danny was in a great deal of pain, assumed to be from his ankle injury, and the nurses tried to make him comfortable while the doctor dealt with some other patients. After about 20 minutes the doctor arrived and sent Danny for an X-ray of his ankle. While in the X-ray department, Danny became unresponsive and died within half an hour. Danny's post-mortem report showed massive abdominal bleeding from a ruptured spleen. He also had a fracture to his ankle.

There are important messages to learn from Danny's story; these are:

- All injuries have the potential to be life- or limb-threatening.
- It is essential that problems are anticipated, rather than reacted to once they develop.

Activity 10.1 asks you to use critical thinking and decision-making skills using our case study patient Danny.

Activity 10.1   Critical thinking

What assessment should have been carried out in Danny's case and what are you looking for in such an assessment, and why?

An outline answer to this activity is given at the end of the chapter.

Primary and secondary surveys

The chapter will now go on to offer an overview of the primary and secondary surveys. For a detailed assessment of cardiogenic and distributive shock (including sepsis and septic shock), please refer to Chapters 4, 6, and 7.

The primary survey

The ATLS approach to the management of the seriously injured trauma patient starts with a rapid primary survey, using the ABCDE approach. This allows life-threatening injuries to be identified in a prioritised sequence and treated accordingly. The objective of this phase is to identify and correct any immediately life-threatening conditions, including the airway, breathing, circulation, disability, and exposure (ABCDE). To do this, the activities in Table 10.1 need to be carried out. The survey follows a simple mnemonic of A, B, C, D, E. These should be worked through in sequence and any issues resolved before proceeding to the next stage of the survey.

Airway and control of cervical spine	Must be considered in conjunction with each other as interventions performed on the airway will impact on the c-spine and vice versa. If no concern for trauma: open airway using head tilt chin lift manoeuvre. If trauma suspected: maintain cervical spine immobilisation and open the airway using jaw thrust manoeuvre. The mental status of the patient should be quickly assessed, and a GCS score of 8 or less usually requires the placement of a definitive airway.
Breathing	During the immediate assessment of breathing, it is vital to diagnose and treat immediately life-threatening situations such as airway obstruction, noisy breathing or narrowing of the airway (see Chapter 2). Note rate, rhythm, and depth of respirations and listen for normal breath sounds. How is the gas exchange? You may be able to make a quick assumption of this initially from signs of cyanosed skin or laboured breathing although urgent arterial blood gas confirmation will be required. Arterial blood gas analysis and, where appropriate, carboxyhaemoglobin levels would provide interim information until formal blood results are available.
Circulation	Establishing reliable venous access is a priority at this point in order to carry out any subsequent treatment as you continue with your primary survey. Delays in gaining venous access may make obtaining access more problematic as the patient progresses into shock. Diagnostic blood tests should be taken for full blood count, coagulation, cross match, and electrolytes. Haemorrhage control should be established and treatment for shock initiated with fluid resuscitation. Examination of chest, abdomen, and pelvis should be carried out at this stage (NICE, 2016). Look for both external AND internal bleeding, including bleeding: into chest; into abdomen; from stomach or intestine; from pelvic or femur fracture; from wounds. Look for hypotension, distended neck veins, and muffed heart sounds that might indicate pericardial tamponade.
Disability	Patient responsiveness should be assessed using the GCS, check for pupil size, whether the pupils are equal, and if pupils are reactive to light. Check movement and sensation in all four limbs and look for abnormal repetitive movements or shaking on one or both sides of the body (seizure/convulsion). Blood sugar measurements should be taken at this time.
Exposure	The patient should be undressed for a full body examination, but hypothermia must also be prevented as acutely ill patients have difficulty regulating body temperature. If cause unknown, remember the possibility of trauma: log roll if suspected spinal injury. Any wounds should be assessed for further management.

Table 10.1 The primary survey

On admission to the ED, the ATLS assessment will primarily be the physician's responsibility. However, all members of the team should be able to contribute to patient safety by being aware of the framework in use. When the primary survey has been completed it should be repeated before proceeding to the secondary survey to ensure that new problems have not arisen and that nothing important has been missed. If **one or more Red Flags** are present in the ABCDE assessment, the patient should be **treated for sepsis.**

The secondary survey

Once life-threatening conditions have been treated, or excluded, then you can carry out the secondary survey. This is a comprehensive head-to-toe examination of the patient, which provides the basis of the admission documentation. You need to pay close attention to the history of this accident and of previous medical history so that important details that may suggest other injuries or complicating factors are not overlooked. You will take a detailed history of the accident from the patient, witnesses, relatives, GP, or medical alert jewellery, if worn. If attending paramedics are present, it is essential to gain information from them before they leave (Cole, 2009).

The mnemonic AMPLE will help you to remember what information you need to obtain during the assessment.

- **A**llergies.
- **M**edication.
- **P**ast medical history.
- **L**ast meal/fluid.
- **E**vents relevant to injury.

The secondary survey should revisit all elements of the primary survey in ABCDE priority order, and you should pay attention to important information that may have had to be deferred while the primary survey was establishing the basis of patient survival.

The secondary survey is one of time and detail as an in-depth assessment of each body region is warranted. You must monitor vital signs and examine your patient's head/skull for irregularity or scalp wound, check the ears for blood or CSF leaks, and check eyes for pupil size and reaction (PEARL – Pupils Equal and Reactive to Light). Observe the thorax for bruising and possible fracture. All four limbs need to be checked for irregularity, deformity, and fractures; compare limbs with each other and look for shortening and rotation. Logrolling should be adopted until the c-spine is cleared by the physicians and documented in the medical notes. Once the primary and secondary surveys have been completed by the medical team, unconscious or confused patients are generally reliant on the nurse to anticipate and identify any deterioration in their condition. Thus, the principles of the primary survey ABCDE can be utilised in everyday practice to provide structure to your own assessment of the patient.

Activity 10.2 focuses upon your own experiences in the clinical setting.

Activity 10.2   Reflection

Try to identify examples of situations when you had to complete primary and secondary surveys. Below are some cues to help you with the exercise.

- In the primary survey, what were the main priorities for the patient and why?
- In the secondary survey, what clinical signs and features were present and did this affect your prioritisation of care?

These reflective questions will help you to practise linking the importance of treating problems as they are found. The ABCDE order of treatment reflects the importance of treatment priority.

As this answer is based on your own reflection, there is no outline answer at the end of the chapter.

Before moving on to each section of the secondary survey, remember to go back and keep checking the patient's ABCDEs. Avoid the common error of being distracted before the whole body has been inspected, as potentially serious injuries can be missed, especially in the unconscious patient. For example, the clinical staff may have noted that the patient was wearing rings that were compromising the circulation to the digits during the primary survey, but this would be of little consequence if the patient was not breathing at that time.

In the next section we will consider the clinical features of the metabolic response to trauma, and we will explore how you can assess and manage the patient to provide clinically effective care.

Metabolic response to trauma

When the body sustains a traumatic injury, an inflammatory response starts from the site of tissue damage as chemical mediators are released. (Mediators are signalling chemical molecules involved in transmitting information between cells.)

The inflammatory mediators involved are:

- histamine;
- kinins (polypeptides);
- prostaglandins (fatty acids);
- **leukotrienes.**

All these mediators in turn cause local vasodilation and subsequently increased blood flow, which brings phagocytes and leukocytes to the original injury to deal with infections or foreign agents and to begin repairing the injury. **Vascular permeability** is enhanced by the mediators, which in turn permit clotting proteins such as fibrin, the enzymatic serum protein complement, kinins, and white blood cells to reach the tissue.

Once the clotting proteins have moved from the blood into the tissues, an osmotic change occurs and oedema forms in the tissue at the site of injury. The clotting proteins then isolate any abnormal agents such as particles or bacteria at the source of the injury by forming an encasing clot to isolate it from the surrounding normal tissue.

Now let us consider some minor trauma, which will make it easier for you to understand how the body responds to major trauma.

Case study

Lily, a hardworking student nurse, has decided to attend a ward night out. She has been saving for some lovely shoes, which don't really fit properly but look fantastic. As the evening progresses, the shoes start to rub her heels and they begin to look red. Lily realises that the trauma she is experiencing is **abrasive trauma**.

Lily is not in a position to change her shoes, so they continue to rub until a blister starts to form as fluid leaks into the tissues from the vasodilation that the inflammatory mediators cause as they rush to the injured area. The pain she experiences is caused by localised swelling from the inflammatory response and by mechanical means as the shoes continue to rub. Eventually, the blister breaks, leaving an open wound and a portal for bacterial entry. Nerve endings are now exposed as the top of the blister bursts, causing further pain.

Monitoring the critically ill patient

We will now move on to review the importance of monitoring the critically ill patient.

Critical care units (ICU/CCUs) are specialist hospital wards that treat patients who are seriously ill and need constant monitoring. These patients might, for example, have problems with one or more vital organ or be unable to breathe without support. The NHS has different levels of critical care, based on the clinical needs of patients ranging from level 1 to level 3 (Chapter 1).

The critical care setting can be a daunting environment to those unfamiliar with caring for such sick patients. Many pieces of previously unseen equipment are in use for monitoring and treating the patient: for example, blood pressure may be recorded continuously on-screen via an arterial line, giving a blood pressure that varies from beat to beat rather than via a cuff measurement that gives a random, one-off blood pressure reading. Many patients will be assisted with bodily functions that are normally autonomic, such as breathing or renal filtration by machinery. Multiple intravenous infusions may be in progress at the same time.

However, as with the patient's initial assessment after injury, the primary survey can be adapted and should be continuously revisited by the nurse caring for the patient to ensure the safety of the patient. Once the primary and secondary surveys have been completed by the medical team, unconscious or confused patients are generally reliant on the nurse to anticipate and identify any deterioration in their condition.

Activity 10.3 focuses upon your own experiences in a critical care clinical setting.

Activity 10.3   Reflection

These reflective questions will help you prioritise your patient care through examining the means of clinically monitoring and continuously assessing the major trauma patient. Think back to how you dealt with major trauma in a critical care setting and what were your nursing priorities with regards to care delivery and best practice?

As this answer is based on your own reflection, there is no outline answer at the end of the chapter.

In the scenario below we will explore Mrs Sharon Bowen's primary assessment.

Case study

Mrs Sharon Bowen, aged 25, sustained a 60% flame burn to her upper body from a witnessed suicide attempt in her parked car after suffering from post-natal depression. She was intubated by the paramedics and 100% oxygen was administered prior to arrival at A&E, as smoke contains dangerous gases such as carbon monoxide that need to be addressed by administering high concentrations of oxygen even before confirmation from blood results (Herndon, 2007).

The c-spine had not been immobilised as Mrs Bowen's accident did not involve any impact and the witnesses to the accident were able to state the mechanism of the injury. Lily, the student, is on duty when Mrs Bowen arrives. She observes the primary survey being undertaken by the medical and nursing staff.

Airway is assessed and managed by the insertion of an endotracheal tube. The effectiveness of ventilation is measured by:

- assessing the symmetrical rise and fall of the chest;
- assessing air entry to the left and right side of the chest (see Chapter 2);
- assessing oxygen saturation;
- assessing carbon dioxide in the patient's expired volume (American College of Surgeons, 2018).

Breathing is occurring with assistance, but manually inflating the chest using an ambubag is difficult and the chest is not rising much with each breath delivered. ABG analysis reveals significant respiratory and metabolic acidosis. Lily notes that Mrs Bowen's trunk is burned circumferentially, and the anaesthetist explains that therefore it is difficult to ventilate the patient. An emergency **escharotomy** is performed on the spot by the doctors to release the taut burned skin that is restricting chest movement. This involves making an incision with a sterile blade through the depth of the burned tissue and extending into unburned skin. This results in an immediate improvement in chest expansion as the patient is easier to ventilate with better oxygenation and gas exchange evident on the next ABG. Escharotomies are performed under general anaesthetic except in an emergency such as this where time delays could mean that the patient will not survive.

Mrs Bowen's ABGs were as follows.

Prior to escharotomy	1 hour post escharotomy
pH 7.05	pH 7.30
pCO_2 9.0 kPa	pCO_2 7.0 kPa
pO_2 10.5 kPa	pO_2 14 kPa
HCO_3 20 mmol/L	HCO_3 27 mmol/L

Note the rapid improvement in Mrs Bowen's ABGs following escharotomy once she can fully expand her chest and exhale carbon dioxide more efficiently. While the blood gases have not yet reached normality, you will recognise a significant improvement from the earlier blood gas analysis.

Blood gas analysis may be measured in millimetres of mercury or kilopascals depending on the blood gas analyser (see Table 10.2).

Kilopascal measurements	Millimetres of mercury measurement
pH 7.35–7.45	pH 7.35–7.45
pO_2 11.5–13.5 kPa	pO_2 80–100 mmHg
pCO_2 4.5–6 kPa	pCO_2 35–45 mmHg
HCO_3 25–30 mmol/L	HCO_3 25–30 mmol/L
Base excess –2 to +2	Base excess –2 to +2

Table 10.2   Normal values for ABGs

Only once the airway, breathing, and cervical spine elements of the primary survey have been addressed, should consideration be given to the other elements of the primary survey such as circulation, disability, and exposure. Initially, the circulation component of the survey will be concerned with checking that the pulse is present and noting whether it is strong and bounding or weak and thready. Then capillary refill can be checked by applying pressure to an area of skin (unburned area in this patient). The skin should blanch and return to normal within two seconds. If it does not, then you may have a hypovolaemic patient.

However, other limbs should be tested to exclude a localised problem with the circulation. For example, if the limb has a circumferential burn, circulation may be sluggish locally but fine generally. Excluding the possibility of major haemorrhage is the immediate priority. Establishing venous access, while important, should not come before first aid for bleeding. Direct pressure should be applied where serious bleeding occurs. Commencing intravenous fluid resuscitation can be dealt with during the secondary survey, provided access has already been established. If access cannot be gained intravenously, then intraosseous access may have to be considered. When these have been addressed, other factors such as disability can be considered. As Mrs Bowen has already been intubated, this could prove to be difficult as the normal ACVPU measures of Alertness, new Confusion, Vocal stimulus, response to Painful stimuli, and Unresponsiveness may be affected by sedatives. However, the aim is to exclude signs of head injury and maxillofacial trauma, and in this situation pupil reaction to light would need to be assessed before proceeding to complete exposure of the patient to ensure that no other life-threatening injuries have been missed. Care must be taken to keep the patient warm during this part of the assessment. If a warm environment cannot be provided, then the patient may have to be exposed in stages to prevent hypothermia. Jewellery should be removed and kept safe at this stage.

With all forms of major trauma, regardless of cause, the risk of hypovolaemic shock is present, along with sepsis either from the original injury or the invasive devices used to monitor the patient's condition. These risk factors may perpetuate the inflammatory response in a negative way, so that it moves from being beneficial to becoming detrimental to the patient.

Case study

Mr David Jones is a 31-year-old man who sustained a crush injury to his abdomen from heavy machinery at work. Primary and secondary surveys are conducted in A&E and he is taken straight to theatre to explore an open abdominal wound. Lily, the student, is working under supervision with her mentor, who is allocated as Mr Jones's nurse when he arrives from theatre. He has multiple injuries including pelvic fractures. The peritoneum has been found to be intact, but a vacuum-assisted closure (VAC) drain is in situ due to a large surface of skin loss over the abdomen with a small but steady drainage of **haemoserous fluid**. On arrival from theatre Mr Jones's vital signs are remarkably stable. He appears pale, but he is prescribed a further two units of red blood cells post-operatively that were not completed in theatre, and these are in the process of being ordered. He has intravenous fluid running and a patient-controlled analgesia (PCA) pump for pain relief but is not dependent on inotropic support. Mr Jones's family have been spoken to by the surgeon as Mr Jones remains on a ventilator in ITU. Lily's mentor starts the admission paperwork after setting up the first unit of blood. As Lily begins to document the patient's observations, the VAC begins to alarm.

Lily checks the cause of the alarm and notices that the 1-litre VAC chamber has filled with frank blood. Mr Jones remains pale but otherwise does not appear to have deteriorated drastically. His heart rate has increased a little and he is now mildly tachycardic. Blood pressure is not yet affected. Lily draws the mentor's attention to the situation. Another nurse is asked to contact the medical staff as Lily and her mentor reassess the patient.

Using the primary survey as a framework, Lily realises that airway and breathing are secure and stable as Mr Jones remains on the ventilator but is able to initiate his own breaths. There is a slight rise in respiratory rate from 16 bpm previously to 24 bpm. Circulation has become a concern due to the blood loss into the VAC, and closer inspection of the patient reveals a significant amount of blood in the bed underneath the patient, although the abdominal dressing does not appear unduly saturated with blood as the fluid has leaked downwards under the dressing as the patient has been lying in a semi-recumbent position. Lily realises the importance of exposure of the patient as one of the components of the primary survey, as some issues may not be obvious initially. As the medical staff arrive, Mr Jones becomes hypotensive with a blood pressure of 83/50. An arterial blood sample is taken for arterial blood gas analysis, and haemoglobin levels. The results indicate the presence of a slight metabolic acidosis and a haemoglobin of 6.8 g/dl (normal 11–15 g/dl). The medical team request that the unit of blood in progress is given at a faster rate and the next unit is ordered immediately. Venous blood samples are taken to confirm U&E and Hb levels.

Arrangements are made for Mr Jones to return to theatre for exploration of the source of the bleeding. Mr Jones returns from theatre before the end of the shift. The second surgery identified that a small artery in the existing abdominal wound was bleeding. This was repaired and Mr Jones made good progress, culminating in his discharge from the critical care unit several days later.

In Activity 10.5 we look at decision making and critical thinking using our case studies of Mrs Sharon Bowen and Mr David Jones.

Activity 10.4   Critical thinking

In the case scenario of Sharon Bowen, what things could be overlooked and what are the consequences of this?

Regarding David Jones, what clinical signs would indicate that his condition is deteriorating and what do you think could be the possible causes for his metabolic acidosis and the consequences of this is not being promptly treated.

An outline answer to this activity is given at the end of the chapter.

Chapter summary

Looking back over this chapter and the scenarios we hope you take away from it several key messages, remembering every patient has differing needs and requires nurses to approach the ABCDE assessment in an innovative, safe, and proactive manner. The aim of this chapter was to help you to assess, recognise, and respond to patients who sustain physiological trauma. In this chapter we have focused on the assessment and management of primary and secondary surveys and the metabolic response to trauma. In all the clinical examples illustrated, the key responsibilities of the nurse are the same:

- The ABCDE is a systematic approach to assessment.
- Problems are treated as they are found – if a problem is found and treated and the patient deteriorates, you start again and work through ABCDE.
- Knowledge about a pattern of injury is helpful as a discovery of one injury should prompt you to search for a related injury.

Below are brief outline answers to the activities listed in the chapter.

Activities: brief outline answers

Activity 10.1: Critical thinking (page 261)

Missed intra-abdominal injuries and concealed haemorrhage are frequent causes of increased morbidity and mortality, especially in patients who survive the initial phase after an injury. Danny's abdomen should have been exposed and examined during the primary and secondary surveys, which was not completed as Danny did not appear to have life-threatening injuries. Inspection of the abdomen would have revealed distension associated with bleeding and may have saved his life.

Activity 10.4: Critical thinking (page 269)

Things that can be overlooked in this situation are airway burns, major trauma, and inhalation exposure to carbon monoxide. Mrs Bowen's scenario represents a textbook situation in which the principles of the ATLS have been utilised to their full potential. Mrs Bowen will remain very ill for many more weeks, but giving the patient the best possible start on their road to recovery begins at the scene of the accident and continues through the emergency unit and onto specialist services such as the burns centre.

Mr Jones would have an increased respiratory rate, increased heart rate and decreasing blood pressure as the body attempts to compensate for the sudden blood loss.

The main cause of his metabolic acidosis would be hypovolaemia due to the excessive hydrogen ions produced in shock. This causes volume depletion due to dehydration.

Mr Jones's story demonstrated to Lily the importance of checking a patient thoroughly (exposure), and she also learned how quickly a seemingly stable patient can deteriorate after major trauma and major surgery. It is essential to keep utilising the principles of the primary and secondary surveys even when a patient may seem to be on the road to recovery.

Further reading

Herndon, D. (2017) *Total Burn Care.* Fifth edition. Edinburgh: Elsevier.

Total burn care guides you in providing optimal burn care and maximising recovery from resuscitation through to reconstruction and rehabilitation.

Mackway-Jones, K, et al. (2013) *Emergency Triage: Manchester Triage Group.* 3rd edition. Chichester: Wiley-Blackwell.

This practical handbook will be an essential purchase for all health service staff who deal with emergencies. It guides the user through the basic methodology of triage, and then demonstrates how to apply the principles of all the major emergency presentations using easy-to-follow flow charts.

Woodrow, P (2018) *Intensive Care Nursing: A Framework for Practice.* Fourth edition. Routledge.

This textbook offers chapters on the assessment, monitoring, and transfer of critically ill patients.

Useful websites

www.nice.org.uk/

This website allows you to access a series of national clinical guidelines to secure consistent, high-quality, evidence-based care for patients using the National Health Service.

www.nice.org.uk/guidance/qs166/chapter/Quality-statement-1-Airway-management

This website is an example of the quality standards set for people with trauma and focuses on the importance of airway management in ensuring survival.

Chapter 11

The patient with altered consciousness

Jane James and Desiree Tait

NMC Future Nurse: Standards of Proficiency for Registered Nurses

This chapter will address the following platforms and proficiencies:

Platform 3: Assessing needs and planning care

At the point of registration, the registered nurse will be able to:

3.2 demonstrate and apply knowledge of body systems and homeostasis, human anatomy and physiology, biology, genomics, pharmacology, and social and behavioural sciences when undertaking full and accurate person-centred nursing assessments and developing appropriate care plans.

3.3 demonstrate and apply knowledge of all commonly encountered mental, physical, behavioural and cognitive health conditions, medication usage and treatments when undertaking full and accurate assessments of nursing care needs and when developing, prioritising and reviewing person-centred care plans.

3.5 demonstrate the ability to accurately process all information gathered during the assessment process to identify needs for individualised nursing care and develop person-centred evidence-based plans for nursing interventions with agreed goals.

3.9 recognise and assess people at risk of harm and the situations that may put them at risk, ensuring prompt action is taken to safeguard those who are vulnerable.

Annex B Nursing Procedures

This chapter will address the following nursing procedures:

2. Use evidence-based, best practice approaches to undertake the following procedures:

2.7 undertake a whole-body systems assessment including respiratory, circulatory, neurological, musculoskeletal, cardiovascular, and skin status.

Chapter aims

By the end of this chapter, you should be able to:

- identify causes of altered consciousness;
- describe the clinical features of altered consciousness in relation to trauma, toxicity, cerebrovascular, and neurological problems, and the clinical implications for the patient;
- undertake a neurological assessment;
- diagnose and differentiate between possible causes of patient deterioration and identify the most appropriate nursing interventions;
- relate the clinical examples in the chapter to your own practice.

Introduction

Consciousness is not fully understood; however, we use the term generally in relation to awareness, responsiveness, and control of ourselves and our environment. In a review of definitions of consciousness, Vimal (2010, p17) concludes a general definition to be:

'consciousness is a mental aspect of an entity (system or process) that is a conscious experience, a conscious function, or both depending on the context,' where the context or metaphysical view of investigation is an important factor. In other words, 'a system or a process is conscious iff [if and only if] its mental aspect is composed of conscious experiences, conscious functions, or both depending on the context'.

Different areas of the cerebral cortex on the surface of the brain are responsible for interpreting awareness of different sensations, such as sight, sound, smell, touch, and taste. We also have awareness of self and our own thoughts. This is cognition and is represented by mental activity. Awareness of self, thoughts, and sensations enables us to respond through controlled activities such as thinking, talking, looking, and moving. Other parts of the brain (the brain stem, diencephalon, and cerebellum) work subconsciously, meaning that we are not aware of them and we cannot control them (Fairley, 2017).

To process information accurately and to elicit appropriate controlled responses, the cerebral cortex relies upon information being sent from, or received by, the subconscious parts. This means that full consciousness is only possible when the brain stem, diencephalon, cerebellum, and cerebrum are working properly. Different levels of consciousness are seen depending upon the area of the brain affected, but loss of awareness and control are always evident to some extent. It is the nurse's responsibility to recognise these signs and to assess, report, and act appropriately.

This chapter gives an overview of the possible causes of altered states of consciousness. It examines in detail the care of three patients with altered consciousness resulting from head injury, stroke, and seizure. It looks at the underlying physiology, social psychology, and ethical implications of all three patients in the context of risk assessment and collaborative management and care. This chapter focuses on disorders of consciousness that have an acute onset that may or may not lead to what the Royal College of Physicians (RCP) (2020) describe as a prolonged disorder of consciousness from which a person may or may not recover.

The chapter begins with a case study followed by an explanation of unconsciousness. An overview of the knowledge and skills required to recognise, assess, prioritise, and manage care for patients with altered consciousness is given. Neurological assessment skills are explored based upon the requirements of the GCS (Teasdale et al., 2014). Acute confusion and delirium are seen in this chapter as examples of altered consciousness but are discussed in detail in Chapter 8.

Case study: Mark is found in the park; he is unconscious

Julia, a student nurse, was walking through the park with her friend on a cold wintry morning when they found a young man lying on the path. Julia approached with caution while calling to him. As she got closer, she could see that his eyes were closed, and he was clearly breathing. He was snoring loudly, and his breath smelled of alcohol, his face was bloodied and bruised. Julia assessed his responsiveness using ACVPU (alert, confusion, responsive to voice or pain, or unresponsive) and was unable to rouse him by speaking loudly to him, by shaking him gently or by pinching his trapezius muscle. While Julia continued her assessment, her friend used her mobile phone to call for an ambulance. To open his airway, Julia lifted the young man's chin and tilted his head back until he stopped snoring. Julia was aware that use of an excessive head tilt could aggravate a possible cervical injury and she maintained manual in-line stabilisation to provide stability to the cervical spine until help arrived. She watched and listened to his breathing and counted his pulse rate before looking in his eyes and using sound and pressure to stimulate him to respond. Starting at his head, Julia and her friend quickly looked and felt for visible injury on the parts of his body that were accessible. They found bruises and swelling on his head, face, and abdomen, and his skin was cold to touch. A wallet was found nearby that contained photographic identification of the young man and the name Mark Spencer on it.

There are many possible reasons why Mark was lying on the ground, and it was most important for Julia and her friend not to put themselves at risk. After excluding any danger, Julia recognised her professional obligation to help, knowing it was important to assess Mark's condition quickly using ACVPU followed by ABCDE (see Chapter 1) and to get help. She knew of several reasons for unresponsiveness, and that more detailed assessment would yield clues as to what had happened to Mark.

Julia's experience highlights the fact that people with altered consciousness may not be able to give information to help with their assessment. People with altered conscious states are vulnerable and at risk of deterioration, and even death, from untreated causes as well as being unable to protect themselves from other harm. Mark's unconsciousness might not have been due to alcohol. Any additional findings that Julia noted on her assessment could be significant, and it was most important for Julia to keep Mark safe from further harm. She could do this by getting expert help, by ensuring his airway, breathing, and circulation were protected (ABC), and by looking for any additional disabilities (D) and any other environmental factors (E).

In summary, what Julia's story highlights are the following points:

- In emergency situations, always ensure that you do not put yourself or others in danger.
- Use a systematic approach to assess the situation and look for clues as to the causes of the problem.
- Be non-judgemental and continue your assessment to the end as there may be more than one problem.
- Organise the people around you and get professional help.
- You may not be able to do anything other than keep the patient safe in the short term, but this can reduce risk of long-term complications.

What are the causes of unconsciousness?

Unconsciousness is a state of unrousable unresponsiveness where the victim is unaware of their surroundings and no purposeful response can be obtained (Martin, 2010). The brain requires a constant supply of oxygenated blood and glucose to function. Interruption of this supply can be sudden, causing unconsciousness within a few seconds. If the interruption is prolonged to ten minutes or more, permanent brain damage occurs as the brain tissue becomes ischaemic and dies. Other causes of unconsciousness can manifest more slowly as the severity of the problem progresses. Even with a gradual decline in consciousness, if the cause is left unattended, unconsciousness will eventually result, and the likelihood of permanent disability increases with the period of unconsciousness (Woodward and Waterhouse, 2009). Cooksley et al. (2018) argue that unconsciousness, regardless of cause, is a time-sensitive emergency where ABCDE assessment and management to achieve physiological stability are essential to promote an effective outcome for the patient. Cooksley et al. (2018) categorise the causes of unconsciousness into four groups including neurological, metabolic, diffuse physiological brain dysfunction, and psychiatric. In this chapter we will focus on neurological, metabolic, and diffuse physiological brain dysfunction, which are detailed in Table 11.1.

Julia had no way of knowing whether Mark's unconsciousness was sudden or gradual but, to assess Mark effectively, she had to consider all possible causes of unconsciousness. She must also be mindful that combinations of different causes may be present – for example, a head injury as well as the influence of alcohol or drugs.

General cause	Possible root cause	Clinical examples
Neurological	1. Asphyxiation/drowning/asthmatic attack/smoke inhalation/anaphylaxis.	1. Liz had a severe asthma attack, and the bronchospasm restricted the flow of air through her airways – she was irritable and restless.
	2. Trauma/injury to lungs/pneumothorax.	2. Peter sustained broken ribs when a tree fell on him, causing pneumothorax and precluding him from taking deep breaths – he couldn't remember his phone number.
	3. Chest infection – sputum retention. Infection increases oxygen consumption and can lead to hypoxaemia and cerebral hypoxia.	3. Sally has pneumonia and secretions have consolidated the bases of both lungs – she was confused and disorientated.
	4. Occlusion of carotid artery by a thrombotic plaque, clot, or embolism.	4. Audrey suffered a transient ischaemic attack – she was incoherent, and her face was drooping on the left, but 30 minutes later she feels things are coming back to normal.
	5. Occlusion of vertebral arteries due to hyperextension of the head.	5. Bill collapsed in the library when he was looking up to get a book from the top shelf. He recovered almost immediately.
	6. Rupture of cerebral vessels as in subarachnoid haemorrhage.	6. Katherine felt an explosion in her head like an elastic band snapping. She had a massive headache and is now responding only to sound.
	7. Hypotension/low cardiac output or slow heart rate that results in reduced cerebral perfusion.	7. Jennifer feels dizzy every time she stands up. Yesterday she fainted at work when she was rushing.
	8. Increased intracranial pressure caused by cerebral oedema, tumour, bleed, hydrocephalus causing reduced cerebral perfusion.	8. Andrew has a shunt for drainage of hydrocephalus. He is becoming increasingly drowsy; his eyes are half closed, and he doesn't seem to be able to concentrate – the doctor thinks his shunt is blocked.
	9. Injury or insult to brain tissue.	9. Diane was hit by a car some weeks ago and sustained brain stem injury. She is now breathing spontaneously, yawns a lot, and makes moaning sounds. She opens her eyes but doesn't look at you and she goes rigid when stimulated.
	10. Meningitis or encephalitis.	10. Ruby's lumbar puncture shows meningitis. She is photosensitive, has a severe headache and is confused, irritable, and just wants to sleep.
Metabolic	11. Hypoglycaemia.	11. Shanta is a diabetic. She is shopping with her friend and is being uncharacteristically aggressive to everyone and cannot be consoled.
	12. Electrolyte imbalance.	12. Sheilagh has had copious diarrhoea. She complained of thirst and headaches, became restless and agitated and has just had a fit – her blood results show high sodium levels.
	13. Sepsis.	13. Hugh was admitted with confusion and a urine infection. He is now hypotensive, tachycardic, and responding only to sound.
Diffuse physiological brain dysfunction	14. Epilepsy – convulsions (post-ictal).	14. Robin had his medication changed and has had violent fits. He is now very sleepy and responding only to pressure stimuli.
	15. Overdose of drugs/alcohol.	15. Ian drank a bottle of whisky and now his friends can't wake him up.
	16. Carbon monoxide poisoning – inhalation of noxious gases.	16. Bob's gas fire was faulty, and he suffered carbon monoxide poisoning – he was unresponsive when found.

Table 11.1 Causes of diminished consciousness, after Cooksley et al. (2018)

Activity 11.1   Critical thinking

Look again at the case study with Mark Spencer. What possible causes of Mark's unconsciousness can you identify from those shown in Table 11.1?

An outline answer to this activity is given at the end of the chapter.

Quickly recognising signs of deteriorating consciousness, and understanding the possible underlying causes, allows early detection of physiological problems and early instigation of correct treatment and care. This can prevent the development of unconsciousness and further risk. Mark's most immediate risk was obstruction of his airway and respiratory arrest, leading to cardiac arrest. Julia recognised this and acted immediately by performing the head tilt, chin lift manoeuvre. She then continued with a more detailed neurological assessment.

Assessing consciousness level

The two aspects of consciousness generally considered when assessing an individual's level of consciousness are arousal, which indicates function of the reticular activating system (RAS) in the brain stem, and awareness or cognition, which indicates function of the cerebral hemispheres. Varying degrees of unconsciousness can occur depending upon the cause and extent of brain dysfunction. Julia used ACVPU as a rapid initial assessment to determine any reduced responsiveness (RCP, 2017), followed by the more detailed GCS (Teasdale et al., 2014). The GCS helped to establish Mark's degree of unconsciousness and which neurological responses were affected. The ACVPU assessment findings can be loosely equated to ranges of the GCS score (see Table 11.2), indicating the urgency for more detailed neurological assessment.

The GCS is a widely used neurological assessment tool recommended by Teasdale et al. (2014) to assess patients with altered consciousness and for use in adults and children over five years of age. The tool, first developed in 1974 has been subject to scrutiny and

ACVPU score	Approximate GCS score
Alert	14–15
(New) Confusion	13–14 (please refer to Chapters 1 and 8)
Responds to voice	9–13
Responds to pain	4–8
Unresponsive	3

Table 11.2   ACVPU and equivalent GCS scores

Source: Romanelli and Farrell, 2021; RCP, 2017.

controversy in relation to clinical reliability. A systematic review by Reith et al. (2016) on the reliability of the GCS did indicate that in clinical settings reliability was adequate, with scope to optimise its use in practice through education and training.

The GCS measures three indicators of neurological function.

- eye opening response (E);
- verbal response (V);
- motor response (M).

Scores are attributed to each indicator (Table 11.3) and should be considered separately, but may also be combined to give the overall coma score. The highest possible score is 15 and the lowest 3. Because Mark did not respond to painful stimulus when Julia did the ACVPU score, it suggested his GCS was dangerously low, indicating a state of coma. NICE (2014b [updated in 2019]) recommend that if a person has a GCS of 8 or less they are at risk of airway obstruction and airway management is required.

Indicator	Score	If the patient ...	When you ...	Because ...
Eye opening	4	Opens eyes spontaneously, without stimulation.	Approach your patient or gently touch them if there is a known hearing impairment.	This demonstrates arousal or wakefulness, which is dependent upon the reticular activating system (RAS: a dense network of neurons) within the brain stem being fully functional. Spontaneous eye opening should **not** be equated to alertness or awareness.
	3	Opens eyes to sound.	Make a noise or say something loud enough to elicit a response (e.g. their name). Or touch your patient's hand, arm, or shoulder and shake gently.	Trauma or increased intracranial pressure could impair neuron pathways within the RAS, requiring increased sensory stimulation to evoke eye opening. Speech is used, then touch, and lastly pain.
	2	Opens eyes in response to pressure.	Exert graded painful peripheral stimuli by first using the side of a pen or pencil to apply pressure to the fingertip for a short time, then exerting painful central stimulus by pinching the trapezius muscle, and finally applying supraorbital notch pressure. Only if there is no response to the previous, lesser stimulus, and there are no fractures in this region.	A central painful stimulus may result in the patient grimacing, thus closing their eyes. An initial peripheral stimulus could avoid misleading results if there is no response to sound or touch. Alternate the finger tested to minimise damage. It is important to elicit the best response, so central stimuli may be applied.

Indicator	Score	If the patient ...	When you ...	Because ...
	1	Does not open eyes to stimuli.	Apply painful central stimulus (supraorbital pressure). If eye opening is not possible due to orbital swelling, you need to note this and write 'C' against 'none' on the neurological observation chart. This assessment should not be attempted unless facial fractures have been excluded.	Intracranial pressure or neural damage due to trauma could be severely impairing the function of the RAS.
	NT	Eyes are closed by a local factor such as eye swelling, possible facial fracture, or surgery.	Find that eye opening is Not Testable (NT).	In this instance the combined score of all three components of the GCS will be invalid and scores in the sub-scales must be considered separately.
Verbal response	5	Is orientated.	Ask questions about the time, place, and person, e.g., what the month or year is, where they are and who they are. Avoid questions requiring only yes/no answers. If the patient is expressively dysphasic, write 'D' instead. It is not essential to know the exact day, date, or location due to the disorientating effect of prolonged hospital stays and hospital transfers.	The highest level of consciousness requires a person to be totally aware of their surroundings, being orientated to time, place, and person. Questions requiring only yes/no answers are not conclusive as answers can be predicted. It is important to be able to recognise and distinguish between **receptive and expressive dysphasia** as these can detract from accurate assessment for orientation. More detailed observation may be required.
	4	Is confused.	Ask the questions above and the patient cannot answer correctly but is able to converse through coherent phrases or sentences.	Deterioration of consciousness begins with impaired ability to think clearly, repetition, impaired perception, and responsiveness with reduced memory of current stimuli relating to time, place, and person in that order.
	3	Uses words.	Ask the questions above. Single-worded answers or the inability to make a sentence of words are classed as words.	The cerebral hemispheres of the brain are most susceptible to damage and are responsible for verbal and analytical abilities, perception of language, and performance of speech. Poor comprehension and impaired ability to express thoughts into words could indicate reduced cerebral function.

(Continued)

Table 11.3 (Continued)

Indicator	Score	If the patient ...	When you ...	Because ...
	2	Makes sounds.	Apply graded stimuli (noise to supraorbital pressure). Noises such as moans or grunting sounds are classed as sounds.	This is a sign of further deterioration of cerebral function extending to deeper structures of the brain. There is usually associated psychomotor impairment at this stage.
	1	Makes no attempt at verbal response to stimuli.	Apply graded stimuli (noise to supraorbital pressure).	Stupour and coma are indicated by little or no spontaneous activity and by being unrousable and unresponsive to external stimuli. These are signs of advanced brain failure.
	NT	Has local factors that interfere with communication.	Find that no verbal response is possible due to an endotracheal tube or tracheostomy (without a speaking valve), write 'T' against 'none'.	Intubated patients cannot speak although they may be conscious. They may attempt to mouth words, which are often very difficult to determine, so alternative scores may be misleading, unless by written test of orientation.
Best motor response	6	Obeys commands.	Give the patient a two-part command to squeeze and release your hand, raise and lower their arm or leg, or put out and pull back their tongue. If there are varying responses from the different limbs you must note the best limb response and record the appropriate score for the response. Deficits in individual limbs will be recorded separately under 'limb movement'.	This indicates how well the brain is functioning as a whole by testing the areas of brain that precipitate motor responses to sensory stimuli. Following commands indicates the ability to process instructions. Grasping is a primitive reflex that may happen spontaneously, thus giving misleading scores if a one-part only command is used. One limb responding worse than the other gives indication of the site of focal brain damage, so is worth noting.
	5	Is localising to stimuli.	Apply a graded pressure stimulus on the head or neck (trapezius pinch or supraorbital notch pressure) if there is no motor response to speech or touch.	Central stimulus used as peripheral pain may evoke a spinal reflex action. Purposeful or semi-purposeful movements are known as localising and the hand must be brought above the clavicle toward the stimulus. Localising may be asymmetrical and when associated with clouding of consciousness because of the RAS being squeezed, can indicate increased intracranial pressure.

Indicator	Score	If the patient …	When you …	Because …
				This causes downward displacement of the cerebral hemispheres and structures of the upper brain to the level of the tentorium cerebelli, a transverse fold in the meninges that separates the structures of the upper and lower brain. The oculomotor nerve emerges to control pupillary constriction around the mid brain and can become trapped if the pressure continues to increase. It is at this point when changes in pupil reactions to light might begin.
	4	Displays normal limb flexion.	Apply a graded pressure stimulus on the head or neck (trapezius pinch to supraorbital notch pressure) if there is no motor response to speech or touch.	Flexion of limbs in response to pain is less well targeted to the stimulus than localisation and indicates advancing brain dysfunction. Fluctuating respiratory function may be noticed at this point, identified by yawning or irregular breathing patterns.
	3	Displays abnormal limb flexion.	Apply a graded pressure stimulus on the head or neck (trapezius pinch to supraorbital notch pressure) if there is no motor response to speech or touch.	Abnormal flexion or decorticate rigidity (see Figure 11.1) may indicate a lesion in the cerebral hemisphere or internal capsule where motor neurons originate.
	2	Displays limb extension.	Apply a graded pressure stimulus on the head or neck (trapezius pinch to supraorbital notch pressure) if there is no motor response to speech or touch.	Extension or decerebrate rigidity (see Figure 11.1) can be an indication of a lesion in the diencephalon, mid brain, or pons. It can also result from severe metabolic disorders, hypoxia, or hypoglycaemia.
	1	Does not respond.		
	NT	Is paralysed or has other limiting factors.	Find that limb response is not testable.	In this instance the combined score of all three components of the GCS will be invalid and scores in the sub-scales must be considered separately.

Table 11.3 Glasgow Coma Scale: how to score

Source: based on information from Teasdale et al., 2014.

Activity 11.2   Evidence-based practice and research

Visit the web link **www.glasgowcomascale.org/what-is-gcs** to see information and guidance on how to conduct a GCS assessment and to rate your findings. Follow the links to the video for a demonstration.

Try to check, observe, stimulate, and rate your patients in this way when you next need to conduct a neurological assessment.

As this is your own research, there is no answer to this activity at the end of the chapter.

In addition to noting GCS, it is important to assess respiratory rate and oxygen saturations; pupil size, shape, and reaction to light; limb response to stimulus; and vital signs including pulse, blood pressure, and temperature. Together these will give more accurate indications of your patient's neurological deficits and degree of risk of further neurological deterioration.

Activity 11.3   Evidence-based practice and research

Take some time to read about the anatomy and physiology of the central nervous system. Make a note of the main structures of the brain and identify the parts that contribute to the neurological functions tested by the three indicators used in the GCS assessment in Table 11.3.

Because you will find this in your anatomy and physiology textbooks, there will be no answer provided for this activity. However, you may find Table 11.3 useful in linking the pathophysiology to your practice.

Let us return to Mark's story and to explore what data Julia was able to collect during her assessment of Mark's condition.

Case study: Returning to Mark's story

When Julia assessed the three indicators of Mark's GCS, he did not open his eyes to central pressure stimulus, nor did he make any vocal sounds. Julia noticed some flexion in response to trapezius pinch when Mark seemed to move his left arm upwards toward her hand. Checking a second time, she could also see that his left knee rose slightly. She considered his best motor response to be normal flexion because his hand did not reach above his clavicle, but he moved one side of his body, thus scoring E1, V1, M4 (see Table 11.3).

This gave a total score of 6 out of 15, confirming that Mark's consciousness level was dangerously low, and he was at risk of obstructing his airway.

Julia had noted bruising and swelling of Mark's face but was still able to lift his eyelids to look at the size and shape of his pupils. She opened both Mark's eyes simultaneously to compare the pupil size and shape. Both were round, although the left pupil looked slightly larger than the right. Julia used her friend's mobile phone to shine a light directly at each pupil in turn. She moved the light across Mark's left eye, from the outer aspect to rest over the pupil, then back again and repeated this on the right side to check the right pupil. Noting each pupil response, Julia could see that the left pupil was slower to constrict than the right pupil, which moved so quickly that she could only really see it dilating when she took the light away. Julia made a point of repeating the observation, looking at the non-stimulated pupil, and noted that the right pupil still constricted quickly when light was shone into the left eye, but the left pupil remained sluggish in response when light was shone into the right eye.

In Table 11.3, reference is made to abnormal flexion and limb extension. These are referred to as decorticate and decerebrate rigidity and are examples of 'abnormal posturing'. They are involuntary flexion or extension of the arms and legs, indicating severe brain injury. They occur when one set of muscles becomes incapacitated while the opposing set is not, and an external stimulus such as pain causes the working set of

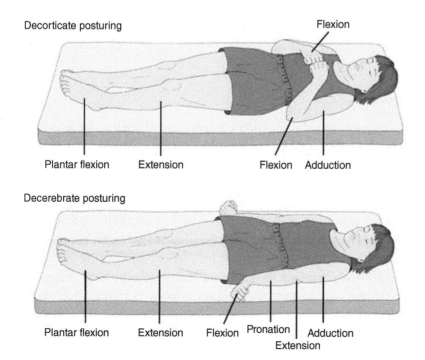

Figure 11.1   Decorticate and decerebrate posturing

muscles to contract. These types of posturing are indicators of the amount of damage that has occurred to the brain and are used to measure the severity of a coma with the GCS (Knight and Decker, 2021). Figure 11.1 presents a diagrammatic illustration of decorticate and decerebrate posturing.

Returning to Mark's story, when the paramedics arrived, Julie was able to update them and they quickly undertook a further ABCDE assessment including GCS and secured Mark's airway with an endotracheal tube (see Chapter 3). This would allow them to administer oxygen and assist with his respirations should his consciousness deteriorate further, affecting the central areas of the brain that control the vital functions. Julia had kept Mark safe until professional help arrived. Activity 11.4 offers an opportunity for you to rehearse assessing pupil reaction with your peers.

Activity 11.4   Evidence-based practice and research

Take a torch with a bright white light and narrow beam and ask a friend to allow you to shine it in their eyes, using the same technique as Julia.

1. Note what happens.
2. What are the difficulties in this technique of pupil assessment?
3. Look at Table 11.3. What might be happening to Mark to elicit the pupil response Julia noted? What might happen next?

An explanation of what you might notice and the answers to the questions can be found at the end of the chapter.

In the A&E department, Mark's GCS was reassessed within 15 minutes according to the guidelines (NICE, 2014b [updated in 2019]). Blood tests and radiological investigations enabled the medical and nursing team to eliminate many of the causes of unconsciousness that you may have identified earlier. For patients with GCS less than 13 on initial assessment in the A&E department, a CT scan should be performed within one hour and provisional results available within a further hour (NICE, 2014b [2019]). It later emerged that Mark had been assaulted and kicked repeatedly in the head after leaving the pub where he had been for a drink with his friend the previous evening to celebrate his twenty-third birthday. Even though there was no evidence of intracranial haematoma or skull fracture on the CT scan, Mark had suffered head trauma, causing obvious external bruising and swelling. His neurological assessment suggested changes to the cerebral hemispheres and oculomotor nerve that could be due to intracranial bruising and cerebral oedema (swelling of his brain tissue).

What are the nursing priorities of the unconscious patient?

Case study: Mark is transferred to intensive care

David is a third-year student nurse on critical care placement in the intensive care unit. Penny, his mentor, agreed that he should look after a newly admitted patient to focus on priorities of care. They prepare a bed area for Mark, who was in A&E having suffered a closed head injury following assault. He is to be sedated, ventilated, and closely monitored for 24 hours. While Mark is being prepared for transfer, Penny asks David to identify the nursing priorities when caring for Mark.

David was aware that he and Penny would need to work collaboratively with the medical team to reduce the risk of death or long-term brain damage for Mark. Any initial damage to Mark's brain (primary damage) was irreversible, but the main objective was to prevent further (secondary) damage resulting mainly from a rising intracranial pressure (ICP). This was the biggest threat to Mark's recovery.

Activity 11.5 Communication

Imagine you are Mark's nurse in the A&E department. Using the SBAR communication tool (see pages 33–34), make a note of the content and sequence of your handover to David and Penny in ICU.

A plan of Mark's handover can be found at the end of this chapter.

A quick ABCDE assessment and response (see Chapter 1) would address any immediate dangers, but David really needed to know which aspects of care could affect Mark's ICP. He was unsure how to prevent further increase and how best to aid reduction of ICP. Penny points out some important specific nursing considerations to help with reducing the risk of secondary damage. These are identified in Table 11.4.

Problem	Intervention	Rationale
Cerebral oedema may increase during first 24–48 hours, causing ICP to rise further.	1. Keep sedated and minimise stimulation. 2. Nurse in a 15–30° head-up tilt.	1. Prevents coughing, sneezing, and straining, which temporarily increase ICP. 2. To optimise cerebral venous drainage.

(Continued)

Table 11.4 (Continued)

Problem	Intervention	Rationale
	3. Keep head in neutral alignment with body. Ensure ET tube ties are not tight around neck. 4. Avoid hip flexion.	3. Avoids obstructing jugular veins, which would prevent cerebral venous drainage. 4. Prevents raised intra-abdominal pressure leading to raised intra-thoracic pressure, which in turn impedes cerebral venous drainage.
Inadequate oxygen delivery to the brain tissues will cause further cerebral damage and exacerbate oedema.	1. Care of ET tube. Perform endotracheal suction to remove secretions if needed. 2. Titrate inspired oxygen and ventilator settings against ABG and SpO$_2$ results to keep PaO$_2$ normal. 3. Keep sedated – monitor sedation score (see Chapter 3).	1. Ensures airway remains patent and optimises gaseous exchange. 2. Optimises ventilation and avoids increased blood flow to the brain which takes up space and increases ICP. 3. Reduces cerebral oxygen demand.
Risk of infection.	1. Avoid infection – use aseptic techniques, monitor body temperature, and aim to keep it normal.	1. Raised body temperature increases O$_2$ demand and CO$_2$ production, thus increasing cerebral oxygen use. Patients with head injury are susceptible to chest infection, which can lead to sepsis. High ICP can squeeze the hypothalamus, causing temperature regulation to be lost.
Inadequate cerebral perfusion pressure (CPP) will compromise oxygen delivery to the brain, exacerbating cerebral oedema. Good perfusion is needed to help to reduce the cerebral oedema.	1. Monitor heart rate. 2. Monitor fluid input and output – replace fluids to prevent hypotension. 3. Keep MAP >70 mmHg and CPP >60 mmHg. 4. Titrate prescribed inotropic drugs to correct hypotension. 5. Keep PaCO$_2$ on low side of normal range. 6. Use correct patient positioning and care of ET tube ties.	1. Changes in heart rate can indicate early BP compensating mechanisms, increasing ICP or inadequate sedation, which may need to be acted upon. Cardiac dysrhythmias need correcting. They reduce efficiency of the heart, causing hypotension. 2. Ensures adequate circulating volume. Gives early identification of excessive diuresis (diabetes insipidus) resulting from pituitary gland being squeezed. Gives indication of renal function.

Problem	Intervention	Rationale
		3. MAP counteracts rise in ICP to allow adequate cerebral perfusion pressure (CPP = MAP – ICP).
		4. Higher CO_2 levels cause cerebral vasodilation. This increases cerebral blood volume. ICP. Increased ICP reduces CPP.
		5. Aids cerebral venous drainage, thus reducing cerebral vascular congestion.
Head injury can cause hyperglycaemia and increase metabolism.	1. Monitor and correct glucose levels as per policy. 2. Commence enteral feeding as soon as possible.	1. Reduces mortality. 2. Prevents catabolism (breakdown of complex substances to produce energy), which creates more CO_2.

Table 11.4   Priorities of care to prevent secondary damage in head injury (after Fairley, 2017)

How can secondary brain injury be prevented?

Secondary brain injury is an indirect result of primary brain injury and is associated with the action of systemic and cerebral processes that can occur following the primary injury (Boss and Huether, 2019). Preventing secondary brain damage depends upon the quality and quantity of circulation to the brain. For Mark, this means having adequate oxygenation and blood pressure, and maintenance of normal ABGs and blood glucose levels. Increases in ICP result from cerebral oedema, infection, haematoma, tumour, or hydrocephalus taking up space within the skull (Boss and Huether, 2019). Because the skull is rigid, the increase in contents causes them to become compressed with a resultant increase in ICP. Mark's raised ICP was due to cerebral oedema, which can subside naturally as healing processes take place. Sometimes intravenous infusion of hypertonic sodium chloride solution or mannitol may be prescribed, to reduce intracranial pressure following traumatic brain injury (Chen et al., 2020). These drugs use the process of osmosis to draw water from an area of high concentration to an area of low concentration, thus drawing fluid from the swollen brain tissue into the cerebral circulation. It is then returned to the central circulation and excreted by the kidneys.

Whether natural process or medical interventions are employed, the injured tissue requires a good blood supply for the swelling to reduce. ICP and arterial blood pressure work in opposition, so cerebral perfusion (blood flow to the cerebral circulation) depends on the blood pressure being higher than the ICP. Cerebral perfusion pressure

(CPP) is the pressure required to maintain cerebral blood flow: CPP = mean arterial pressure – intracranial pressure (CPP = MAP – ICP). Thus, if Mark's ICP rises, his MAP must also rise by the same amount as his ICP. If Mark's MAP dropped too low, cerebral circulation would be compromised and his brain tissue would be poorly perfused. Poor perfusion leads to cerebral vasodilation and further swelling, thus compounding the problem. Other factors that can affect CPP leading to cerebral vasodilation include high arterial $PaCO_2$ above 6 kPa, and pH lower than 7.35. Conversely, a low $PaCO_2$ (below 4 kPa), a high pH (above 7.45), or high CPP will trigger cerebral vasoconstriction and reduce blood flow to the brain. Nursing assessment and care must therefore focus on continuous assessment and monitoring of Mark with the aim of achieving homeostasis. Table 11.4 summarises the management principles to facilitate homeostasis.

Case study: Mark's continuing care in ICU

David and Penny prioritised Mark's care for the next 24 hours. Mark remained stable but his repeat CT scan showed evidence of cerebral oedema. It was agreed that he should be kept sedated and ventilated for a further 24 hours to allow this to settle down. When Mark's sedation was reduced, he was restless and agitated, requiring re-sedation. One day later, Mark developed sepsis, secondary to pneumonia. On day seven, Mark's sedation was stopped and he was extubated successfully. He was not agitated, but his GCS remained low at 9 (E3, V2, M4) indicating residual brain damage. Mark's recovery from this point was very uncertain, and it was impossible to know whether the brain damage resulted from primary or secondary injury.

Being alert to subtle changes in patient behaviour

In the next section of the chapter, we will explore and discuss the importance of continuing observation and monitoring of all aspects of neurological assessment including behaviour and limb movement.

Case study: Pam suffered a haemorrhagic stroke ten days ago

Imagine you are working on the rehabilitation ward and looking after Mrs Pam Green, who suffered a haemorrhagic stroke ten days ago. This morning when you woke her, she resisted getting out of bed and did not appear to be making her usual effort with her exercises. Communication can be difficult because of her expressive dysphasia, but today she did not appear to be concordant, and she was yawning, so you left her in bed. You return two hours later to find Pam slumped in her bed. On assessment of her GCS, she scores 5 (E1, V1, M3), and her pupils are fixed and dilated. There is no response to light.

Activity 11.6 Critical thinking

Consider Pam's scenario and answer the following questions.

- What signs of altered consciousness were missed?
- What could these signs have indicated?
- What could have been done?
- Why do you think Pam did not get the required attention?

Answers to these questions can be found at the end of this chapter.

Pam's deterioration appeared to be a sudden event, but clues were evident some time before she became unresponsive. You should make objective assessments despite communication difficulties and avoid any preconceptions. You will experience situations like Pam's in all spheres of nursing. It is important to be aware of the subtle changes in patient behaviour as these are the earliest indicators of altered consciousness. If you are alert to these changes then, in many cases, early intervention can prevent deterioration.

Because Pam had previously suffered a stroke and had some residual neurological deficits, continued assessment using the GCS would not only identify any deterioration but could also be used to measure progress. Limb assessment may be specifically useful in this instance.

Limb assessment

Limb assessment usually forms part of the overall neurological assessment with the GCS, pupil responses, and vital signs. Changes in limb movements can help to pinpoint more specifically the area and degree of brain injury, although it is important to eliminate any pre-existing conditions that may affect limb movement, such as previous stroke or injury (Woodward and Waterhouse, 2009). Ideally, the patient should be able to obey commands, despite expressive dysphasia, Pam should have been able to respond. Some patients with receptive dysphasia (difficulty with understanding written or spoken language) may benefit from a demonstration of what is expected of them.

It is important to compare left side with right side of arms and then legs, rather than assessing each limb independently, although results for each limb should be recorded separately. Pam could have been asked to lift her limbs against gravity or slight resistance. This is more useful than asking her to squeeze your hands, as grasping is a primitive reflex and may give misleading results. Deviation from previous recorded findings is most significant and this may well have been revealing in Pam's scenario.

Spontaneous or involuntary movement should be recorded, as well as limb strength, which is classified as:

- normal: usual power and strength;
- mild weakness: inability to fully lift limbs or difficulty in moving against resistance;
- severe weakness: unable to lift limbs but can move them laterally.

Patients who are unable to obey commands can be assessed for limb movement in response to pressure, as in the motor response section of the GCS. Any difference between responses in left and right must be noted in the limb movement assessment.

When Pam seemed to be resisting care, her condition was deteriorating. A thorough GCS, including limb assessment, would have revealed that she opened her eyes to voice (E1), made sounds or words (V2 or 3), and localised to pressure (M5), but that her best motor response was weaker than her last limb assessment had shown. With this information, medical attention could have been summoned much earlier. Unfortunately, it is likely that Pam suffered another intracerebral bleed, and prognosis in this instance is extremely poor.

Seizure: what action is needed?

Seizures are transient episodes of neurological deficit and take many different forms depending upon their origin and cause. They are often associated with epilepsy, but can be triggered by drugs, alcohol, metabolic disorders, pre-eclampsia, head injury or cerebral hypoxia, and pyrexia in children (Boss and Huether, 2019). Abnormal electrical activity can start in one part of the brain and spread, sometimes involving localised areas, and sometimes affecting the whole cerebral cortex. Various symptoms result, depending upon the area and location of brain involvement.

Case study: Seizure

Student nurse, Claire, was returning to the ward from an errand when she met a young lady in the ward entrance. She seemed to be walking aimlessly, but on approach Claire established that she was Josie Watkins, who was visiting her mother, a patient on the ward. Claire directed Josie to the correct bed but saw her stop. Josie was fiddling with her hands, then collapsed on to the floor. Her arms were jerking and she was making choking sounds. Claire shouted for help and cleared the area of obstacles. She was unsure of what to do next and was relieved when Satya, the ward sister, appeared.

Josie was showing early signs of a generalised seizure when Claire met her. The subtle behaviour that Claire noticed is significant and will be useful for Josie and her family members to recognise in future. The most important and immediate concern was to keep her safe for the duration of the seizure, using the ABCDE approach, and to protect her from injury.

Activity 11.7 Evidence-based practice and research

Visit the International League Against Epilepsy website at **www.ilae.org** to find out more about the classification of seizures, current research, and recommendations. Also refer to the overview at: **www.nice.org.uk/guidance/cg137**

As this is your own research, there is no answer to this activity at the end of the chapter.

It is not recommended, or safe, to open the mouth of someone having a seizure to insert an oropharyngeal airway because of jaw clenching, and stimulation may further exacerbate the seizure. It is usual to allow short seizures to run their course, observing closely, and to intervene once the seizure stops (NICE, 2021c). It is not advisable to restrain the victim. If seizures are continuous, prescribed emergency medication such as diazepam should be administered through an accessible route with quick absorption (NICE, 2021c).

Case study: Seizure (continued)

Satya, the ward sister, removed Josie's neck scarf and cushioned her head with a pillow. She asked Claire to record the duration of the seizure and all the different components, such as noises, movements and progression, skin colour, and injuries. Another nurse brought emergency equipment and positioned it at Josie's head ready for Satya to use if needed. Once Josie seemed to relax (after 75 seconds), Satya asked Claire for help to put Josie into the recovery position. Josie's airway was protected using a head tilt and chin lift, and Satya had oxygen and a face mask ready. Claire carried out a full set of observations including respirations, oxygen saturations, pulse, blood pressure, temperature, and neurological assessment. Josie began to respond after a further two minutes and was helped onto a bed to recover. Satya found out from her mother that Josie suffered with epilepsy and had recently had her medication regime reviewed.

Claire's experience could have happened outside the hospital, where no emergency equipment is available. However, despite the help from experienced healthcare professionals, we can see that the initial actions required only common sense. Claire acted appropriately by:

- noting symptoms leading up to the seizure;
- calling for help;
- preparing a safe environment;
- staying with the patient;
- being prepared to intervene with the ABCDE approach afterwards.

The duration of seizures can vary from two minutes to repeated or prolonged convulsive seizures lasting more than five minutes. Status epilepticus can be described as continuous or recurrent seizure activity that lasts more than five minutes and which requires urgent intervention. These seizures pose increased risk of hypoxia to the patient as cerebral oxygen consumption increases and there may be insufficient oxygen supply. This is a life-threatening situation and demonstrates why it was important for the ward sister to have oxygen ready to administer to Josie if she needed it. Seizures lasting longer than 60 minutes can lead to acidosis, dehydration, hypoglycaemia, possible fractures, and muscle breakdown, which in turn can cause AKI (Opdam, 2019). It is important to respond quickly to support airway, breathing, and circulation in this instance and to summon urgent expert and medical help in order that appropriate medical treatment can be given (NICE, 2021c). Keep a record of the phases of the seizure and time the duration of the seizure to determine the severity of the situation. The patient may not remember events, so information is useful for them and their families for future management and care. It is important to reassure the patient and to be able to provide accurate and reliable information regarding the cause and possible triggers of their seizures and their likely course. The nurse has a role in patient education and health promotion, as well as recognising signs of impending and actual problems.

In patients not known to have epilepsy, alternative causes of seizure should be considered and subsequently treated to avoid further seizures.

Chapter summary

This chapter highlights the nursing responsibilities of rapid and accurate neurological assessment and subsequent prioritisation of care for patients with altered consciousness and at risk of deterioration. Nurses can come across patients with altered consciousness in all clinical settings, and early intervention and prioritisation of care can reduce complications. Outcomes are not always good, but increased understanding of neurological problems will enable you to make evidence-based clinical judgements.

Activities: brief outline answers

Activity 11.1: Critical thinking (page 277)

Several of the causes identified in Table 11.1 could apply to Mark: alcohol intoxication; drug overdose; head injury; hypoglycaemia; hypotensive episode such as fainting; hypoxia; infection such as meningitis or encephalitis; post-ictal (post-fit); spontaneous intracranial bleed such as subarachnoid haemorrhage.

Activity 11.4: Evidence-based practice and research (page 284)

1. Normally, when a bright narrow beam of light is shone into one eye and held there, the pupil of that eye constricts briskly to a pinpoint size of about 1 mm. The pupil dilates again, usually back to its original size, when the light is removed. To avoid misleading results in

pupil size difference, it is important to check equality of pupil sizes prior to subjecting them to light stimulus. Normally, both pupils respond when light is shone in only one of them – this is the consensual response that helps to test the oculomotor nerve.

2. Difficulties with this technique.
    *   You may find some healthy people have unequal pupils ordinarily.
    *   With brown eyes it is sometimes difficult to determine the margin of the pupil from the iris, so the motor response may need to be noted from the dilation of the pupil on removing the light rather than looking for constriction on applying the light stimulus.
    *   The brightness of light in the room, and the width and strength of the light beam, affect starting pupil size and may hinder response.
    *   Moving the light stimulus across the bridge of the patient's nose can hinder response, so it is better to introduce the light from the outer aspect of the eye.
    *   Patients who are photosensitive (for example, secondary to meningitis) will find this very uncomfortable and may resist the assessment.
    *   Likewise, orbital oedema that precludes eye opening hinders assessment in the patients who may need to be monitored.

3. Mark's direct pupil responses indicated that his optic and oculomotor cranial nerves were functioning. The fact that his left pupil was slow to constrict suggests that either the left optic nerve had impaired sensitivity to light, or that the conduction pathway of the left oculomotor nerve was impeded. The brisk consensual response of the right pupil when light was shone into the left eye demonstrates that the left optic nerve was sensing the light. These findings give strong clues as to the extent of intracranial pressure increase (see Table 11.3) and suggest that Mark's left oculomotor nerve was getting squeezed, and the intracranial pressure was such that the cerebral hemispheres were being pushed down toward the tentorium cerebelli. If the pressure continued to rise, the next sign would be a change in left pupil shape to oval due to compression of the oculomotor nerve, then a fixed and dilated left pupil, accompanied by reduced motor responses to painful stimuli and haemodynamic changes as the diencephalon and brain stem start to get squeezed. This is a dangerous situation for Mark.

Activity 11.5: Communication (page 285)

Introduce self and department.

Patient's name: Mark Spencer, 23-year-old male.

Situation

*   Unconscious closed head injury.
*   Intubated and ventilated.
*   Bruising and swelling to head, face, and abdomen.
*   No other injuries.

Background

*   Give home situation if known.
*   Went out for a drink last night.
*   Assaulted – kicked repeatedly in the head.
*   Found unconscious in park this am – give original GCS – and has been unconscious since.
*   No significant past medical history.
*   Usually fit and well.
*   Takes no medication.

Assessment

*   Airway: intubated by paramedics at the scene.
*   Breathing: spontaneously on admission, now sedated and ventilated. Give breathing rate, % oxygen delivered, and oxygen saturations readings.

- Circulation: give heart rate, blood pressure, temperature measured and peripheral temperature to touch, fluid input and output.
- Disability: give latest GCS score and pupil assessment, blood glucose result, CT scan and X-ray results. Summarise blood results and give any significant deviations from normal. Give information relating to medication and fluid administered and diuretic response to hypertonic saline if given.
- Exposure: if not already mentioned, give urine output and state whether catheterised. Indicate other injuries and how they have been treated.

Response

Outline proposed plan

- Keep sedated and ventilated for next 24 hours.
- Repeat CT scan tomorrow to check for reduction in cerebral oedema.
- Repeat ABGs one hour after transfer.
- Keep PaO_2 normal and $PaCO_2$ on low side of normal.
- Give any information regarding family, police, and property.
- Agree a time for transfer.

Activity 11.6: Critical thinking (page 289)

First, Pam may not have been asleep, but she opened her eyes to sound. Resisting getting out of bed and lack of effort and concordance may not have been stubbornness but due to reduced awareness, cognition, and control. Early signs of deterioration in consciousness include decreased concentration, agitation, dullness, and lethargy. These fit with Pam's changed behaviour, but because of her usual expressive dysphasia, her falling GCS went unnoticed. Depending upon the degree of Pam's expressive dysphasia, it may be difficult to ascertain confusion and words lacking order from sounds not resembling words. Yawning is an early respiratory indicator of rising ICP (Aksoy Gündoğdu et al., 2020).

Had Pam's GCS been thoroughly assessed, it should have been possible to note that she could not obey commands and that she was losing control of motor function. Assessment of vital signs, limb movement, and pupil reactions may have helped to conclude findings.

It is not clear whether the course of Pam's deterioration could have been prevented.

It is not safe to assume that recovering patients are safe from deterioration.

Further reading

Heimgartner, N, Rebar, C and Gersch, C (2019) *Emergency Nursing Made Incredibly Easy!* Third edition. Wolters Kluwer Health.

This book gives easy-to-understand explanations of emergency care and includes a specific chapter dedicated to neurological problems.

Goulden, I and Clarke, D (2016) Traumatic brain injury, in Clarke, D and Ketchell, A (eds) *Nursing the Acutely Ill Adult: Priorities in Assessment and Management.* 2nd edition. London: Palgrave Macmillan.

This chapter deals with traumatic brain injury, considering medical and surgical interventions in a clearly laid out format.

NICE (2014 [updated 2019]) *Head Injury: Triage, Assessment, Investigation and Early Management of Head Injury in Infants, Children, Young People and Adults.* London: NICE.

This gives comprehensive guidance on care of patients with head injury. Nurses involved in caring for acutely ill patients should have this information.

Useful websites

www.ilae.org

The International League Against Epilepsy website presents a wealth of information about epilepsy. The different classifications and manifestations are explained. There are presentations, research papers, and practice guidelines.

www.stroke.org.uk

The Stroke Association website gives information for patients and professionals about the different stages of stroke. There are links to research articles as well as information and advice that you can pass on to your patients.

www.glasgowcomascale.org/

This website explains the rationale for the Glasgow Coma Scale. It explains how to conduct an assessment and how to chart responses. There are video links to narrated demonstrations.

Chapter 12 The patient with an endocrine disorder

David Blesovsky and Desiree Tait

Chapter aims

By the end of this chapter, you should be able to:

- demonstrate an understanding of the causes of endocrine problems with reference to diabetes, adrenal, and thyroid disorders;
- identify the three main reasons for emergency admission of the person with diabetes mellitus;
- describe the role of the nurse in caring for people diagnosed with an endocrine emergency;

- demonstrate how to assess, record, and respond to people experiencing endocrine emergencies in a timely manner;
- reflect on the case studies in the chapter to enhance your own clinical skills.

Introduction

This chapter aims to give you an understanding of the most common acute emergencies encountered by people living with endocrine disorders. These will include those associated with diabetes mellitus: hypoglycaemia, diabetic ketoacidosis (DKA), and hyperosmolar hyperglycaemic syndrome (HHS). Rarer endocrine emergencies include those associated with the adrenal gland, thyroid gland, and pituitary gland. These are summarised in Table 12.1 and some are discussed in more detail later in the chapter.

In a study of emergency admissions in England (Steventon et al., 2018), it has been identified that there has been an increase in the age of the admission population and an increase in the complexity of their health conditions, including co-morbidities related to endocrine disorders. The most common of these are related to diabetes mellitus, with the other endocrine conditions accounting for only around 100 emergency admissions a year.

This chapter will begin by tabulating a brief overview of common endocrine emergencies and proceed to examine in detail those related to diabetes mellitus and provide an overview of the priorities of care for people experiencing adrenal and thyroid disorders. When a person presents with an endocrine emergency the nurse needs to be able to rapidly assess them so that early identification and treatment can occur. Table 12.1 provides a summary of the main endocrine problems by identifying the hormone and the disease caused by either under- or over-production of the specific hormone.

Endocrine emergencies associated with diabetes mellitus

Endocrine emergencies associated with diabetes mellitus may be associated with several biopsychosocial factors that influence behaviour and wellbeing. The three emergency problems associated with diabetes mellitus are:

- **hypoglycaemia** where blood glucose levels fall below the normal range of 4 mmol/L and is generally associated with people who take insulin and/or a group of drugs known as sulphonylureas (BNF, 2021);
- **hyperglycaemia** in the form of diabetic ketoacidosis (DKA) and associated with insulin dependent diabetics where the glucose level is above 11 mmol/L, plasma ketones of more than 3 mmol/L and acidosis with a pH of less than 7.3 (JBDS, 2021);
- **hyperglycaemia** in the form of HHS characterised by a plasma glucose of above 30 mmol/L, plasma ketones of less than 3 mmol/L, pH of more than 7.3 and serum osmolarity of more than 20 omol/kg (JBDS, 2012).

Endocrine problem	Hormone(s) involved	Specific disease	Population affected	Treatment
Diabetes mellitus	Insulin	Type 1 diabetes: absolute insulin deficiency. Onset: acute.	Usually, children and young people at onset and diagnosis. 10% of the total population of people with diabetes in the UK have type 1 (Diabetes UK, 2020a).	Insulin therapy by injection (NICE, 2015a [updated 2021]).
		Type 2 diabetes: insulin resistance and with varying degrees of insulin deficiency. Onset: insidious.	Until a few years ago, this was a disease of adults aged 40+. However, increasing obesity levels and sedentary lifestyles worldwide have resulted in younger people – even some children – being diagnosed. 90% of people with diabetes in the UK have type 2 and of those 20–30% use insulin to control their diabetes (Diabetes UK, 2020a).	Treatment is progressive starting with: 1. diet and exercise 2. diet, exercise, and medications 3. diet, exercise, medications, and insulin (NICE, 2015b [updated 2021]).
		Gestational diabetes: glucose intolerance occurring during pregnancy. Onset: during antenatal period.	Women during pregnancy.	Combination of diet control, oral therapy, and sometimes insulin (NICE, 2015c [updated 2020]).
Adrenal disorders	Aldosterone and cortisol produced in the cortex of the adrenal glands	Addison's disease occurs because of destruction of the adrenal cortex. Addisonian crisis occurs when a person with Addison's disease experiences severe physiological stress where the adrenal gland is unable to provide the extra cortisol needed.	Can affect people of any age from childhood to adult, although most seen between ages 30–50 years and more common in women.	Addisonian crisis can result in severe dehydration, hypotension, shock, altered consciousness, seizures, hypoglycaemia, cardiac arrest. Monitor ABCDE and GCS closely, rapid fluid replacement (5% dextrose in normal saline), monitor blood glucose and rapidly treat hypoglycaemia, cortisol administration (IV hydrocortisone), identify and treat cause of crisis (infection, surgery, trauma) (NICE, 2020b).

Endocrine problem	Hormone(s) involved	Specific disease	Population affected	Treatment
	Adrenaline and noradrenaline produced in the medulla of the adrenal gland	Pheochromocytoma (very rare tumour of adrenal gland).	Can occur at any age but, as above, peak incidence is between 30 and 50 years.	Rapid blood pressure stabilisation and then prepare for surgery for tumour removal (Lenders et al, 2014).
Thyroid disorders	Thyroid hormones T_3 and T_4 produced and released from the thyroid gland	Hyperthyroidism (overactive thyroid and production of thyroid hormones). Thyrotoxic crisis/thyroid storm can occur when hyperthyroidism is complicated by stressors such as trauma or infection.	Can occur at any age, more common in women: 8% compared to 1% of men developing the disease.	Reduction of the effects of raised hormone levels until stable. Close monitoring of ABCDE (see Chapter 1). Treat with drug therapy that includes beta-blockers, sedatives, hydrocortisone, and specific anti-thyroid drugs such as carbimazole (NICE, 2019c).
		Myxoedema (including Hashimoto's disease) underactive thyroid. Myxoedema coma (decompensated hypothyroidism often associated with infection).	Can be a rare congenital problem, far more common in women than men and in people over the age of 60. Hashimoto's disease is an autoimmune disease with strong familial links and commonly seen in women after having their first baby.	ABCDE assessment and management of respiratory depression, bradycardia and reduced cardiac output, paralytic ileus, reduced urine output, loss of consciousness, hypothermia. Management of coma is around organ support and addressing the cause and administration of thyroxine (Gish et al, 2016).
Pituitary disorders	Antidiuretic hormone	Diabetes insipidus (DI) characterised by an absolute or relative inability to concentrate urine, presenting as thirst (polydipsia), polyuria, and hypotonic urine (copious amounts of dilute urine).	An acquired disorder: 30% **idiopathic**, 25% brain or pituitary tumour, 20% cranial surgery, and 16% head trauma. Can be a rare congenital problem. Some people can have kidneys that are insensitive to ADH (nephrogenic DI) although this is very rare.	Rapid administration of desmopressin (DDAVP) and close monitoring of ABCDE (BNF, 2021).
		Syndrome of inappropriate antidiuretic hormone hypersecretion (SIADH). The body makes too much antidiuretic hormone leading to fluid retention.	Can affect any age group, but more common in the elderly and hospitalised patients. Some evidence that menstruating women are more at risk.	Initial close monitoring of ABCDE with concurrent fluid restriction and monitoring.

Table 12.1 Disorders of the endocrine system: a summary based on NICE guidelines

In the following sections we explore each of these in more detail and look at how they can be associated with biopsychosocial factors and clinical diagnosis. Table 12.2 provides a summary of the key differences between the main types of diabetes with data on diabetes prevalence provided by Diabetes UK (2020b).

Type 1 diabetes mellitus	Type 2 diabetes mellitus	Gestational diabetes mellitus
• Less common at around 8–10%. • Sudden onset at any age, but more common in the young (<40 years). • Usually underweight at diagnosis. • Caused by cessation of insulin production from the beta cells of the pancreatic islets. Thought to be an immune response frequently following an infection. • Manifested as absolute insulin deficiency. • Treatment is insulin injections for life.	• Most common form of diabetes mellitus seen, accounting for 90% of all cases. • Gradual onset over weeks or months. More common in the elderly, or overweight and sedate adults. • Combination of insulin resistance at cellular level and reduction in insulin production at the beta cells of the pancreatic islets. • Treatment is lifestyle change, diet, oral agents, and in later life insulin therapy.	• Diabetes that occurs during pregnancy and with an incidence of 2–5%. • Closely resembles type 2 diabetes mellitus. • Frequently self corrects following childbirth. • Mothers have an increased risk of developing type 2 diabetes mellitus in later life (50%).

Table 12.2   Differences between types of diabetes mellitus, informed by JBDS (2021) and Diabetes UK (2020b)

Hypoglycaemia

For the person with diabetes mellitus, hypoglycaemia is the most frightening side effect of having the disease and can be associated with suboptimal diabetes management (Liu et al., 2020). Hypoglycaemia can be characterised by a blood glucose of less than 4 mmol/L and occurs more frequently in people who manage their diabetes with insulin injections. The person will show signs of autonomic (neurogenic) effects caused by elevated levels of adrenaline in the system and neuroglycopenic symptoms (see Table 12.3), which occur because of glucose-deprived brain cells. The symptoms in Table 12.3 are not definitive as symptoms vary from patient to patient.

Assessment	Observation	Hypoglycaemia
Airway	• Airway patent.	• Most commonly normal.
Breathing	• Respiratory rate and pattern. • O_2 saturations.	• Normal respiratory rate and pattern.

Assessment	Observation	Hypoglycaemia

Circulation	• Blood pressure.
	• Pulse.
	• Capillary refill time (CRT).
	• Skin.
	• Central venous pressure (CVP).
	• Urine output.
		• Autonomic effects:
		  o sweating
		  o palpitations
		  o dry mouth.
		• CRT normal.
		• Skin clammy.

Disability	• AVPU/GCS.
	• Pain assessment.
	• Blood glucose.
		• Anxiety (autonomic).
		• Neuroglycopenic symptoms:
		  o irritability
		  o difficulty thinking and speaking
		  o tiredness
		  o poor coordination
		  o visual problems
		  o shakiness
		  o drowsiness
		  o confusion
		  o seizures
		  o coma
		  o GCS <15.

Exposure	• Other. • Temperature.	• Nausea (autonomic). • Paraesthesia (neuroglycopenic). • Normal temperature.

Table 12.3 ABCDE assessment of hypoglycaemia

As can be seen from Table 12.3 the symptoms of hypoglycaemia are many and varied and patients need to learn the signs so that they can recognise the symptoms and treat themselves before collapse occurs. There are three levels of hypoglycaemia:

- Mild: recognised symptoms, these tend to be autonomic in nature, and self-treated (blood glucose of 3–4 mmol/L); no assistance required. Treated with dextrose tablets or refined carbohydrates, the patient will know what works for them, followed by long-acting carbohydrate (unless they are on an insulin pump). Repeat blood glucose 10–15 minutes later (BNF, 2021).
- Moderate: recognition of symptoms, but symptoms are neuroglycopenic in nature (blood glucose of 2.5–3.5 mmol/L). The patient could be confused and irritable and have difficulty concentrating; they may need help. Give dextrose tablets if the patient can swallow or 30% glucose gel (hypo stop) applied to the buccal mucosa. Repeat blood glucose 10–15 minutes later and if no increase then give more dextrose and contact doctor (this intervention can be applied three times in order to achieve a response (BNF, 2021).

- Severe: hypoglycaemia which does not respond to interventions after 30–45 minutes of treatment or the person is drowsy or unconscious. Assistance is required urgently (blood glucose <2.5 mmol/L). Medical interventions will include an intramuscular injection with glucagon (1 mg) or glucose 10% by IV infusion (BNF, 2021). A blood glucose of less than 1.5 mmol/L is a medical emergency and if action is not taken rapidly, then there is serious risk of brain damage occurring. The person will need rapid and continuous assessment using ABCDE until medical help arrives.

Hypoglycaemia is caused by either too much insulin being administered, too much exercise or not enough food eaten, or a combination of these. The patient needs to learn how their body reacts to exercise and work out how to reduce insulin and/or increase carbohydrate intake. Unfortunately, iatrogenic hypoglycaemia is not uncommon; the National Diabetes Inpatient Audit (Health and Social Care Information Centre, 2014) identified that 25% of patients with diabetes made medication errors. This suggests that there is a need for nurses to be able to recognise hypoglycaemia in their patients.

Activity 12.1 Evidence-based practice and research

Go to the InDependent Diabetes Trust website (**www.iddt.org**) and investigate the incidence of medication errors related to diabetes. What do you think can be done to reduce this major problem?

An outline answer to this activity is given at the end of the chapter.

Hyperglycaemia

Hyperglycaemia is classified as blood glucose above the normal level (4–7 mmol/L), but it is not uncommon for patients with diabetes mellitus to run their blood glucose levels between 5–10 mmol/L, particularly those with type 1 diabetes who have suffered frequent hypoglycaemic attacks (Lui et al., 2020). The biopsychosocial triggers for hyperglycaemia can include:

- being newly diagnosed with diabetes;
- physiological stress including infection, physical trauma, the presence of acute co-morbid conditions (Brashers et al., 2019);
- fear of hypoglycaemia (Lui et al., 2020);
- psychological distress including anxiety and/or depression (Stahl-Pehe et al., 2019);
- difficulty with coping and poor adherence to insulin treatment.

Acute hyperglycaemia has two presentations: diabetic ketoacidosis (DKA) and HHS. Both DKA and HHS are initiated post infection but can occur through non-compliance with treatment and following other major medical events such as MI (see Table 12.4). DKA and HHS are two acute complications of diabetes that can result in increased ill health and death if not competently and effectually treated. Mortality rates for DKA and HHS have been declining in the last 20 years due to improvements in the assessment and standardisation of management, with DKA estimated at 1% and up to 20% for HHS, where mortality rates for HHS are associated with co-morbid conditions and old age (Gosmanov et al., 2021). Table 12.4 summarises the presenting features and signs and symptoms.

Condition	Biochemical conditions	ABCDE: Signs and symptoms	Demographics
Diabetic ketoacidosis (DKA)	**D:** • Blood glucose >11.1 mmol/L. • **Or** known to have type 1 diabetes. **K:** • Ketonaemia ≥3.0 mmol/L **A:** pH <7.3 Bicarbonate bicarbonate <15 mmol/L.	• Rapid onset. **Airway and breathing** • Rapid panting breaths (Kussmaul respirations) • Fruity or acetone odour on the breath **Circulation** • Tachycardia • Hypotension • Dry mouth • Nausea/vomiting • **Polyuria** • **Polydipsia** • Negative fluid balance related to dehydration. **Disability and Exposure** • Headache • CNS depression/ confusion/ drowsiness • Possible signs of infection, trauma, recent illness	• Most commonly younger, slimmer patients with type 1 diabetes. • Mortality 1% but still the most common cause of death in young people with diabetes.
Hyperosmolar hyperglycaemic syndrome (HHS)	Plasma glucose >30 mmol/L (frequently much higher). pH normal 7.35–7.45. Serum bicarbonate >15 mmol/L. Serum osmolality >320 micro-osmole/kg	• Insidious onset (several days or weeks). **Airway and Breathing** • Central nervous system depression may be associated with an increased risk to airway. **Circulation** • Tachycardia	• Most commonly older, obese patients with type 2 diabetes. • Mortality rate: 20%. • Recent history of physiological stress.

(Continued)

Table 12.4 (Continued)

Condition	Biochemical conditions	ABCDE: Signs and symptoms	Demographics
		• Hypotension • Dry mouth • Nausea/vomiting • **Polyuria** • **Polydipsia** • Negative fluid balance related to dehydration. **Disability and Exposure** • Headache • CNS depression/ confusion/ drowsiness/coma • Evidence of infection.	

Table 12.4 Presenting features and signs and symptoms of DKA and HHS, using an ABCDE approach and based on diagnostic criteria by JBDS (2012, 2021)

Diabetic ketoacidosis

DKA is a life-threatening complication of type 1 diabetes, although it is seen in type 2 diabetes during acute illnesses. Presenting features and signs and symptoms can be found in Table 12.4. The underlying cause for most patients is an infection and because of this it is more commonly seen during the winter months. Also, it is commonly seen as the presenting problem of patients newly diagnosed with type 1 diabetes. Other factors are poor compliance with treatment and psychological stress; a combination of these factors have been identified in young women with type 1 diabetes, who think that it will help them lose weight quickly, which rapidly leads to DKA (Martinez et al., 2016; Umpierrez et al., 2002).

DKA is caused by an absolute deficiency of circulating insulin with the subsequent increase in glucagon, catecholamines, cortisol, and growth hormone, all of which raise the glucose levels in the blood through **glycogenolysis** (splitting up of glycogen) in the liver. The body starts to digest its own fat stores and muscle mass through the digestion of amino acids and glycerol, the waste products of which are ketones (Nyenwe and Kitabchi, 2016). Ketones are acids and so acidaemia occurs.

Once DKA is identified, the diabetes specialist team must be involved with the management of every patient admitted (JBDS, 2021). All care needs to be in line with local and national clinical guidelines and nurses need to be aware of these to provide the high standards of safe care required (JBDS, 2021).

Case study: Tim Brown (age 19 years) lives with type 1 diabetes; he has been found by his mother in a drowsy state with an elevated blood glucose

Situation

Tim was brought in by ambulance to ED at 19.00 hours after his mum found him in his bedroom very drowsy, slightly confused, and vomiting. She did his blood sugar and found that it was high. On assessment in ED, he was diagnosed with DKA. (D) plasma glucose: 18.4 mmol/L; (K) ketones: 6.4 mmol/L; (A) pH: 6.9; and HCO_3: 8.0 mmol/L.

Background

Tim was diagnosed with type 1 diabetes at the age of 14. He takes insulin twice a day and self-monitors his glucose/insulin requirement. He has an active social life and since starting his studies at university has been going out partying, not taking his usual insulin or monitoring his blood glucose levels, feeling like he just wants to be like everyone else. He lives at home with his mum.

Assessment on admission:

Airway:

- Tim can maintain his own airway and is able to cough but continues to feel nauseated. He is drowsy but responding to voice.

Breathing:

- R: 28/minute; SpO_2: 90%; receiving oxygen to maintain his saturations 94–96%. He has rapid, panting respirations (Kussmaul respirations) and his breath smells of ketones. Arterial blood gases:
  - pH: 6.9
  - PaO2: 8.2 kPa
  - PaCO2: 2.8 kPa
  - HCO3: 8.0 mmol/L
  - Lactate: 3.1 mmol/L

Circulation:

- P: 108/minute and regular; ECG confirms tachycardia; BP: 100/40; temperature: 37.0 °C.
- Biochemistry results:
  - WCC: 12.5×10^9/L
  - Na: 136 mmol/L
  - K: 4.8 mmol/L
  - Urea: 8.2 mmol/L
  - Creatinine: 135 micromole/L

(Continued)

(Continued)
- o   Blood glucose: 18.4 mmol/L
- o   Blood ketones: 6.4 mmol/L
- Insulin infusion: 50 units (IU) of actrapid made up to 50 ml with 0.9% sodium chloride. Administered 0.1 units/kg/hr has been commenced at 7 ml/hr (weight 70 kg)
- Infusion of 1 L 0.9% sodium chloride to run over 1 hour
- Urine: passed on admission 680 ml
- Urinalysis: ketones high
- Urinary catheterisation was refused

Disability:
- Tim is drowsy and listless but responds to commands
- Blood glucose: 18.4 mmol/L
- GCS: 13
- He is not complaining of pain

Exposure:
- Skin and mucus membranes dry and intact
- There is no sign of a rash or injuries

Tim is critically ill and requires a multidisciplinary approach to his assessment, management, and recovery. In DKA the risk of mortality is associated with electrolyte imbalance, severe metabolic acidosis, and cerebral oedema. The nurse's role is based around ongoing clinical assessment and observation of vital signs using the ABCDE rapid assessment process. The JBDS (2021) recommend management should be aimed at:

1. immediate management in the first hour;

2. management from 60 minutes to 6 hours;

3. management from 6 to 12 hours;

4. management beyond 12 hours.

Table 12.5 summarises the priorities of management during stages 1 to 4.

Stage 1: Immediate management of DKA in the first hour (JBDS, 2021)	Rationale
Confirm diagnosis of DKA • Plasma glucose >11.1 mmol/L or known type 1 diabetic • Ketonemia ≥3.0 mmol/L • Metabolic acidosis (pH of <7.3; bicarbonate of <15 mmol/L)	It is essential to confirm the diagnosis of DKA before initiating treatment as the management of hyperglycaemia associated with HHS has a different management approach and any delay in interventions could make the patient's situation critical.

Stage 1: Immediate management of DKA in the first hour (JBDS, 2021)	Rationale
Continuous ABCDE assessment is required. *Assess electrolyte balance, renal function, venous blood gases/or arterial blood gases depending on the acuity of the patient, screen for sepsis, CXR, MSU, and other precipitating factors.* *Assess circulation: is patient in shock?* • If systolic (S) BP <90 mm Hg: fluid challenge of 500 ml NaCl in 15 min followed by a second bolus if SBP is <100 mmHg. • If no shock present infuse 1000 ml NaCl over 1 hour. *Assess severity:* • If severe DKA: (Ketones >6, pH <7.1, HCO$_3$ <15, K$^+$ <3.5, GCS <12, SpO$_2$ <92%, SBP 90, HR >100/<60/min) CALL ITU team. *Administer a fixed rate of insulin:* • Commence a fixed rate of insulin via infusion at 0.1 unit/kg/hr (maximum 15 ml/hr starting dose). *Assess and monitor potassium replacement and initiate cardiac monitoring.* • > 5.5 mmol/L: no K replacement • 3.5–5.5 mmol/L: 40 mmol potassium replacement by infusion • <3.5 mmol/L: seek ITU advice *Reassess patient for signs of respiratory failure, AKI, persistent vomiting, persistent acidosis, declining GCS.*	A person with DKA is at risk of hypovolaemic shock (Chapter 6) related to the osmotic diuresis that accompanies hyperglycaemia, nausea and vomiting, and reduced oral intake of fluids as a consequence. Strict assessment of fluid balance is required to manage this. If the patient's condition becomes critical a higher level of care is required (Chapter 1). The primary aim of managing DKA is to correct the metabolic abnormalities that occur. The use of a fixed rate insulin infusion will: suppress ketogenesis; reduce blood glucose; correct electrolyte disturbance. Should the blood glucose fall below 14 mmol/L a 10% glucose infusion can be commenced to facilitate the continued steady resolution of metabolic imbalance or consider reducing insulin to 0.05 units/kg/hr. Hypokalaemia and hyperkalaemia are potentially life-threatening conditions associated with DKA. A risk of pre-renal AKI is associated with hypovolaemic shock, and hyperkalaemia especially in a severely acidotic patient where potassium ions have shifted from the intracellular to extracellular space to accommodate hydrogen ions (acidic) moving from extracellular to intracellular for buffering by intracellular proteins. As the acidosis is gradually corrected the acidic hydrogen ions can return to the extracellular space (blood) and potassium ions will return to the intracellular space. Thus, a drop in plasma potassium will be observed. Hyper- and hypokalaemia are associated with cardiovascular arrhythmias and cardiac arrest (Kjeldsen, 2010).
Stage 2: Management from 60 minutes to 6 hours (JBDS, 2021)	**Rationale**
Airway/Breathing and Circulation: • Monitor capillary blood glucose (CBG) and plasma ketones hourly using a bedside monitor. • Consider reducing the insulin to 0.05 units/kg/hr if glucose falls below 14 mmol/L or commencing 10% glucose. • Monitor venous blood gases at 2 hrs, 4 hrs, 6 hrs, 12 hrs, and 18 hrs. • Monitor urea and electrolytes at 6 hrs, 12 hrs, and 24 hrs. • Hourly monitoring of ABCDE and NEWS2.	Continue ABCDE monitoring to assess and interpret the patient's condition and work collaboratively with the multidisciplinary team to manage any signs of deterioration in the patient's condition. Fluid resuscitation and monitoring of electrolytes to maintain homeostasis. Monitor the progression toward treatment targets to ensure the patient's progress toward recovery.

(Continued)

Table 12.5 (Continued)

Stage 2: Management from 60 minutes to 6 hours (JBDS, 2021)	Rationale
Fluid resuscitation and potassium replacement according to blood levels of potassium as above. (KCl: potassium chloride) • 1 L 0.9% NaCl over 2 hrs (+/– KCl) • 1 L 0.9% NaCl over 2 hrs (+/– KCl) • 1 L 0.9% NaCl over 4 hrs (+/– KCl) • When CBG is <14.0 mmol/L add 125 ml/hr of 10% glucose together with the saline *Review fluid balance and circulation and manage fluid resuscitation according to co-morbidity and severity of the patient's condition.* *Review achievement of treatment targets:* • Fall in CBG of >3 mmol/L until <14 mmol/L • Fall in capillary blood ketones of >0.5 mmol/L/hr • Rise in venous H_2CO_3 of 3.0 mmol/L	
Stage 3: Management from 6 to 12 hours (JBDS, 2021)	**Rationale**
Continue ABCDE assessment including monitoring of blood results according to Stage 2. *Continue with fluid resuscitation and potassium management.* • 1 L 0.9% NaCl over 4 hrs (+/– KCl) • 1 L 0.9% NaCl over 6 hrs (+/– KCl) • If CBG <14.0 mmol/L add 10% glucose at 125 ml/hr via a different infusion.	Continue ABCDE monitoring to assess and interpret the patient's condition and work collaboratively with the multidisciplinary team to manage any signs of deterioration in the patient's condition. Fluid resuscitation and monitoring of electrolytes to maintain homeostasis. Monitor the progression toward treatment targets to ensure the patient's progress toward recovery.
Stage 4: Management beyond 12 hours (JBDS, 2021)	**Rationale**
Resolution of DKA is defined as: • pH >7.3 • Blood ketones <0.3 mmol/L *Always assess ABCDE and monitor the underlying cause of the DKA.* *Refer to the specialist diabetic team.*	Monitor the progression toward treatment targets to ensure the patient's progress toward recovery. The patient's underlying biopsychosocial triggers for DKA should be assessed and managed, supported by the diabetic specialist team.

Table 12.5 Priorities of multidisciplinary management of DKA, informed by JBDS (2021).

Two hours after Tim's diagnosis and commencement of the recommended management as in Table 12.5, a review of his condition identified a steady improvement. Tim's oxygen saturation had improved to 94% and his respirations had fallen to 24 breaths per minute. His BP and heart rate had stabilised following the regime of fluid resuscitation and his plasma pH had increased from 6.9 to 7.1. Tim's ketone levels had fallen by 0.9 mmol/l over the first two hours, indicating safe and steady resolution of ketones toward the desired target of <3 mmol/L. A review of his plasma glucose indicated a fall from 18.4 to 12.2 mmol/L and, in line with JBDS (2021) guidance, an infusion of 10% glucose was commenced in addition to his IV fluid regime and the medical team considered reducing the insulin infusion to 0.05 units/kg/hr, to be reviewed in one hour. Tim also required the addition of 40 mmol KCl to the 0.9% saline infusion prescribed for fluid resuscitation as his plasma potassium levels fell from 4.8 to 3.4 mmol/L (Table 12.5).

Tim's condition continued to improve and, in collaboration with the diabetic nurse specialists, his management and support networks were reviewed to assist him with adapting to university life. Young adults with type 1 diabetes can become overwhelmed by trying to balance the process of living and adapting to becoming an adult with the management of their diabetes; this is referred to as diabetes distress (Stahl-Pehe et al., 2019). In Tim's case his concerns about being part of his group of new friends and management of his diabetes had led to diabetes-related distress, and a loss of optimal management of his diet, insulin regime, and blood sugar levels. Hyperglycaemia increases the risk of serious infection, and findings by Carey et al. (2018) support a requirement for further research in this area, particularly in relation to hyperglycaemia in people living with type 1 diabetes.

Hyperosmolar hyperglycaemic state

HHS is classed as a medical emergency and is different to DKA, as is the required treatment. HHS differs from DKA in the following ways:

- the degree of insulin deficiency (DKA – absolute insulin deficiency, HHS – insulin resistance and reduced insulin availability);
- the degree of elevation of glucose levels, which is higher in HHS;
- the degree of fluid deficiency, which is more severe in HHS (Brashers et al., 2019).

HHS is far more common in the older adult, but as younger people and teenagers develop type 2 diabetes they can also present with HHS (JBDS, 2012). Underlying infections are the most common precipitating cause for the development of HHS. It has a higher mortality rate than DKA and patients are more likely to present with co-morbidities such as cardiovascular and circulatory disease (Gosmanov et al., 2021). Seizures and cerebral oedema are uncommon but recognised complications of HHS, and can take many days to develop, resulting in more severe dehydration and metabolic disturbances. Table 12.4 shows the presenting features and signs and symptoms of HHS and as soon as they are identified, the diabetes specialist team should be informed and involved in the management of the patient. The key role of the nurse is the rapid assessment of the patient using the ABCDE approach (see Table 12.4) and recording observations according to the degree of deterioration (RCP, 2017) from admission and during treatment to stabilise symptoms.

In HHS, relative insulin deficiency leads to reduced uptake of glucose in cells over time and cellular starvation. The presence of some insulin means that lipolysis (the metabolism of fats to release glucose) is prevented and thus normal or minimally elevated plasma ketones are found together with no corresponding metabolic acidosis. According to Brashers et al. (2019), cellular starvation in the presence of infection and/or other co-morbidities triggers the release of the stress hormones glucagon, catecholamines, cortisol, and growth hormone, together with increased **gluconeogenesis** and proteolysis. Correspondingly pro-inflammatory mediators promote further insulin resistance, and the net effect is hyperglycaemia of >30 mmol/L and hyper-osmolarity of >320 mosmol/kg, polyurea due to osmotic diuresis, and dehydration.

The characteristic features of a person with HHS (JBDS, 2012) include:

- hypovolaemia;
- hyperglycaemia (>30 mmol/L) WITHOUT hyperketonaemia (i.e., <3.0 mmol/L) or acidosis (i.e., pH >7.3 or bicarbonate >15 mmol/L);
- osmolarity >320 mosmol/kg.

The multidisciplinary treatment goals for HHS are to treat the underlying cause and gradually (JBDS, 2012):

- normalise the osmolality;
- replace fluid and electrolyte losses;
- normalise blood glucose.

Other goals include the prevention of complications related to clinical deterioration, including:

- arterial or venous thromboses;
- other potential complications, e.g. cerebral oedema;
- foot ulceration.

The multidisciplinary management of HSS is illustrated in Table 12.6 and can be applied to Sangit's story.

Multidisciplinary management of HHS, after JBDS (2012, 2021)	Rationale
Ensure the diagnostic criteria have been met following a full ABCDE assessment and diagnosis of underlying pathophysiology, and initial safety needs have been met. • Marked hyperglycaemia of >30 mmol/L **without** significant ketonaemia (<3.0 mmol/L) and **without** acidosis (pH >7.3) • Venous osmolarity >320 mosmol/kg • No evidence of acidosis or ketonaemia confirmed.	It is important to identify: • Underlying pathophysiology and initiate treatment to break the chain of stress and inflammatory responses. • Whether the hyperglycaemia is caused by HHS or DKA as this will direct the correct treatment protocol.

Multidisciplinary management of HHS, after JBDS (2012, 2021)	Rationale
Commence fluid resuscitation in accordance with co-morbidity assessment: • 1 L 0.9% NaCl over 1 hr • 1 L 0.9% NaCl over 2 hrs (check potassium level) • 1 L 0.9% NaCl over 2 hrs (check potassium level) • 1 L 0.9% NaCl over 4 hrs (check potassium level) • 1 L 0.9% NaCl over 4 hrs (check potassium level) • NB: When capillary blood glucose <14 mmol/L, commence 10% dextrose at 125 ml/hr alongside the saline infusion.	• If a person is presenting with myocardial infarction and/or is a risk of heart failure, fluid resuscitation will need to be assessed under specialist medical direction to reduce the risk of further heart failure and deterioration. • In HHS, although the onset of the condition is slower and more insidious, the measure of hyperglycaemia is higher with an associated risk of hyperosmolarity and a risk of cerebral oedema. • The effect of increased serum osmolarity on the brain cells can be severe, as the intracellular fluid leaves the cells toward the extracellular fluid. To preserve the intracellular volume the brain produces its own osmotic solutes to maintain a safe balance. However, if the blood glucose level of a patient with HHS is reduced too quickly this can have a rebound effect on the brain leading to a higher osmolarity in the brain and brain swelling (Adeyinka and Kondamudi, 2021). A slow and controlled reduction in blood glucose is therefore required.
Only commence IV insulin therapy is the patient has ketonaemia >1.0 mmol/L.	• Insulin therapy should not be required except in the presence of elevated ketones and ketoacidosis. This facilitates a controlled reduction in blood glucose and reduces the risk of cerebral oedema.

Table 12.6 Priorities of multidisciplinary management of HHS informed by JBDS (2012, 2021).

Case study: Sangit – HHS

Harry is a third-year student nurse on placement in A&E. One Saturday morning, a young man, Ashya Gupta, comes in with his father, Sangit. The older man seems to have trouble staying awake and does not appear to know where he is or why.

Carole, the triage nurse, asks Ashya how long his father has been unwell. Ashya replies that he has been running a temperature for a couple of days. He phoned his GP, who advised him to take a few days rest and drink plenty of fluids as the problem was likely to resolve itself. Sangit did as advised but this morning he was incoherent and drowsy. The family did not want to phone an out-of-hours GP, but they were sure that Sangit needed urgent medical attention.

(Continued)

(Continued)

Harry is surprised when Carole asks Ashya what Sangit has been drinking. Sangit said his father has a lot of tea (black, with two sugars) as well as plenty of orange juice. It also transpires that Sangit has been needing to pass urine often. However, when asked if his father suffers from diabetes, Sangit replies that he does not.

To Harry's surprise, Carole tests Sangit's blood sugar level and finds it to be 42 mmol/L. She explains to Ashya that his father is suffering from severe dehydration and a high level of glucose in the blood, which will need to be treated with intravenous fluids in hospital.

Later, when Carole and Harry are eventually able to take a break, Carole explains that Sangit is very likely to have HHS and that he has underlying type 2 diabetes, which will need ongoing treatment once his acute condition has been managed.

Once on the ward, the priorities of care for Sangit are initially to manage the HHS as set out in Table 12.6. Once his condition and possible trigger factors have been stabilised, the next phase is to facilitate and support education and self-management in collaboration with the diabetic specialist team. Harry returned to the ward to visit Sangit a few days later. He seemed a different person; alert and aware of what was going on around him. He shared his worries with Harry about his ability to cope with his diagnosis of type 2 diabetes and the impact on his family.

Activity 12.2   Communication

Put yourself in Harry's shoes. Imagine you are a nurse on the medical ward with responsibility for Sangit's care. What advice can you give to Ashya and Sangit to help Sangit live safely with type 2 diabetes?

How would you:

a. reassure him about his treatment and medication?
b. advise him about any lifestyle changes that will help to ensure he stays as healthy as possible?

An outline answer to this activity is given at the end of the chapter.

Other acute endocrine problems

Addison's disease

Addison's disease is a chronic condition where there is a deficiency of the cortical hormones, cortisol, and aldosterone. The patient will be on hormone replacement therapy for life. Your role in caring for a patient with this condition is one of prevention through close monitoring and strict administration of steroid therapy. Omission of just one dose can cause steroid deprivation and push the patient into crisis. It is not uncommon for these patients to suffer more than one endocrine problem and if they have type 1 diabetes mellitus, then the combination of steroid therapy and insulin becomes time-specific: they must be administered at the exact time required. An acute or critical episode is described as an adrenal or Addisonian crisis and can be precipitated by a concurrent illness or failure to take replacement medication (Venkatesh and Cohen, 2019). Addisonian crisis can occur when demand for cortisol cannot be met; this is frequently triggered by a gastric infection and is the most important predictor of impending Addisonian crisis (White and Arlt, 2010). Eight per cent of patients with Addison's disease will fall into crisis and this is invariably through poor management. You need to use your rapid assessment skills to fully monitor the patient and any changes that may occur, making sure that you provide full holistic care and give medication at the correct times. It is advisable to listen to the patient as he or she will often be the expert on their disease. Table 12.7 summarises the symptoms related to deficiencies in the cortical hormones.

Symptoms related to a deficiency in cortisol	Symptoms related to a deficiency in aldosterone
• Muscle weakness • Fatigue • Hypoglycaemia • Ileus and vomiting • Reduced immunity • Low cardiac output	• Polydipsia • Polyuria • Dehydration • Hypovolaemia • **Hyponatraemia** • Hyperkalaemia • Postural hypotension • Arrhythmias

Table 12.7 Symptoms related to deficiencies in the cortical hormones (informed by Venkatesh and Cohen, 2019)

Case study: Linda – Addison's disease

Linda is a 42-year-old marketing executive who has Addison's disease. This means her body is unable to produce adequate levels of the hormones aldosterone and cortisol. She is admitted to hospital following a period of diarrhoea and vomiting accompanied by pain and fever.

On admission, Linda is found to have the following:

• BP: 95/60 mmHg

(Continued)

(Continued)

- Blood glucose level: 4.1 mmol/L
- Temperature: 38.6 °C

The immediate management of the patient is rapid ABCDE assessment, prompt rehydration, and correction of the hypoglycaemia. IV hydrocortisone should be administered and then a full history taken to identify the trigger for this crisis event. Antibiotic therapy will have to be considered if the underlying problem is an infection. You will need to assess, record, and report findings according to the NEWS2 score and escalation plan to prevent this problem worsening.

Thyroid storm

Thyroid storm (thyrotoxic crisis) is a rare acute, life-threatening, hypermetabolic state associated with an excessive release of thyroid hormones. It is, arguably, the most serious complication of hyperthyroidism, and mortality rates can range from 10% to 75% (Handy and Li, 2019). While the condition is associated with high levels of thyroid hormones, there is no definitive test to determine a trigger value and diagnosis of thyroid storm is measured by the severity of clinical signs and symptoms (Handy and Li, 2019). The clinical presentation on ABCDE assessment can include the following:

- Airway and Breathing: dyspnoea, hypoxia associated with increased oxygen demand from the hypermetabolic state. There may be evidence of pulmonary oedema associated with cardiac failure.
- Circulatory: tachycardia, atrial fibrillation, ventricular arrhythmias, hypertension during the early phase of the state but hypotension in the latter stages, heart failure. Gastrointestinal symptoms may include nausea and vomiting, and diarrhoea. Fever is the most common characteristic sign and may be >41 °C.
- Disability: tremor and hyperreflexia are common early signs of thyroid storm as well as anxiety and agitation. If left untreated the person can progress to thyroid encephalopathy and coma.
- Exposure: goitre.

In many cases precipitating factors may be present, but not always. Some factors identified include:

- infection, sepsis;
- severe illness including DKA, cardiovascular or circulatory disease, or physiological trauma;

Respiratory	Cardiovascular	Gastrointestinal	Renal	Metabolic	Neurological
• Hypoxia.	• Bradycardia.	• Anorexia.	• Fluid retention.	• Hypothermia.	• Confusion.
• Hypercarbia.	• Hypotension.	• Nausea.	• Hyponatraemia.	• Hypoglycaemia.	• **Obtundation**.
• Pneumonia.	• Low cardiac output.	• Abdominal pain.	• Oedema.		• Lethargy.
	• Cardiogenic shock.	• Constipation.			• Seizures.
		• Paralytic ileus.			• Coma.
	• Metabolic acidosis.				

Table 12.8 Signs and symptoms of myxoedema coma

- withdrawal of anti-thyroid treatment or overdose of thyroxine.

Management is aimed at reducing the effects of thyroid hormones, T_3 and T_4, until the patient is stable and comfortable. There are some drug therapies that are used and these include sedatives, beta blockers, hydrocortisone, and specific anti-thyroid drugs such as Lugol's iodine and carbimazole (Handy and Li, 2019). Through good assessment, observation, recording and reporting of findings, the priorities of nursing care for this group of patients include:

- reducing metabolic demands and supporting cardiovascular function;
- providing psychological support;
- preventing complications;
- providing information about disease process/prognosis and therapy needs.

Myxoedema coma

Myxoedema coma is a rare life-threatening form of hypothyroidism, commonly seen in untreated patients. It is a medical emergency and, even with early diagnosis and best possible treatment, has a high mortality rate of 60% (Vivek et al., 2011). Causes are usually associated with those who have hypothyroidism, who are then faced with additional trauma or stress. Most cases appear in winter and hypothermia may play a part, although infections are seen as a predisposing factor. The discontinuation of thyroid supplements needs to be closely managed and sudden discontinuation can be a factor. Symptoms are those of decreased thyroid hormone secretion and hypometabolic state and are listed in Table 12.8.

Management is aimed at organ support and identifying what has caused the problem, such as administering thyroxin (Handy and Li, 2019). Nursing care involves rapid assessment of the person's clinical signs and symptoms using the ABCDE approach (Chapter 1). Patients are usually transferred to ICU for advanced respiratory and cardiovascular support.

Chapter summary

This chapter has outlined the most common endocrine problems likely to be seen in clinical practice, and explored the skills needed for assessing, recognising, and responding to patients presenting with these problems. It has concentrated on the conditions most likely to present as emergencies, primarily complications of diabetes mellitus: hypoglycaemia, DKA, and HHS. The nurse's responsibilities are similar in all of these problems, but as the causes are different, health professionals need to be alert to the possible meaning of different clusters of symptoms. Nurses can come across patients with diabetes mellitus in any clinical specialty but, with effective ABCDE assessment and early recognition, prioritisation, and management, problems can be minimised. This chapter has also touched upon the assessment and management of rarer endocrine disorders that may be encountered, and discussed the priorities of assessment and management of people experiencing these situations to promote safety and recovery.

Activities: brief outline answers

Activity 12.1: Evidence-based practice and research (page 302)

This is predominantly a discussion issue, but from the work of the NDIA errors in insulin prescribing, medication, and administration keep occurring at an alarming level. The key to preventing this is continuous education at all clinical levels from nursing staff through to consultants. By mining into the data that the NDIA provide, it can be seen that a lot of the problem is in the prescription, where new doctors have written up the insulin in the incorrect way, but it is clear to see that administration errors still occur, and these can only be prevented with good education and awareness of the problem.

Activity 12.2: Communication (page 312)

Advice for Ashya and Sangit should include the following.

- Always take your diabetes medication, even if you feel unwell and can't eat.
- If you monitor your blood glucose, you may need to test more frequently when feeling unwell and contact your healthcare team if your blood glucose levels remain high (>15 mmol/L).
- Drink plenty of unsweetened fluids and, if you can't eat, replace meals with snacks and drinks containing carbohydrate.

If the above advice is followed, then control of Sangit's blood glucose will stabilise. He will have to balance his dietary habits, eating more complex carbohydrates, non-starchy vegetables, less fat, and protein and increase his exercise. Do be aware that people don't always remember information that is given to them by word of mouth, especially if they are unwell or upset at the time they are told it. So, make sure you have leaflets and other written materials to give the family to take away.

Further reading

Bilous, R and Donnelly, R (2021) *Handbook of Diabetes*. Fifth Edition. London: Wiley-Blackwell.

See especially Chapter 1 (Introduction to diabetes), Chapter 12 (Diabetic ketoacidosis, hyperglycaemic hyperosmolar state and lactic acidosis) and Chapter 13 (Hypoglycaemia).

White, K and Arlt, W (2010) Adrenal crisis in treated Addison's disease: a predictable but undermanaged event. *European Society of Endocrinology*, Jan 1, 162: 115–20.

Useful websites

www.diabetes.org.uk

Diabetes UK has a very informative website, with pages for professionals and pages for patients. There are also a lot of resources and information sheets to download or purchase. As well as exploring the site yourself, you should also make sure any patients with diabetes, and their family members, know about it.

www.Idf.org

International Diabetes Federation.

www.iddt.org

Independent Diabetes Trust.

Chapter 13 Conclusion

Lessons learned – an action plan for practice

Desiree Tait

The chapters in this book have provided an opportunity for you to explore the clinical assessment and rapid decision-making skills required to manage acute and critically ill patients. The case studies and scenarios used in the book are fictional, but the physiological and psychological data used are based on real situations. Reading the scenarios and working through the activities in each chapter have given you an opportunity to rehearse situations in a safe environment and reflect on their outcome. The key messages that have emerged from this book can be summarised as follows:

- Always use a comprehensive, systematic, and holistic approach to nursing assessment.
- Always interpret the findings from your assessment and determine a diagnosis of the current situation.
- Always respond to your findings in a timely manner, ensuring that you communicate your concerns and review the situation.
- Always provide support and protection for vulnerable people in your care.
- Always provide a person-centred approach to care and ensure that you acknowledge and communicate the wishes and concerns of the patient and families when delivering nursing care.
- Always demonstrate a collaborative approach to care.

Within the chapters we have discussed the care of acutely ill patients and those at risk of deterioration in acute and critical care settings in both community and hospital settings. It is important to recognise that the rapid decision-making skills we have explored to manage a deteriorating person safely can be used in all settings with the only limitation being the availability of resources. Skilled clinical decision making is a core demonstration of autonomous and professional practice that can be supported by clinical guidelines and professional knowledge and experience.

Developing an action plan for practice

In your role as a senior student and as a registered nurse, your priority will be to ensure that you meet the standards and competencies set by the NMC (2018a). After qualification, these standards will continue to be a basis from which to develop your practice as well as to teach others. According to Benner et al. (2011), rapid assessment and understanding of the patient's condition is based on the nurse's ability to interpret, recognise, and respond to patterns and trends in the patient's behaviour and physiological data. This ability comes from knowledge and experience developed over time, the presence of leadership and organisational skills, and the presence of clinical forethought (the ability to anticipate and act on potential problems). The development toward proficient and expert practice involves the refinement of clinical knowledge and evidence-based practice so that an intuitive and automatic understanding of practice is achieved. To continue to develop and expand your clinical decision-making skills, we have identified five action points that you can use on your journey.

1. *Never lose your willingness to learn.* Nursing and healthcare practice is a dynamic and innovative environment; use every opportunity to reflect on and develop your practice.

2. *Know your patients and always be receptive to their condition.* The patient, or client, is the person who lives with the experience of their condition. They know and sense when something has changed, and it is reasonable to assume that knowing and listening to your patient and their family will help you to interpret their condition quickly and effectively.

3. *Reflect on your nursing experiences and question the issues raised.* When reflecting on your practice, question and challenge your decision making. Can you justify the decisions you made with an evidence base? How strong is that evidence base? Do you need to explore this issue in more detail?

4. *Combine your knowledge from experience with evidence-based practice.* Clinical reasoning and decision making can be guided by an evidence base such as clinical pathways and care bundles, research, and theoretical frameworks. It is also important to remember that each patient is an individual, and the clinical value of all evidence-based interventions needs to be judged in the context of individualised patient care.

5. *Continue to work collaboratively with colleagues and demonstrate emotional intelligence when communicating with others.* To collaborate effectively with others, you need to be aware of your own emotions and their impact on others, know your strengths and limitations, and have a sense of self-worth. You need to have an empathic awareness of others, with political and social awareness, so that you can interpret and manage communication between individuals and groups.

These action points will guide you on the path to professional maturity when involved in direct care and when collaborating with others. Nursing is a dynamic and exciting profession with a continuing demand to question and learn from practice, and is a journey to be enjoyed. Good luck with your future careers.

Glossary

abrasive trauma   a process of wearing away a surface area of the skin/mucous membrane by friction resulting from trauma.

activated partial thromboplastin time (APPT)   a measure of the efficiency of activation and duration of clotting time.

acute pain   pain that is temporary, resulting from surgery, an injury, or an infection.

acute pancreatitis   a sudden and often severe inflammation and swelling of the pancreas. The pancreas is normally protected from the digestive enzymes that it produces; however, during an acute episode the pancreatic enzymes begin to digest the tissue of the pancreas. In severe cases this is described as acute necrotising pancreatitis. The most common cause is alcohol abuse.

adenosine triphosphate (ATP)   a chemical in cells that is able to release energy during a chemical reaction. It is the major source of energy for all the body's cellular functions.

advanced trauma life support   a safe reliable method for immediate management of the injured trauma patient.

aldosterone   a hormone that increases the reabsorption of sodium ions and water. This increases circulating blood volume and blood pressure.

aminophylline   a drug used to prevent and treat wheezing, breathlessness, and dyspnoea associated with asthma and COPD. It works by relaxing and dilating the bronchi in the respiratory system and making it easier for the patient to breathe. Side effects include an increase in heart rate and risk of cardiac arrhythmias, restlessness, and irritability.

angiotensin I   an inactive chemical that is triggered by the release of renin and activated by an enzyme to produce angiotensin II.

angiotensin II   once activated by the renin angiotensin system, angiotensin II exerts a vasoconstrictor effect, increases a sensation for thirst, and ultimately increases blood pressure.

angiotensin converting enzyme (ACE)   an enzyme secreted by the pulmonary endothelial cells to act as a catalyst in the conversion of angiotensin I to angiotensin II.

antidiuretic hormone (ADH)   a hormone that increases the concentration of urine (osmolarity) and reduces the excretion of water by the kidneys. It also has a powerful vasopressor effect, thus increasing peripheral resistance and blood pressure; also known as vasopressin.

benzodiazepines a group of drugs that have a number of sedative, muscle relaxant, and amnesic effects. They are prescribed to relieve anxiety, induce sleep, as an anticonvulsant in the management of seizures, to relieve muscle spasm, and to manage alcohol withdrawal.

beta agonist a group of drugs that include salbutamol and are effective in causing bronchodilation. They relieve bronchospasm, wheezing, and breathlessness. They are most frequently administered by the inhalation route and can have an effect in just a few minutes. Side effects include an increase in heart rate and risk of cardiac arrhythmias, restlessness, anxiety, and shaking/tremor in the limbs. The side effects usually last for only a few minutes.

bradykinin a protein found in the body that, when released, causes vasodilation during the inflammatory response and, when systemic, can lead to a reduction in blood pressure.

carbon monoxide poisoning occurs following enough inhalation of carbon monoxide gas (CO). CO is a colourless, odourless, and tasteless toxic gas found in appliances such as gas boilers and in exhaust fumes from older vehicles. CO poisoning is potentially fatal because of the ability of the CO to bind to haemoglobin. As a result, the blood is unable to carry enough oxygen to the tissues and organs.

cardiogenic shock occurs when there is an inadequate circulation of blood to the body's organs and tissues due to primary failure of the ventricles of the heart to function effectively.

central venous pressure the blood pressure in the vena cava, the blood vessel returning to the right atrium of the heart. Measuring the CVP allows you to measure the amount of blood returning to the heart and is an indication of fluid balance in the circulation. When the CVP is low, the patient may be suffering from hypovolaemia; when it is high, the patient may be fluid overloaded or suffering from right-sided cardiac pump failure leading to a backlog of blood in the venous circulation.

cerebrospinal fluid a bodily fluid that occupies the subarachnoid space and the ventricular system around and inside the brain and spinal cord.

chronic pain pain that lasts longer than three months. It is different from acute pain in that it is not easy to find the cause, and diagnosis can reveal no injury in the body at all, yet the patient can be experiencing very debilitating pain.

clotting time the time required for blood to form a clot.

Colles fracture a fracture of the distal radius in the forearm with dorsal (posterior) displacement of the wrist and hand. The fracture is sometimes referred to as a 'dinner fork' or 'bayonet' deformity due to the shape of the resultant forearm.

compensatory stage of shock the second stage of shock, which occurs when the body has triggered compensatory mechanisms to improve blood supply to organs and tissues in order to maintain homeostasis.

complement system a system made up of plasma proteins that react with one another to make pathogens, such as a bacterial infection, easier to break down and digest. Overall, the system induces a series of inflammatory responses that help to fight infection.

CRP a blood test to measure the levels of C-reactive protein in the blood. This gives information about the presence of infection.

distributive shock occurs when there is inadequate circulation of the blood to the body's organs and tissues due to the systemic dilation of blood vessels. This is found, for example, in anaphylactic shock and septic shock.

dobutamine a drug that stimulates the beta receptors of the sympathetic nervous system. It is used to improve cardiac output in patients with cardiogenic shock.

dopamine a neurotransmitter acting on receptors in the brain. It acts on the sympathetic nervous system to increase heart rate and blood pressure.

dysoxia see tissue dysoxia.

dyspnoea a term that is used to describe difficult or laboured breathing and is often associated with breathlessness.

empirical antibiotic therapy refers to the commencement of treatment before a firm diagnosis is reached. In the case of infection, patients are prescribed broad spectrum antibiotics until the microorganisms are cultured and diagnosed. The antibiotics may then be changed if the microorganisms are not sensitive to the prescribed medication.

escharotomy provides a release of tissue constriction that compromises the underlying structures, whether those are circulatory or respiratory structures. Untreated, the tissue constriction will lead to loss of limbs by compromising the circulation, or death by constricting chest movement and preventing lung expansion.

expressive dysphasia a language disorder that occurs when the part of the brain responsible for converting our thoughts to language is damaged, resulting in the person having difficulty with expressing their thoughts verbally.

FBC full blood count – a test to discover whether the different elements of a person's blood are in the correct proportions.

gate control theory a theory proposed by Ronald Melzack and Patrick Wall in 1965 to explain the multidimensional nature of pain. The theory explains that an individual's pain experience can be modulated by stimulating neural gates in the spinal cord to open or close. Thus, the pain experience can be moderated by, for example, rubbing it better or diversionary therapy.

glomerular filtration rate (GFR) the number of millilitres of blood the kidneys are able to filter in one minute. The lower the rate, the less effectively the kidneys are working.

glucogenolysis the splitting up of glycogen in the liver, yielding glucose.

gluconeogenesis the synthesis of glucose from non-carbohydrate sources, such as amino acids and glycerol. It occurs primarily in the liver and kidneys whenever the supply of carbohydrates is insufficient to meet the body's energy needs.

Guillain-Barré syndrome a neurological disorder that occurs when the body's immune system attacks part of the peripheral nervous system. This can lead to symptoms such as muscle weakness, paralysis, breathing difficulties, and an unstable heart rate and blood pressure. Most people who get the disease can make a complete recovery although initially the disorder is considered a medical emergency.

haemoserous fluid   blood-stained fluid that is leaking from the wound (haemoserous means 'stained with blood').

histamine   chemical released by the mast cells as part of the inflammatory response. Its action is to dilate blood vessels and increase capillary permeability to white blood cells in order to fight the pathogens in infected tissues.

hyperkalaemia   the medical term that describes a potassium level in the blood that's higher than normal. The blood potassium level is normally 3.6 to 5.2 millimoles per litre (mmol/L).

hyperlipidaemia   refers to raised blood levels of cholesterol. Raised levels of cholesterol, in combination with other risk factors, can increase the risk of stroke and/or heart disease.

hyponatraemia   the medical term for low sodium levels in the blood. The normal range is 135–45 mEq/L. Many medical illnesses, such as congestive heart failure, liver failure, renal failure, diabetes, or pneumonia, may be associated with hyponatraemia.

hypovolaemic shock   occurs when there is inadequate circulation of the blood to the body's organs and tissues due to loss of blood or body fluids.

idiopathic   relating to or denoting any disease or condition which arises spontaneously or for which the cause is unknown.

inflammatory mediators   various chemicals that, when released by immune cells, cause vasodilation and bring about an inflammatory response.

initial stage of shock   the first stage of shock, which occurs when the body begins to recognise and respond to a reduction in blood flow to the organs and tissues.

inotropic therapy   includes the use of drugs that improve the force of muscle contraction and are said to have a positive inotropic effect.

interleukins   a family of proteins that control some aspects of the immune response. They do this by conveying signals between white blood cells.

intubated (intubation)   the placement of a flexible, cuffed tube into the trachea in order to maintain an open airway and facilitate processes such as assisted ventilation, administering anaesthesia during surgical procedures, and to prevent airway obstruction and/or accidental inhalation of toxic substances; referred to as tracheal intubation.

invasive ventilation   intubation and respiratory support provided either to assist normal breathing or, in some cases, to replace normal breathing. Patients usually require sedation when receiving invasive ventilation.

iron lung   a large cylindrical steel chamber. Patients lay in the chamber with only their head and neck free. The chamber was airtight, and at set intervals the atmospheric pressure inside the chamber was reduced to lower than atmospheric pressure. This change in pressure reduced the work of breathing for the patient and the patient was able to take a deeper breath (increase their TV). When the interchamber pressure returned to normal, the patient exhaled normally.

ischaemia   a restriction in blood supply, and therefore in the supply of oxygen, to tissues.

kinins   any of a group of substances formed in body tissue in response to injury.

Kussmaul breathing   a very deep, repetitive, gasping respiratory pattern associated with profound acidosis (e.g., diabetic ketoacidosis).

laparoscopic cholecystectomy   the surgical removal of the gall bladder using a minimally invasive technique.

leukotrienes   any of a group of physiologically active substances that possibly function as mediators during acute inflammatory responses.

lymphocytes   a family of white blood cells that are responsible for defending the body against infection and damage. They include B lymphocytes that attack bacteria and toxins, and T lymphocytes which attack cells that have been taken over by a damaging organism such as a virus or by cancerous cells.

mandibular   refers to any tissue or bony structure that makes up the lower jaw.

midazolam   a short-acting drug of the benzodiazepine family. It is used to induce sedation and amnesia before and during medical procedures, to treat acute seizures, and as sedation in the management of ventilated patients.

monocyte   a type of white blood cell that plays a role in the inflammatory and immune response. Monocytes can develop either into dendritic cells that play a role in the antibody antigen response or into macrophages, which are cells that eat other damaged cells.

muscarinic antagonist   a group of drugs, also known as anticholinergic drugs, and include ipratropium bromide (atrovent). They cause bronchodilation in the lungs and are used to treat asthma and COPD. They are administered by inhalation and patients may complain of a dry mouth when taking these drugs.

nephrotoxic   the poisonous effect of medication on the kidneys.

neutrophil   the most common type of white blood cell that acts as the first line of defence when the inflammatory response is triggered. Neutrophils will recognise anything that should not be present in the body as an invader and destroy it.

nitric oxide   a compound that acts as a vasodilator, helps to regulate the uptake of oxygen in cells, and can destroy viruses and cancer cells as part of the immune system.

nitrous oxide   a colourless, non-flammable chemical compound used in medicine for its analgesic, anaesthetic, and anxiolytic effects, usually administered by inhalation and distributed through the lungs by diffusion.

nociceptive pain   is caused by stimulation of peripheral nerve fibres that respond only to stimuli approaching or exceeding harmful intensity, the most common categories being thermal, mechanical, and chemical.

nociceptors   sensory neurons that are found in any area of the body that can sense pain either externally or internally.

non-steroidal anti-inflammatory drugs (NSAIDs)   a group of drugs that have analgesic, anti-inflammatory, and antipyretic effects. These drugs can cause dyspepsia and gastric ulceration.

obstructive shock   occurs when there is inadequate circulation of the blood to the body's organs and tissues due to physical obstruction of blood flow from the heart or aorta, such as in cardiac tamponade when the pericardial sac fills with blood and squashes the ventricles.

obstructive sleep apnoea   a condition characterised by repeated intermittent obstruction or collapse of the upper airways during sleep, often accompanied by loud snoring. The patient experiences periods of apnoea (no breathing), tiredness, and lethargy.

obtundation   less than full alertness.

oedema   an excessive accumulation of serous fluid in the intercellular spaces of tissue.

osmolarity   the measure of the concentration of solute particles in a solution.

pathogen   a microorganism that can cause disease.

phagocytosis   the process that cells such as neutrophils use to destroy dead or foreign cells by ingesting or engulfing them.

phlebitis   the inflammation of the walls of the vein.

pneumothorax   a collection of air that has leaked into the space between the layers of the lung sac. The lung is contained in two sacs: the visceral and parietal layers of the pleura. The parietal layer lines the thoracic wall, and the visceral layer covers all the surfaces of the lungs. Leakage of air into the pleural space can build up and cause the lung to collapse. When this happens, the patient is unable to take a deep breath and becomes breathless and dyspnoeic.

polydipsia   abnormally great thirst as a symptom of disease (such as diabetes) or psychological disturbance.

polyuria   production of abnormally large volumes of dilute urine.

primary survey   a methodical process used to quickly identify immediate life-threatening injuries and conditions that require immediate attention.

progressive stage of shock   the third stage of shock, which occurs when the underlying cause of the shock has not been corrected and the body is no longer able to compensate for the reduction in blood flow. Cell damage becomes more severe over time and can be irreversible.

prostaglandins   a group of substances that influence a number of body functions such as the dilation and constriction of blood vessels, control of blood pressure, and the inflammatory response. They are also influential in the promotion of uterine contractions during childbirth.

prothrombin time (PT)   a blood test that measures how long it takes blood to clot. It is also known as an INR test (international normalised ratio) when the results are standardised to facilitate wider standard interpretation.

pulmonary embolism   occurs when a blood vessel supplying blood to the lungs becomes clogged by a blood clot or embolus. This prevents an amount of blood from perfusing the alveoli and, as a result, the body receives a reduced supply of oxygenated blood.

receptive dysphasia   is a language disorder that occurs when the part of the brain responsible for processing our understanding of written and spoken words is damaged, resulting in the person having difficulty with understanding written or spoken language.

refractory stage of shock   the fourth and final stage of shock, which occurs when the body's organs begin to fail due to a sustained lack of oxygen and nutrients; eventually the organs completely fail and this leads to death.

renin-angiotensin-aldosterone mechanism   a hormone system that helps to regulate fluid balance and blood pressure. The system forms part of the body's response to shock.

respiratory depression   a respiration that has a rate below 12 breaths per minute or that fails to provide full ventilation and perfusion of the lungs.

revascularisation   restoration of circulation to tissues after this has been compromised by accident or ischaemia.

secondary survey   a complete examination of the patient from top to toe, both front and back.

septic shock   shock caused by decreased tissue perfusion and oxygen delivery as a result of severe infection and sepsis. It can cause multiple organ dysfunction syndrome (formerly known as multiple organ failure).

somatic pain   pain arising from tissues such as skin, muscle, tendon, joint capsules, fasciae, and bone.

ST segment   this is the normally flat line between the s and t segments of the pqrst waveform found in an electrocardiograph (ECG). The ECG records the electrical wave pattern of conduction as the message for the heart muscle to contract spreads through the heart, recording the pattern of a person's heartbeat.

STEMI   this is an abbreviation of 'ST elevation myocardial infarction'. The ST segment located over the damaged area of the heart in a 12-lead ECG becomes elevated as part of the inflammatory response and indicates an area of muscle that has been starved of a blood supply.

tachypnoea   rapid breathing or respiration.

tissue dysoxia   a very low concentration of oxygen in the body tissues.

tumour necrosis factor (TNF)   one of the cytokines that is influential in the inflammatory response. TNF induces cell death in cancer cells and is involved in stimulating the inflammatory response.

U&E   a blood test to measure the levels of urea and electrolytes in a person's blood. This can give valuable information about the person's kidney function.

vascular permeability   the degree to which one substance allows another substance to pass through it.

vasodilation   the widening of blood vessels resulting from the relaxation of the muscular wall of the blood vessels.

vasopressin   *see* antidiuretic hormone (ADH).

ventilation   a method used to assist spontaneous breathing. The techniques available include non-invasive ventilation where respiratory support is provided through a tight-fitting mask and the patient continues to breathe with support.

visceral pain   pain arising from the internal organs; patients state the pain feels like squeezing, cramping, or pressure.

References

Abbey, JA, Piller, N, De Bellis, A et al. (2004). The Abbey pain scale: a 1-minute numerical indicator for people with end-stage dementia. *International Journal of Palliative Nursing*, 10(1): 6–13. doi:10.12968/ijpn.2004.10.1.12013.

Abdo, W and Heunks, L (2012) Oxygen-induced hypercapnia in COPD: myths and facts. *Critical Care*, 16(5): 323.

Adam, S, Odell, M and Welch, J (2010) *Rapid Assessment of the Acutely Ill Patient*. Oxford: Wiley Blackwell.

Adeyinka, A and Kondamudi, N (2021) Hyperosmolar hyperglycaemic nonketotic coma. Accessed at: https://europepmc.org/books/n/statpearls/article-23198/?extid=290837 07&src=med#, on 17/10/21.

Aiken, L, Sloane, D, Griffiths, P et al. (2017) Nursing skill mix in European hospitals: a cross-sectional study of the association with mortality, patient ratings, and quality of care. *British Medical Journal of Quality and Safety*, 26: 559–68.

Aksoy Gündoğdu, A, Özdemir, A and Özkan, S (2020) Pathological yawning in patients with acute middle cerebral artery infarction: prognostic significance and association with the infarct location. *Balkan Medical Journal*, 37(1): 24–8.

Alce, T, Page, V and Vizcaychipi, M (2014) Delirium, in Bersten, A and Soni, N (eds) *Oh's Intensive Care Manual*. Seventh edition. Oxford: Butterworth Heinemann Elsevier.

Aldemir, M, Ozen, S, Kara, O et al. (2001) Predisposing factors for delirium in the surgical intensive care unit. *Critical Care*, 5: 265–70.

Alencar Neto, J (2018) Morphine, oxygen, nitrates, and mortality reducing pharmacological treatment for acute coronary syndrome: an evidence-based review. *Cureus*, 10(1): e2114.

American Association of Critical Care Nurses (2015) *Implementing the ABCDE Bundle at the Bedside*. Accessed at: www.aacn.org/wd/practice/content/actionpak/withlinks-ABCDE-ToolKit.content?menu=practice

American College of Surgeons (2018) *Advanced Trauma Life Support: Student Course Manual*. Tenth edition. Chicago: American College of Surgeons.

American Psychiatric Association (2013) *Diagnostic and Statistical Manual of Mental Disorders (DSM-5)*. Fifth edition. Virginia: The American Psychiatric Association.

Amsterdam, E, Wenger, N, Brindis, R et al. (2014) 2014 AHA/ACC guideline for the management of patients with non-ST-elevation acute coronary syndromes: executive summary. *Circulation*, 130(25): 2354–94.

Arend, E and Christensen, M (2009) Delirium in the intensive care unit: a review. *Nursing in Critical Care*, 14(3): 145–54.

Ashelford, S, Raynsford, J and Taylor, V (2019) *Pathophysiology and Pharmacology in Nursing*. Second edition. London: SAGE/Learning Matters.

Babaev, A, Frederick, P, Pasta, D, Every, N, Sichrovsky, T and Hochman, J for the NRMI Investigators (2005) Trends in management and outcome of patients with acute myocardial infarction complicated by cardiogenic shock. *Journal of the American Medical Association*, 294(4): 448–54.

Balas, M, Vasilevskis, E, Burke, W et al. (2012) Critical care nurses' role in implementing the 'ABCDE bundle' into practice. *Critical Care Nurse*, 32(2): 35–48.

Bellelli, G, Morandi, A, Davis, D, et al. (2014) Validation of the 4AT, a new instrument for rapid delirium screening: a study in 234 hospitalised older people, *Age and Ageing*, 43(4): 496–502. Accessed at: https://doi.org/10.1093/ageing/afu021

Bellomo, R (2019) Renal replacement therapy, in Bersten, A and Handy, J (eds) *Oh's Intensive Care Manual*. Eighth edition. Oxford: Butterworth Heineman Elsevier, pp617–25.

Benner, P, Hooper-Kyriakidis, P and Stannard, D (2011) *Clinical Wisdom and Interventions in Critical Care*. Second edition. Philadelphia, PA: WB Saunders Company.

Bersten, A (2019) Respiratory monitoring, in Bersten, A and Handy, J (eds) *Oh's Intensive Care Manual*. Eighth edition. Elsevier, pp492–501.

Bersten, A and Bihari, S (2019) Acute respiratory distress syndrome, in Bersten, A and Handy, J (2019) *Oh's Intensive Care Manual*. Eighth edition. Elsevier, pp428–38.

Bersten, A and Handy, J. (eds) (2019) *Oh's Intensive Care Manual*. Eighth edition. Oxford: Butterworth Heinemann Elsevier.

Best Practice in the Management of Epidural Analgesia in the Hospital Setting (2020) https://fpm.ac.uk/sites/fpm/files/documents/2020-09/Epidural-AUG-2020-FINAL.pdf

Bilben, B, Grandal, L, and Sovik, S (2016) NEWS as an emergency department predictor of disease severity and 90 day survival in the acutely dyspneic patient: a prospective observational study. *Scandinavian Journal of Trauma, Resuscitation and Emergency Medicine*, 24: 80.

BNF (2021) *British National Formulary, NICE*. London: BMA and Royal Pharmaceutical Society. Accessed at: https://bnf.nice.org.uk/ on 23/08/21.

Bone, R, Balk, R, Cerra, F et al. (1992) Definitions for sepsis and organ failure and guidelines for the use of innovative therapies in sepsis. The ACCP/SCCM Consensus Conference Committee. American College of Chest Physicians/Society of Critical Care Medicine. Chest, 101(6): 1644–55. doi: 10.1378/chest.101.6.1644. PMID: 1303622

Borthwick, M, Bourne, R, Craig, M, Egan, A and Oxley, J (2003) *Evolution of Intensive Care in the UK*. Intensive Care Society. Accessed at: www.ics.ac.uk/ics-homepage/guidelines-and-standards

Borthwick, M, Bourne, R, Craig, M et al. (2006) *Detection, Prevention and Treatment of Delirium in Critically Ill Patients*. Leicester: United Kingdom Clinical Pharmacy Association.

Boss, B and Huether, S. (2019) Alterations in cognitive systems, cerebral haemodynamics, and motor function. In McCance, K and Huether, S (2019) *Pathophysiology: The Biological Basis of Disease in Adults and Children.* Eighth edition. St Louis, MO: Elsevier Mosby, pp504–49.

Brashers, V (2019) Alterations of cardiovascular function. In McCance, K and Huether, S *Pathophysiology: The Biological Basis of Disease in Adults and Children.* Eighth edition. St Louis, MO: Elsevier Mosby, pp1059–114.

Brashers, V and Huether, S (2019) Alterations in pulmonary function. In McCance, K and Huether, S (2019) *Pathophysiology: The Biological Basis of Disease in Adults and Children.* Eighth edition. St Louis, MO: Elsevier Mosby, pp1163–201.

Brashers, V, Jones, R and Huether, S (2019) Alterations of hormonal regulation. In McCance, K and Huether, S *Pathophysiology: The Biological Basis of Disease in Adults and Children.* Eighth edition. St Louis, MO: Elsevier Mosby, pp669–712.

Bray, K, Hill, K, Robson, W et al. (2004) British Association of Critical Care Nurses' position statement on the use of restraint in adult critical care units. *Nursing in Critical Care,* 9(5): 199–212.

Bridges, E and Dukes, S (2005) Cardiovascular aspects of septic shock: pathophysiology, monitoring and treatment. *Critical Care Nurse,* 25(2): 14–40.

British Geriatric Society (2020) *Delirium.* Accessed at: www.bgs.org.uk/topics/delirium, on 26/08/21.

British Medical Association (BMA), Resuscitation Council (UK) and RCN (Royal College of Nursing) (2016) *Decisions Relating to Cardiopulmonary Resuscitation.* London: British Medical Association.

BTS (British Thoracic Society) (2015) *Annotated BTS Guideline for the Management of Community Acquired Pneumonia in Adults* (2009). Accessed at: file:///D:/Downloads/Annotated%20BTS%20CAP%20Guideline%20Summary%20of%20Recommendations%20(1).pdf, on 07/08/21.

BTS and ICS (2016) *BTS/ICS Guidelines for the Ventilatory Management of Acute Hypercapnic Respiratory Failure in Adults.* Accessed at: www.brit-thoracic.org.uk/quality-improvement/guidelines/niv/ on 23/08/21.

BTS and SIGN (Scottish Intercollegiate Guidelines Network) (2019) *British Guidelines on the Management of Asthma.* Accessed at: www.brit-thoracic.org.uk/quality-improvement/guidelines/asthma/

Butterfield, J et al. (2003) *Collins English Dictionary.* Glasgow: Collins.

Carey, I, Critchley, J, DeWilde, S et al. (2018) Risk of infection in type 1 and type 2 diabetes compared with the general population: a matched cohort study. *Diabetes Care,* (3): 513–21. doi: 10.2337/dc17-2131. Epub 12 Jan 2018. PMID: 29330152.

Carville, S, Wonderling, D and Stevens, P (2014) Early identification and management of chronic kidney disease in adults: summary of updated NICE guidance. *British Medical Journal,* 349: g4507.

Cecconi, M, De Backer, D, Antonelli, M et al. (2014) Consensus on circulatory shock and haemodynamic monitoring. Task force of the European Society of Intensive Care Medicine. *Intensive Care Medicine,* 40(12): 1795–815.

Chen, H, Liu, J, Chen, L and Wang, G (2014) Effectiveness of daily interruption of sedation in sedated patients with mechanical ventilation in ICU: a systematic review. *International Journal of Nursing Sciences*, 1(4): 346–51.

Chen, H, Song, Z and Dennis, J (2020) Hypertonic saline versus other intracranial pressure-lowering agents for people with acute traumatic brain injury. *Cochrane Database of Systematic Reviews*. Issue 1. Art. No.: CD010904. DOI: 10.1002/14651858.CD010904. pub3.

Churpek, M, Snyder, A, Han, X et al. (2017) Quick sepsis related organ failure assessment, systemic inflammatory response syndrome, and early warning scores for directing clinical deterioration in infected patients outside the intensive care unit. *American Journal of Respiratory and Critical Care Medicine*, 195(7): 906–11.

Cleeland, CS and Ryan, KM (1994) Pain assessment: global use of the Brief Pain Inventory. *Annals of the Academy of Medicine* (Singapore), 23(2): 129–38.

Cole, E (2009) *Trauma Care: Initial Assessment and Management In the Emergency Department.* Oxford: Blackwell Publishing.

Cooksley, T, Rose, S and Holland, M (2018) A systematic approach to the unconscious patient. *Clinical Medicine*, 18(1): 88–92. Accessed at: https://doi.org/10.7861/clinmedicine.18-1-88.

Coulter Smith, MA, Smith, P and Crow, R (2014) A critical review: a combined conceptual framework of severity of illness and clinical judgement for analysing diagnostic judgements in critical illness. *Journal of Clinical Nursing*, 23(5–6): 784–98.

Creed, F and Spiers, C (eds) (2010) *Care of the Acutely Ill Adult: an Essential Guide for Nurses.* Oxford: Oxford University Press.

Creed, F, Dawson, J and Looker, K (2010) Assessment tools and track and trigger systems, in Creed, F and Spiers, C (eds) *Care of the Acutely Ill Adult: an Essential Guide for Nurses.* Oxford: Oxford University Press.

Cretikos, M, Bellomo, R, Hillman, K et al. (2008) Respiratory rate: the neglected vital sign. *Medical Journal Australia*, 188(11): 657–9.

Dalton, M, Harrison, J, Malin, A and Leavey, C (2018) Factors that influence nurses' assessment of patient acuity and response to acute deterioration. *British Journal of Nursing*, 27(4): 212–18.

Daniels, R and Nutbeam, T (2019) *The Sepsis Manual.* Fifth edition. Birmingham: UK Sepsis Trust. Accessed at: https://sepsistrust.org/professional-resources/education-resources/, on 26/08/21.

Dayton, E and Henriksen, K (2007) Communication failure: basic components, contributing factors and the call for structure. *Joint Commission Journal on Quality and Patient Safety*, 33(1): 34–47.

De Daudio, R and Romagnoli, S (2019) Sepsis and septic shock, in Bersten, A and Handy, J (2019) *Oh's Intensive Care Manual.* Eighth edition. Elsevier, 836–48.

Diabetes UK (2020a) *Diabetes Statistics.* Accessed at: www.diabetes.org.uk/professionals/position-statements-reports/statistics, on 28/08/21.

Diabetes UK (2020b) *Differences between Type 1 and Type 2 Diabetes.* Accessed at: www.diabetes.org.uk/diabetes-the-basics/differences-between-type-1-and-type-2-diabetes, on 28/08/21.

Dixon, M (2018) Assessment and management of older patients with delirium in acute settings. *Nursing Older People*, 30(4): 35–42. doi: 10.7748/nop.2018.e969. Epub 2 May 2018. PMID: 29717845.

Dougherty, L and Lister, S (2020) *The Royal Marsden Hospital Manual of Clinical Nursing Procedure.* Tenth edition. Professional Edition Wiley.

Downey, C, Tahir, W, Randell, R, Brown, J and Jayne, D (2017) Strengths and limitations of early warning scores: a systematic review and narrative synthesis. *International Journal of Nursing Studies*, 76: 106–19.

Duffield, C, Roche, M, Diers, D, Catling-Paull, C and Blay, N (2010) Staffing, skill mix and the model of care. *Journal of Clinical Nursing*, 19: 2242–51.

Duke, G and Bersten, A (2019) Non-invasive ventilation, in Bersten, A and Handy, J *Oh's Intensive Care Manual.* Eighth edition. Elsevier, 483–91.

Edvardsson, D, Watt, E and Pearce, F (2017) Patient experiences of caring and person-centredness are associated with perceived nursing care quality. *Journal of Advanced Nursing*, 73(1): 217–27.

Elliot, M, Worrall-Carter, L and Page, K (2014) Intensive care readmission: a contemporary review of the literature. *Intensive and Critical Care Nursing*, 30: 121–37.

Ely, E (2014) *Confusion Assessment Method for the ICU (CAM-ICU): The Complete Training Manual.* Vanderbilt University Medical Centre. Accessed at: www.icudelirium.org/docs/CAM_ICU_training.pdf

Ely, E, Margolin, R, Francis, J et al. (2001) Evaluation of delirium in critically ill patients: validation of the confusion assessment method for the intensive care unit (CAM-ICU). *Critical Care Medicine*, 29(7): 1370–9.

Ely, E, Truman, B, Shintani, A et al. (2003) Monitoring sedation status over time in ICU patients: reliability and validity of the Richmond Agitation-Sedation Scale (RASS). *Journal of the American Medical Association*, 289(22): 2983–91.

Eom, J, Lee, M, Chun, H et al. (2014) The impact of a ventilator bundle on preventing ventilator-associated pneumonia: a multi-centre study. *American Journal of Infection Control*, 42: 34–7.

Etkind, S, Daveson, B, Kwok, W et al. (2015) Capture, transfer and feedback of patient-centred outcomes data in palliative care populations: does it make a difference? A systematic review. *Journal of Pain and Symptom Management*, 49(3): 611–24.

European Delirium Association and American Delirium Society (2014) The DSM-5 criteria, level of arousal and delirium diagnosis: inclusiveness is safer. *Biomed Central Medicine*, 12(141): 1–4.

Faculty of Pain Medicine of the Royal College of Anaesthetists (2020) *Best Practice in the Management of Epidural Analgesia in the Hospital Setting.* Accessed at: https://fpm.ac.uk/sites/fpm/files/documents/2020-09/Epidural-AUG-2020-FINAL.pdf

Fairbrother, G, Jones, A and Rivas, K (2010) Changing model of nursing care from individual patient allocation to team nursing in the acute inpatient environment. *Contemporary Nurse*, 35(2): 202–20.

Fairley, S (2017) Neurological problems, in Adam, S, Osborne, S and Welch, J (eds) *Critical Care Nursing Science and Practice*. Oxford: Oxford University Press, 277–322.

Field, T, Tjia J, Mazor K, et al. (2011) Randomized trial of a warfarin communication protocol for nursing homes: an SBAR-based approach. *American Journal of Medicine*, 124(179): e1–7.

Fliser, D, Laville, M and Covic, A (2012) A European Renal Best Practice (ERBP) position statement on the Kidney Disease Improving Global Outcomes (KDIGO) clinical practice guidelines on acute kidney injury: part 1 – definitions, conservative management and contrast-induced nephropathy. *Nephrology Dialysis Transplant*, 27(12): 4263–72.

Francis, R (2013) *Report of the Mid Staffordshire NHS Foundation Trust Public Inquiry: Executive Summary*. London: The Stationery Office.

Franklin, C and Matthew, J (1994) Developing strategies to prevent in hospital cardiac arrest: analysing responses of physicians and nurses in the hours before the event. *Critical Care Medicine*, 22: 244–7.

GAIN (2014) *Guidelines for the Treatment of Hyperkalaemia in Adults* GAIN. Accessed at: www.gain-ni.org/images/Uploads/Guidelines/GAIN_Guidelines_Treatment_of_Hyperkalaemia_in_Adults_GAIN_02_12_2014.pdf

Gao, H, McDonnell, A, Harrison, DA et al. (2007) Systematic review and evaluation of physiological track and trigger warning systems for identifying at-risk patients on the ward. *Intensive Care Medicine*, 33: 667–79.

Garcia, E, Godoy-Izquierdo, D, Godoy, J, Perez, M and Lopez-Chicheri, I (2007) Gender differences in pressure pain threshold in a repeated measures assessment. *Psychology, Health & Medicine*, 12(5): 567–79.

Gibson, V (2015) Recognising and managing community-acquired pneumonia. *Nursing Standard*, 30(12): 53–9.

Gish, D, Loynd, R, Melnick, S et al. (2016) Myxoedema coma: a forgotten presentation of extreme hypothyroidism. *BMJ Case Reports*, bcr2016216225.

Gosmanov, A, Gosmanova, E and Kitabchi, A (2021) Hyperglycemic crises: diabetic ketoacidosis and hyperglycemic hyperosmolar state, in Feingold, KR, Anawalt, B, Boyce, A et al. (eds) *Endotext* [Internet]. South Dartmouth, MA: MDText.com, Inc.; 2000–. Accessed at: www.ncbi.nlm.nih.gov/books/NBK279052/.

Gov.UK (2020) *Opioids: Risk of Dependence and Addiction*. Accessed at: www.gov.uk/drug-safety-update/opioids-risk-of-dependence-and-addiction

Gowda, R, Fox, J and Khan, I (2008) Cardiogenic shock: basics and clinical considerations. *International Journal of Cardiology*, 123: 221–8.

Gregory, J (2012) How can we assess pain in people who have difficulty communicating? A practice development project identifying a pain assessment tool for acute care. *International Practice Development Journal*, 2(2): 1–20. Accessed at: www.fons.org/Resources/Documents/Journal/Vol2No2/IDPJ_0202_06.pdf.

Gregory, J (2019) Use of pain scales and observational pain assessment tools in hospital settings. *Nursing Standard*, e11308.

Greulich, S, Mayr, A, Gloekler, S et al. (2019) Time-dependent myocardial necrosis in patients with ST-segment-elevation myocardial infarction without angiographic collateral flow visualized by cardiac magnetic resonance imaging: results from the multicenter STEMI-SCAR Project. *Journal American Heart Association*, 8(12): e012429.

Griffiths, P, Recio-Saucedo, A, Dall'Ora, C et al. (2018) The association between nurse staffing and omissions in nursing care: a systematic review. *Journal of Advanced Nursing*, 74, 1474–8.

Grossman, S and Porth, CM (2013) *Porth's Physiology: Concepts of Altered Health States*. Ninth edition. Philadelphia, PA: Wolters Kluwer/Lippincott Williams & Wilkins.

Gyawali, B, Ramakrishna, K and Dhamoon, AS (2019) Sepsis: The evolution in definition, pathophysiology, and management. *SAGE Open Medicine*. doi:10.1177/2050312119835043.

Hall, J (2016) *Guyton and Hall: Textbook of Medical Physiology*. Thirteenth edition. Philadelphia, PA: Saunders Elsevier.

Hammer, G and McPhee, S (2014) *Pathophysiology of Disease: An Introduction to Clinical Medicine*. Seventh edition. New York: McGraw Hill Education/Medical.

Handy, J and Li, A (2019) Thyroid emergencies, in McCance, K and Huether, S (eds) *Pathophysiology: The Biological Basis of Disease in Adults and Children*. Eighth edition. St Louis, MO: Elsevier Mosby, 757–66.

Hastings, M (2009) *Clinical Skills Made Incredibly Easy*. Philadelphia, PA: Lippincott Williams & Wilkins.

Health and Social Care Information Centre (2014) *National Diabetes Inpatient Audit*. London: HSCIC.

Hellyer, T, Ewan, V, Wilson, P, et al. (2016) The Intensive Care Society recommended bundle of interventions for the prevention of ventilator-associated pneumonia. *Journal of the Intensive Care Society*, 17(3): 238–43.

Herndon, D (2007) *Total Burn Care*. Third edition. London: WB Saunders.

Higgins, C (2013) *Understanding Laboratory Investigations*. Third edition. Chichester: Wiley-Blackwell.

Hobl, E, Stimpfl, T, Ebneret, J et al. (2014) Morphine decreases clopidogrel concentrations and effects: a randomized, double-blind, placebo-controlled trial. *Journal of the American College of Cardiology*, 63(7): 630–5.

Hølen, J, Saltvedt, I, Fayers, P, et al. (2007) Doloplus-2, a valid tool for behavioural pain assessment? *BMC Geriatrics*, 7, 29. doi:10.1186/1471-2318-7-29.

Hooper, N and Armstrong, T (2021, Jan.) Haemorrhagic shock. In: *StatPearls* [Internet]. Treasure Island, FL: StatPearls Publishing. Accessed at: www.ncbi.nlm.nih.gov/books/NBK470382/, on 25/08/21.

Horner, D and Bellamy, M (2012) Care bundles in intensive care. *Continuing Education in Anaesthesia Critical Care & Pain*, 12(4): 199–202.

International Classification of Disease (ICD-10) (2016) *International Statistical Classification of Diseases and Related Health Problems.* Accessed at: www.who.int/classifications/icd/ICD10Volume2_en_2010.pdf, on 26/08/21.

ICS (Intensive Care Society) (2021) *Levels of Adult Critical Care, Second Edition: Consensus Statement.* London: ICS. Accessed at: www.cc3n.org.uk/uploads/9/8/4/2/98425184/2021-03__levels_of_care_second_edition.pdf

ICSI (Institute for Clinical Systems Improvement) (2009) *Diagnosis and Treatment of Chest Pain and Acute Coronary Syndrome (ACS).* Bloomington, MN: ICSI.

IHI (Institute for Healthcare Improvement) (2009) *Improvement Map: Patient Care Processes – Pressure Ulcer Prevention.* Accessed at: www.ihi.org/offerings/initiatives/improvemaphospitals/Pages/default.aspx

IHI (2011) *Rapid Response Team Data Collection and SBAR Communication Tool.* Accessed at: www.ihi.org/knowledge/Pages/Tools/SBARToolkit.aspx

IHI (2012) *How-To Guide: Prevent Ventilator-Associated Pneumonia.* Accessed at: www.ihi.org/resources/Pages/Tools/HowtoGuidePreventVAP.aspx

IHI (2015) *Implement the IHI Central Line Bundle.* Accessed at: http://app.ihi.org/imap/tool/processpdf.aspx?processGUID=e876565d-fd43-42ce-8340-8643b7e675c7

Innes, J and Tiernan, J (2018) The respiratory system in Innes, J, Dover, A and Fairhurst, K (eds) *Macleod's Clinical Examination.* Edinburgh: Elsevier, 75–92.

International Association for the Study of Pain (2017). *IASP Terminology.* Accessed at: www.iasp-pain.org/Education/Content.aspx?ItemNumber=1698.

Jaakkola, J, Hernberg, S, Lajunen, T et al. (2019) Smoking and lung function among adults with newly onset asthma. *British Medical Journal Open Respiratory Research,* 6: e000377.

Jackson, A (1998) Infection control, a battle in vein: infusion phlebitis. *Nursing Times,* 94(4): 68, 71. PMID: 9510815.

James, J et al. (2010) Vital signs for vital people: an exploratory study into the role of the health care assistant in recognising, recording and responding to the acutely ill patient in the general ward setting. *Journal of Nursing Management,* 18: 548–55.

Jarvis, H (2006) Exploring the evidence base for the use of non-invasive ventilation. *British Journal of Nursing,* 15(14): 756–9.

JBDS (Joint British Diabetes Societies) (2012) *Management of Hyperosmolar Hyperglycaemic State (HHS).* Accessed at: https://abcd.care/resource/management-hyperosmolar-hyperglycaemic-state-hhs, on 28/08/21.

JBDS (2021) *The Management of Diabetic Ketoacidosis (DKA) in Adults.* Accessed at: https://abcd.care/resource/management-diabetic-ketoacidosis-dka-adults, on 28/08/21.

Jeffries, D, Johnson, M and Griffiths, R (2010) A meta-study of the essentials of quality nursing documentation. *International Journal of Nursing Practice,* 16: 112–24.

Jin, J, Sclar, G, Oh, V and Li, S (2008) Factors affecting therapeutic compliance: a review from the patient's perspective. *Therapeutics and Clinical Risk Management,* 4(1): 269–86.

Kane, B, Decalmer, S, Murphy, P et al. (2012) The proposed national early warning system (NEWS) could be hazardous for patients who are at risk of hypercapnic respiratory failure. *Thorax*, 67 (Supplement 2): A16–A17.

Kaplan, J, Eiferman, D, Porter, K et al. (2019) Impact of a nursing-driven sedation protocol with criteria for infusion initiation in the surgical intensive care unit. *Journal of Critical Care*, 50: 195–200.

Karkabi, B, Meir, G, Zafrir, B et al. (2021) Door-to-balloon time and mortality in patients with ST-elevation myocardial infarction undergoing primary angioplasty. *European Heart Journal – Quality of Care and Clinical Outcomes*, 7(4): 422–6.

Katz, S, Arish, N, Rokach, A et al. (2018) The effect of body position on pulmonary function: a systematic review. *BMC Pulmonary Medicine*, 18: 159.

KDIGO AKI Work Group (2012) KDIGO clinical practice guidelines for acute kidney injury. *Kidney International* 2 (Supplement): 1–138.

Keep, J, Messmer, A, Sladden, R et al. (2016) National early warning score at emergency department triage may allow early identification of patients with severe sepsis and septic shock: a retrospective observational study. *Emergency Medical Journal*, 33: 37–41.

Kelly, C and Lynes, D (2011) Best practice in the provision of nebuliser therapy. *Nursing Standard*, 25(31): 50–6.

Kjeldsen, K (2010) Hypokalemia and sudden cardiac death. *Experimental Clinical Cardiology*, 15(4): e96–e99.

Knight, J, Decker, LC (2021, Jan) *Decerebrate and Decorticate Posturing*. [Updated 2021 Aug 9]. In: StatPearls [Internet]. Treasure Island, FL: StatPearls Publishing. Accessed at: www.ncbi.nlm.nih.gov/books/NBK559135/

Kydonaki, K, Hanley, J, Huby, G et al. (2019) Challenges and barriers to optimising sedation in intensive care: a qualitative study in eight Scottish intensive care units. *British Medical Journal Open*, 9: e024549.

Lane, D and Lip, G (2012) Use of the CHA2DS2-VASc and HAS-BLED scores to aid decision making for thromboprophylaxis in nonvalvular atrial fibrillation. *Circulation*, 126: 860–5.

Lassen, HC, Bjorneboe, M, Ibsen, B and Neukirch, F (1954) Treatment of tetanus with curarisation, general anaesthesia and intratracheal positive pressure ventilation. *Lancet*, ii: 1040–4.

Lawrence, P and Fulbrook, P (2011) The ventilator care bundle and its impact on ventilator-associated pneumonia: a review of the evidence. *Nursing in Critical Care*, 16(5): 222–34.

Leander, M, Lampa, E, Rask-Andersen, A et al. (2014) Impact of anxiety and depression on respiratory symptoms. *Respiratory Medicine*, 108: 1594–600.

Lenders, J, Duh, Q, Eisenhofer, G et al. (2014) Pheochromocytoma and paraganglioma: an Endocrine Society clinical practice guideline. *The Journal of Clinical Endocrinology & Metabolism*, 99(6): 1915–42. Accessed at: https://doi.org/10.1210/jc.2014-1498

Levy, M, Evans, L and Rhodes, A (2018) The Surviving Sepsis Campaign Bundle: 2018 update. *Intensive Care Medicine*, 44: 925–8. Accessed at: https://doi.org/10.1007/s00134-018-5085-0

Lewington, A and Kanagasundaram, S (2011) *Clinical Practice Guidelines: Acute Kidney Injury*. Renal Association. Accessed at: www.renal.org/guidelines/modules/acute-kidney-injury#sthash.yn97aOPJ.dpbs

Lim, W, Mohammed Akram, R, Carson, K et al. (2012) Non-invasive positive pressure ventilation for treatment of respiratory failure due to severe acute exacerbations of asthma (review). *Cochrane Database of Systematic Reviews*. Issue 12.

Liu, J, Bispham, J, Fan L et al. (2020) Factors associated with fear of hypoglycaemia among the T1D Exchange Glu population in a cross-sectional online survey. *BMJ Open* 10:e038462. doi:10.1136/bmjopen-2020-038462.

Lotan, M, Moe-Nilssen, R, Ljunggren, A et al. (2009) Measurement properties of the Non-Communicating Adult Pain Checklist (NCAPC): a pain scale for adults with intellectual and developmental disabilities, scored in a clinical setting. *Research Developmental Disability*, 31(2): 367–75. doi: 10.1016/j.ridd.2009.10.008. Epub 8 Nov 2009. PMID: 19900787.

Ludikhuize, J, Smorenburg, SM, de Rooij, SE and de Jonge, E (2012) Identification of deteriorating patients on general wards: measurement of vital parameters and potential effectiveness of the Modified Early Warning Score. *Journal of Critical Care*, 27(4): e7–13.

Maiden, M and Peake, S (2019) Overview of shock, in Bersten, A and Handy, J (eds) *Oh's Intensive Care Manual*. Eighth edition. Oxford: Butterworth Heinemann Elsevier.

Mallett, J, Albarran, J and Richardson, A (2013) *Critical Care Manual of Clinical Procedures and Competencies*. Chichester: Wiley-Blackwell.

Marik, P (2015) *Evidence-Based Critical Care*. Third edition. Cham (Switzerland): Springer.

Mark, B and Harless, D (2011) Adjusting for patient acuity in measurement of nurse staffing: two approaches. *Nursing Research*, 69(2): 107–14.

Martin, EA (ed) (2010) *Oxford Concise Medical Dictionary*. Oxford: Oxford University Press.

Martin, L, Cheek, D and Morris, S (2019) Shock, multiple organ dysfunction syndrome, and burns in adults. In McCance, K and Huether, S (eds) *Pathophysiology: The Biological Basis of Disease in Adults and Children*. Eighth edition. St Louis, MO: Elsevier Mosby, 1543–71.

Martinez, K, Frazer, SF, Dempster, M, Hamill, A, Fleming, H and McCorry, NK (2016) Psychological factors associated with self-management among adolescents with type 1 diabetes: a review. *Journal of Health Psychology*. https://doi.org/10.1177/1359105316669580

Massey, D, Chaboyer, W and Anderson, V (2016) What factors influence ward nurses' recognition of and response to patient deterioration? An integrative review of the literature. *Nursing Open*, 4(1): 6–23.

McCaffery, M and Pasero, C (1999) *Pain: A Clinical Manual*. St Louis, MO: Mosby.

McCance, K (2019) Cellular biology, in McCance, K and Huether, S (eds) *Pathophysiology: the Biological Basis of Disease in Adults and Children*. Eighth edition. St Louis, MO: Elsevier Mosby.

McCance, K and Huether, S (2019) *Pathophysiology: The Biological Basis of Disease in Adults and Children.* Eighth edition. St Louis, MO: Elsevier Mosby.

McGaughey, J, O'Halloran, P, Porter, S and Blackwood, B (2017) Early warning systems and rapid response to the deteriorating patient in hospital: a systematic realist review. *Journal of Advanced Nursing,* 73: 2877–91.

McGloin, H, Adam, S and Singer, M (1999) Unexpected deaths and referrals to intensive care of patients on general wards: are some cases potentially avoidable? *Journal of the Royal College of Physicians of London,* 33: 255–9.

McQuillan, P, Pilkington, S, Allan, A et al. (1998) Confidential inquiry into quality of care before admission to intensive care. *British Medical Journal,* 316(748): 1853–8.

Melzack, R (1975) The McGill Pain Questionnaire: major properties and scoring methods. *Pain,* 1(3): 277–99. doi: 10.1016/0304-3959(75)90044-5.

Melzack, R (1996) Gate control theory: on the evolution of pain concepts. *The Journal of Pain,* 5(2): 128–38.

Melzack, R and Wall, PD (1965) Pain mechanisms: a new theory. *Science,* 150(3699): 971–9. https://doi.org/content/150/3699/971.

Merritt, S (2009) Chronic obstructive pulmonary disease, in Smith, SA, Price, AM and Challiner, A (eds) *Ward-Based Critical Care: A Guide for Health Professionals.* Keswick: M & K Publishing.

Merten, H, van Galen, L and Wagner, C (2017) Safe handover. *British Medical Journal.* Accessed at: www.bmj.com/content/359/bmj.j4328.long

Miller, M, Bosk, E, Iwashyna, T and Krein, S (2012) Implementation challenges in the intensive care unit: the why, who, and how of daily interruption of sedation. *Journal of Critical Care,* 27(2): 218.e1–218.e7.

Mills, N, Japp, A, and Robson, J (2018) The cardiovascular system, in Innes, J, Dover, A and Fairhurst, K (eds) *Macleod's Clinical Examination.* Fourteenth edition. Edinburgh: Elsevier, 39–74.

Mistraletti, G, Pelosi, P, Mantovani, E, Beradino, M and Gregoretti, C (2012) Delirium: clinical approach and prevention. *Best Practice and Research Clinical Anaesthesiology,* 26: 311–26.

Morandi, A, Pandharipande, P, Jackson, J, Bellelli, G, Trabucchi, M and Ely, E (2012) Understanding terminology of delirium and long-term cognitive impairment in critically ill patients. *Best Practice and Research Clinical Anaesthesiology,* 26: 267–76.

Morris, M and Pearson, D (2020) *Asthma.* Accessed at: https://emedicine.medscape.com/article/296301-overview#a1, on 11/08/21.

Mulkey, M, Roberson, D, Everhart, D et al. (2018) Choosing the right delirium assessment tool. *Journal of Neuroscience Nursing,* 50(6): 343–8.

Müller, M, Jürgens, J, Redaelli, M et al. (2018) Impact of the communication and patient hand-off tool SBAR on patient safety: a systematic review. *British Medical Journal Open,* 8: e022202.

Murray, J (2011) Pulmonary oedema: pathophysiology and diagnosis. *The International Journal of Tuberculosis and Lung Disease,* 15(2): 155–60.

Mutschler, M, Nienaber, U, Münzberg, M et al. (2013) The Shock Index revisited – a fast guide to transfusion requirement? A retrospective analysis on 21,853 patients derived from the TraumaRegister DGU. *Critical Care*, 17(4): R172. https://doi.org/10.1186/cc12851.

Namigar, T, Serapa, K, Esraa, A et al. (2017) The correlation among the Ramsay Sedation Scale, Richmond Agitation Sedation Scale and Riker Sedation Agitation Scale during midazolam-remifentanil sedation. *Revista Brasileira de Anestesiologia*, 67(4): 347–54.

Narayan, M (2010) Culture's effects on pain assessment and management. *American Journal of Nursing*, 110(4), 38–47.

National Kidney Foundation (2006) *Updates: Clinical Practice Guidelines and Recommendations.* New York: NKF.

NCEPOD (2009) *Adding Insult to Injury: A Review of the Care of Patients Who Died in Hospital with a Primary Diagnosis of Acute Kidney Injury.* Accessed at: www.ncepod.org. uk/2009report1/Downloads/AKI_report.pdf

NCEPOD (2010) *National Confidential Enquiry into Patient Outcome and Death.* Accessed at: www.ncepod.org.uk/index.htm

NCEPOD (2015) *Just Say Sepsis.* Accessed at: www.ncepod.org.uk/2015report2/ downloads/JustSaySepsis_FullReport.pdf, on 26/08/21.

Ng, K, Shubash, C and Chong, J (2019) The effect of dexmedetomidine on delirium and agitation in patients in intensive care: systematic review and meta-analysis with trial sequential analysis. *Anaesthesia*, 74(3): 380–92. doi: 10.1111/anae.14472. Epub 27 Oct 2018. PMID: 30367689.

NICE (2007) *Acutely Ill Patients in Hospital: Recognition of and Response to Acute Illness in Adults in Hospital, NICE Clinical Guideline CG50.* London: NICE.

NICE (2011) *NICE Pathways.* Accessed at: www.pathways.nice.org.uk

NICE (2014a [updated 2019]) *Pneumonia: Diagnosis and Management of Community – and Hospital-Acquired Pneumonia in Adults, NICE Clinical Guideline CG191.* London: NICE. Accessed at: www.nice.org.uk/guidance/cg191, on 23/08/21.

NICE (2014b [updated 2019]) *Head Injury: Assessment and Early Management, NICE Clinical Guideline CG176.* London: NICE. Accessed at: www.nice.org.uk/guidance/cg176, on 23/08/21.

NICE (2014c) *Pressure Ulcers: Prevention and Management, NICE Clinical Guideline CG179.* London: NICE. Accessed at: www.nice.org.uk/guidance/cg179, on 23/08/21.

NICE (2015a [updated 2021]) *Type 1 Diabetes in Adults: Diagnosis and Management, NICE Guideline NG17.* London: NICE. Accessed at: www.nice.org.uk/guidance/ng17, on 28/08/21.

NICE (2015b [updated 2020]) *Type 2 Diabetes in Adults: Management, NICE Guideline NG28.* London: NICE. Accessed at: www.nice.org.uk/guidance/ng28, on 28/08/21.

NICE (2015c [updated 2020]) *Diabetes in Pregnancy: Management from Preconception to the Postnatal Period, NICE Guideline NG3.* London: NICE. Accessed at: www.nice.org.uk/ guidance/ng3, on 28/08/21.

NICE (2016) *Major Trauma: Assessment and Initial Management, NICE Guideline NG39.* London: NICE. Accessed at: www.nice.org.uk/guidance/ng39.

NICE (2017a) *Sepsis Recognition, Diagnosis and Early Management, NICE Guideline NG51.* London: NICE. Accessed at: www.nice.org.uk/guidance/ng51.

NICE (2017b) *Intravenous Fluid Therapy in Adults in Hospital, NICE Clinical Guideline CG174.* London: NICE. Accessed at: www.nice.org.uk/guidance/cg174, on 23/08/21.

NICE (2018 [updated 2019]) *Chronic Obstructive Pulmonary Disease in Over 16s: Diagnosis and Management, NICE Guideline NG115.* London: NICE. Accessed at: www.nice.org.uk/guidance/ng115, on 15/10/21.

NICE (2019a) *Delirium: Diagnosis, Prevention and Management, NICE Clinical Guideline CG103.* London: NICE. Accessed at: www.nice.org.uk/guidance/cg103, on 26/08/21.

NICE (2019b) *Acute Kidney Injury: Prevention, Detection, and Management, NICE Guideline NG148.* London: NICE. Accessed at: www.nice.org.uk/guidance/ng148, on 23/08/21.

NICE (2019c) *Thyroid Disease: Assessment and Management, NICE Guideline NG145.* Accessed at: www.nice.org.uk/guidance/ng145, on 28/08/21.

NICE (2020a) *Acute Coronary Syndromes, NICE Guideline 185.* London: NICE. Accessed at: www.nice.org.uk/guidance/ng185, on 23/08/21.

NICE (2020b) *Clinical Knowledge Summary: Addison's Disease.* Accessed at: https://cks.nice.org.uk/topics/addisons-disease/ on 28/08/21.

NICE (2021a) *Acutely Ill Patients in Hospital: Overview.* London: NICE. Accessed at: file:///D:/Downloads/acutely-ill-patients-in-hospital-acutely-ill-patients-in-hospital-overview%20(1).pdf, on 25/08/21.

NICE (2021b) *Chronic Pain (Primary and Secondary) in Over 16s: Assessment of all Chronic Pain and Management of Chronic Primary Pain, NICE Guideline 193.* Accessed at: www.nice.org.uk/guidance/ng193.

NICE (2021c) *Epilepsies: Diagnosis and Management, NICE Clinical Guideline 137.* London: NICE. Accessed at: www.nice.org.uk/guidance/cg137.

Nichol, A, Duff, S, Pettila, V et al. (2016) What is the optimal approach to weaning and liberation from mechanical ventilation? In Deutschman, C and Neligan, PJ (eds) *Evidence-based Practice of Critical Care.* Second edition. Elsevier, 52–60.

NMC (Nursing and Midwifery Council) (2018a) *Standards of Proficiency for Registered Nurses.* London: NMC.

NMC (2018b) *Standards of Proficiency for Registered Nurse Associates.* London: NMC.

NMC (2018c) *The Code: Professional Standards of Practice and Behaviour for Nurses, Midwives and Nursing Associates.* London: NMC.

NPSA (National Patient Safety Agency) (2007a) *Recognising and Responding Appropriately to Early Signs of Deterioration in Hospitalised Patients.* London: NPSA.

NPSA (2007b) *Safer Care for the Acutely Ill Patient: Learning from Serious Incidents.* London: NPSA.

Nutbeam T and Daniels R on behalf of the UK Sepsis Trust (2021) *Clinical Tools.* Accessed at: sepsistrust.org/professional-resources/clinical/, on 07/08/21.

Nyenwe, E and Kitabchi, A (2016) The evolution of diabetic ketoacidosis: an update of its etiology, pathogenesis and management. *Metabolism,* (4): 507–21. doi: 10.1016/j.metabol.2015.12.007. Epub 19 Dec 2015. PMID: 26975543.

O'Driscoll, B, Howard, L, Earis, J et al. (2017) BTS *Guideline for Oxygen Use in Adults in Health Care and Emergency Settings.* London: British Thoracic Society; also in *Thorax,* 72 (Supplement 1): i1–i90.

Opdam, H (2019) Status epilepticus. In Bersten, A and Handy, J (2019) *Oh's Intensive Care Manual.* Eighth edition. Elsevier, 642–50.

Ostermann, M, Bellomo, R, Burdmann, E et al. (2020) Controversies in acute kidney injury: conclusions from a Kidney Disease: Improving Global Outcomes (KDIGO) Conference. *Kidney International,* 98: 294–309.

Page, V (2008) *ICU Delirium: Why It Matters.* Accessed at: www.icudelirium.co.uk/why-it-matters

Patschan, D and Müller, G (2015) Acute kidney injury. *Journal of Injury and Violence Research,* 7(1): 19–26.

Patschan, D, Patschan, S and Müller, G (2012) Inflammation and microvasculopathy in renal ischaemia reperfusion injury. *Journal of Transplantation,* 764154: 1–7.

Patton, K, Thibodeau, G and Hutton, A (2016) *Anatomy and Physiology: Adapted International Edition.* Elsevier.

Pirhonen, L, Olofsson, E, Fors, A et al. (2017) Effects of person-centred care on health outcomes: a randomized controlled trial in patients with acute coronary syndrome. *Health Policy,* 121: 169–79.

Polosa, R and Thomson, NC (2013) Smoking and asthma: dangerous liaisons. *European Respiratory Journal,* 41: 716–26.

Prescott, A, Lewington, A and O' Donoghue, D (2012) Acute kidney injury: top ten tips. *Clinical Medicine,* 12(4): 328–32.

Quirke, S, Coombs, M and McEldowney, R (2011) Suboptimal care of the acutely unwell ward patient: a concept analysis. *Journal of Advanced Nursing,* 67(8): 1834–45.

Ramsay, M, Savego, T, Simpson, B and Goodwin, R (1974) Controlled sedation with alphaxolone-alphadolone. *British Medical Journal,* 2(920): 656–9.

RCN (2015) *Pain Knowledge and Skills Framework for the Nursing Team.* www.britishpainsociety.org/static/uploads/resources/files/RCN_KSF_2015.pdf

RCN (2017) *The UK Nursing Labour Market Review 2017.* London: Royal College of Nursing.

RCO (Royal College of Ophthalmologists) and ICS (Intensive care Society) (2017) *Eye Care in the Intensive Care Unit.* Accessed at: www.ics.ac.uk/Society/Guidance/PDFs/Eye_Care_in_ICU on 23/08/21.

RCP (Royal College of Physicians) (2012) *National Early Warning Score (NEWS): Standardizing the Assessment of Acute Illness Severity in the NHS. Report of a working party.* London: RCP.

RCP (2017) National Early Warning Score (NEWS) 2: *Standardizing the Assessment of Acute Illness Severity in the NHS.* Updated report of a working party. London: RCP.

RCP (2020) *Prolonged Disorders of Consciousness Following Sudden Onset Brain Injury: National Clinical Guidelines.* Accessed at: www.rcplondon.ac.uk/guidelines-policy/prolonged-disorders-consciousness-following-sudden-onset-brain-injury-national-clinical-guidelines, on 27/08/21.

RCP, British Geriatrics Society, and British Pain Society (2007) *The Assessment of Pain in Older People: National Guidelines.* Concise Guidance to Good Practice Series, No. 8. London: RCP. Accessed at: www.britishpainsociety.org/static/uploads/resources/files/book_pain_older_people.pdf.

Reith, F, Brennan, P, Maas, A et al. (2016) Lack of standardization in the use of the Glasgow Coma Scale: results of international surveys. *Journal of Neurotrauma*, 33(1): 89–94. doi: 10.1089/neu.2014.3843. Epub 12 Aug 2015. PMID: 25951090.

Renal Association (2013) *Chronic Kidney Disease Stages.* Accessed at: www.renal.org/information-resources/the-uk-eckd-guide/ckd-stages#sthash.PsjK16Qq.dpbs

Resuscitation Council (UK) (2015) *Guidelines and Guidance: A Systematic Approach to the Acutely Ill Patient (ABCDE Approach).* Accessed at: www.resus.org.uk/resuscitation-guidelines/a-systematic-approach-to-the-acutely-ill-patient-abcde

Rhodes, A, Evans, LE, Alhazzani, W et al. (2017) Surviving Sepsis Campaign: international guidelines for management of sepsis and septic shock: 2016. *Intensive Care Medicine*, 43(3): 304–77. doi: 10.1007/s00134-017-4683-6. Epub 18 Jan 2017. PMID: 28101605.

Richardson, A and Whatmore, J (2014) Nursing essential principles: continuous renal replacement therapy. *Nursing in Critical Care*, 20(1): 8–15.

Riker, R, Fraser, G, Simmons, L and Wilkins, M (2001) Validating the sedation agitation scale with the bispectral index and visual analogue scale in adult ICU patients after cardiac surgery. *Intensive Care Medicine*, 27(5): 853–8.

Ritchie, M. (2011) *Mixed Pain.* Accessed at: www.gmjournal.co.uk/media/21867/gmdec2011p624.pdf

Ritter, J, Flower, R, Henderson, G et al. (2020) *Rang and Dale's Pharmacology.* Ninth edition. Edinburgh: Elsevier.

Romanelli, D and Farrell, MW (2021) *AVPU Score.* (Updated 14 Apr 2021). In: *StatPearls* [Internet]. Treasure Island, FL: StatPearls Publishing. Available from: www.ncbi.nlm.nih.gov/books/NBK538431/

RPS (Royal Pharmaceutical Society) (2018) *Royal Pharmaceutical Society.* Accessed at: www.rpharms.com/

Saunderson Cohen, S (2002) *Trauma Nursing Secrets.* Philadelphia, PA: Hanley and Belfus.

Scala, R and Pisani, L (2018) Noninvasive ventilation in acute respiratory failure: which recipe for success? *European Respiratory Review*, 27(149): 180029.

Schofield, P (2018) The assessment of pain in older people: UK national guidelines. *Age and Ageing*, 47(S1): i1–i22. https://doi.org/10.1093/ageing/afx192.

Scott, C (2003) *Setting Safe Nurse Staffing Levels: RCN Research Report*. London: Royal College of Nursing.

Sepsis Alliance (2015) *Life After Sepsis*. Accessed at: www.sepsisalliance.org/life_after_sepsis

Seymour, C, Liu, V, Iwashyna, T et al. (2016) Assessment of clinical criteria for sepsis: for the Third International Consensus Definitions for Sepsis and Septic Shock (Sepsis-3). *JAMA*, 315(8): 762–74. doi:10.1001/jama.2016.0288

Shankar-Hari, M, Phillips, G, Levy, M et al. (2016) Developing a new definition and assessing new clinical criteria for septic shock: for the Third International Consensus Definitions for Sepsis and Septic Shock (Sepsis-3). *JAMA*, 315(8): 775–87. doi:10.1001/jama.2016.0289.

Sharma, S, Jackson, P and Makan, J (2004) Cardiac troponins. *Journal of Clinical Pathology*, 57: 1025–6.

Sharp, S, McAllister, M and Broadbent, M (2015) The vital blend of clinical competence and compassion: how patients experience person centred care. *Contemporary Nurse*, 52(2–3): 300–12.

Silcock, D, Corfield, A, Gowens, P et al. (2015) Validation of the National Early Warning Score in the prehospital setting. *Resuscitation*, 89: 31–5.

Silva, M, Sousa-Muñoz, R, Frade, H et al. (2017) Sundown syndrome and symptoms of anxiety and depression in hospitalized elderly. *Dementia Neuropsychology*, 11(2): 154–61.

Simillis, C and Rashheed, S (2019) Acute gastrointestinal bleeding, in Bersten, A and Handy, J (eds) *Oh's Intensive Care Manual*. Eighth edition. Oxford: Butterworth Heinemann Elsevier.

Sincero, M (2012) *How Does Stress Affect Performance?* Explorable.com. Accessed at: https://explorable.com/how-does-stress-affect-performance, on 19/12/14.

Singer, M, Deutschman, CS, Seymour CW et al. (2016) The Third International Consensus Definitions for Sepsis and Septic Shock (Sepsis-3). *JAMA*, 315(8): 801–10. doi:10.1001/jama.2016.0287.

Skaer, TL (1998) Cancer pain management. *American Journal of Pharmaceutical Education*, 62: 182–9.

Smith, G, Prytherch, D, Meredith, P, Schmidt, P and Featherstone, P (2013) The ability of the National Early Warning Score (NEWS) to discriminate patients at risk of early cardiac arrest, unanticipated intensive care unit admission and death. *Resuscitation*, 84: 465–70.

Smith, J (2009) How to keep score of acuity and dependency. *Nursing Management*, 16(8): 14–19.

Sneyers, B, Laterre, P, Bricq, E, Perreault, M, Wouters, D and Spinewine, A (2014) What stops us from following sedation recommendations in intensive care units? A multi-centric qualitative study. *Journal of Critical Care*, 29: 291–7.

Snow, AL, O'Malley, KJ, Cody, M et al. (2004) A conceptual model of pain assessment for noncommunicative persons with dementia. *The Gerontologist*, 44(6): 807–17. doi:10.1093/geront/44.6.807.

Spapen, H, Jacobs, R and Honoré, P (2017) Sepsis-induced multi-organ dysfunction syndrome – a mechanistic approach. *Journal of Emergency and Critical Care Medicine*, 1(10): 27.

St John Ambulance. (2021) *How to Do the Primary Survey (DRABC)*. Accessed at: www.sja.org.uk/get-advice/first-aid-advice/how-to/how-to-do-the-primary-survey/, on 23/08/21.

Stahl-Pehe, A, Glaubitz, L, Bächle, C et al. (2019) Diabetes distress in young adults with early-onset Type 1 diabetes and its prospective relationship with HbA1c and health status. *Diabetic Medicine*, 36(7): 836–46. doi: 10.1111/dme.13931. Epub 25 Mar 2019. PMID: 30761589.

Stamenkovic, D, Laycock, H, Karanikolas, M et al. (2019) Chronic pain and chronic opioid use after intensive care discharge: is it time to change practice? *Frontiers in Pharmacology*, 10: 23. doi: 10.3389/fphar.2019.00023.

Standl, T, Annecke, T, Cascorbi, I et al. (2018) The nomenclature, definition and distinction of types of shock. *Deutsches Arzteblatt International*, 115(45): 757–68. doi: 10.3238/arztebl.2018.0757. PMID: 30573009; PMCID: PMC6323133.

Stasevic Karlicic, I, Stasevic, M, Jankovic, S, Djukic Dejanovic, S, Dutina, A and Grbic, I (2016) The validation and inter-rater reliability of the Serbian translation of the Richmond agitation and sedation scale in post anesthesia care unit patients. *Hippokratia*, 20(1): 50–4.

Steventon, A, Deeny, S, Friebel, R et al. (2018) *Briefing: Emergency Hospital Admissions in England: Which May Be Avoidable and How?* The Health Foundation. Accessed at: www.health.org.uk/sites/default/files/Briefing_Emergency%20admissions_web_final.pdf, on 28/08/21.

Tait, D (2009) *A Gadamerian Hermeneutic Study of Nurses' Experiences of Recognising and Managing Patients with Clinical Deterioration and Critical Illness in a NHS Trust in Wales.* Unpublished doctoral thesis: University of Wales, Swansea.

Tait, D and White, S (2019) What triggers critical illness? In White, S and Tait, D *Critical Care Nursing: The Humanised Approach*. London: Sage, 35–68.

Taran, Z, Namadian, M, Faghihzadeh, S et al. (2019) The effect of sedation protocol using Richmond Agitation-Sedation Scale (RASS) on some clinical outcomes of mechanically ventilated patients in intensive care units: a randomized clinical trial. *Journal of Caring Science*, 8(4): 199–206. doi: 10.15171/jcs.2019.028. PMID: 31915621; PMCID: PMC6942649.

Teasdale, G, Maas, A, Lecky, F et al. (2014) The Glasgow Coma Scale at 40 years: standing the test of time. *Lancet Neurology*, 13(8): 844–54. doi: 10.1016/S1474-4422(14)70120-6. Erratum in: *Lancet Neurology*, 13(9): 863. PMID: 25030516.

Thomas, D, Cote, T and Lawhorne, L (2008) Understanding clinical dehydration and its treatment. *Journal of the American Medical Directors Association*, 9: 292–301.

Thompson, C and Dowding, D (2002) *Clinical Decision Making and Judgement in Nursing.* Edinburgh: Churchill Livingstone.

Tidswell, R and Singer, M (2018) Sepsis: thoughtful management for the non-expert. *Clinical Medicine,* 18(1): 62–8.

Tirkkonen, J, Tamminen, T and Skrifvars, M (2017) Outcome of adult patients attended by rapid response teams: a systematic review of the literature. *Resuscitation,* 112: 43–52.

Tuxen, D and Hew, M (2019) Asthma and chronic obstructive pulmonary disease in the intensive care unit. *Anaesthesia and Intensive Care Medicine,* 20(11): 651–7.

UK ONS (2016) *24 Hour Triage: Rapid Assessment and Access Tool Kit.* Accessed at: www.ukons.org/site/assets/files/1134/oncology_haematology_24_hour_triage.pdf

UK Sepsis Trust (2020) *Professional Resources.* Accessed at: https://sepsistrust.org/professional-resources/, on 26/08/21.

Umpierrez, GE, Isaacs, SD, Bazargan, N, You, X, Thaler, LM and Kitabchi, AE (2002) Hyperglycemia: an independent marker of in-hospital mortality in patients with undiagnosed diabetes. *The Journal of Clinical Endocrinology & Metabolism,* 87(3): 978–82.

Vahdatpour, C, Collins, D and Goldberg, S (2019) Cardiogenic shock. *Journal of the American Heart Association,* 8: e011991.

Vasilevskis, E, Han, J, Hughes, C and Ely, E (2012) Epidemiology and risk factors for delirium across hospital settings. *Best Practice and Research Clinical Anaesthesiology,* 26: 277–87.

Venkatesh, B and Cohen, J (2019) Adrenocortical insufficiency in critical illness, in Bersten, A and Handy, J (2019) *Oh's Intensive Care Manual.* Eighth edition. Elsevier, 767–74.

Vimal, Ram Lakhan Pandey (2010) On the quest of defining consciousness. *Mind & Matter,* 8: 93–121.

Vincent, J, Jones, G, David, S et al. (2019) Frequency and mortality of septic shock in Europe and North America: a systematic review and meta-analysis. *Critical Care* 23: 196. https://doi.org/10.1186/s13054-019-2478-6

Vivek, M, Raiz, AM, Sujoy, G et al. (2011) Myxoedema coma: a new look into an old crisis. *Journal of Thyroid Research,* 493462.

Wahlin, I (2017) Empowerment in critical care: a concept analysis. *Scandinavian Journal of Caring,* 31: 164–74.

Walker, R, Gebregziabher, M, Martin-Harris, B and Egede, L (2015) Understanding the influence of psychological and socioeconomic factors on diabetes self-care using structured equation modelling. *Patient Education and Counselling,* 98: 34–40.

Warden, V, Hurley, AC and Volicer, L (2003) Development and psychometric evaluation of the Pain Assessment in Advanced Dementia (PAINAD) scale. *Journal of the American Medical Directors Association.* 4(1): 9–15. doi: 10.1097/01.JAM.0000043422.31640.F7.

Wheeldon, A (2013) The respiratory system and associated disorders, in Muralitharan, N and Peate, I (eds) *Fundamentals of Applied Pathophysiology: An Essential Guide for Nursing and Healthcare Students.* Chichester: Wiley-Blackwell.

White, K and Arlt, W (2010) Adrenal crisis in treated Addison's disease: a predictable but undermanaged event. *European Society of Endocrinology,* 162: 115–20.

White, S and Tait, D (2019) *Critical Care Nursing: The Humanised Approach.* London: Sage.

Whitehouse, T, Snelson, C and Grounds, M (2014) *Intensive Care Society Review of Best Practice for Analgesia and Sedation in Critical Care.* London: Intensive Care Society.

Whitlock, J, Rowland, S, Ellis, G and Evans, A (2011) Using the SKIN bundle to prevent pressure ulcers. *Nursing Times,* 107(35): 20–3.

WHO (World Health Organization) (2006) *Cancer Pain Relief.* Second edition. Geneva: WHO.

WHO (2007) *People-Centred Health Care: A Policy Framework.* Geneva: WHO.

WHO (2016) *Global Strategic Directions for Strengthening Nursing and Midwifery 2016–2020.* World Health Organization. Accessed at: www.who.int/hrh/nursing_midwifery/global-strategic-midwifery2016–2020.pdf?ua=1

Wiersema, R, Jukarainen, S, Eck, RJ et al. (2020) Different applications of the KDIGO criteria for AKI lead to different incidences in critically ill patients: a post hoc analysis from the prospective observational SICS-II study. *Critical Care,* 24(164) https://doi.org/10.1186/s13054-020-02886-7.

Williams, B (2019) The National Early Warning Score and the acutely confused patient. *Clinical Medicine Journal,* 19(2): 190–1. doi:10.7861/clinmedicine.19-2-190.

Wilson, B (2007) Nurses' knowledge of pain. *Journal of Clinical Nursing,* 16(6): 1012–20.

Woodrow, P (2019) *Intensive Care Nursing: A Framework for Practice.* Fourth edition. London: Routledge.

Woodward, S and Waterhouse, C (2009) *Oxford Handbook of Neuroscience Nursing.* Oxford: Oxford University Press.

Zhuo-Ying, T, Traub, RJ and Dong-Yuan, C (2019) Epigenetic modulation of visceral pain. *Epigenetics of Chronic Pain,* 7: 141–56. https://doi.org/10.1016/B978-0-12-814070-3.00008-9

Zinchenko, R (2018) *Medical and Surgical Emergencies: The ABCDE Approach.* Tunbridge Wells: Anshan.

Zwarenstein, M, Goldman, J and Reeves, S (2009) *Interprofessional Collaboration: Effects of Practice-Based Interventions on Professional Practice and Healthcare Outcomes (Review).* Accessed at: www.onlinelibrary.wiley.com/doi/10.1002/14651858.CD000072.pub2/pdf/standard

Index

Lightning Source UK Ltd.
Milton Keynes UK
UKHW030658290123
416090UK00001B/7